D0294996

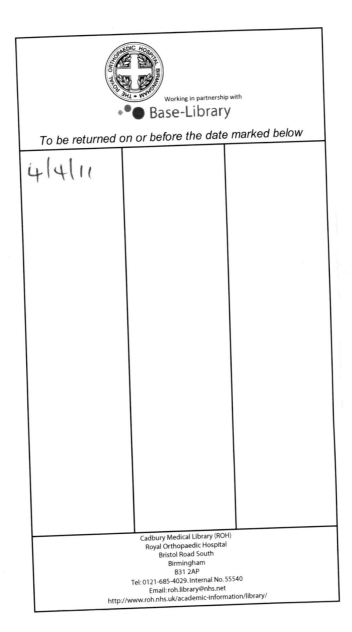

Working in partnership with

Base-Library

To be returned on or before the date marked below

4/4/11

New Avenues for the Prevention of
Chronic Musculoskeletal Pain and Disability

Pain Research and Clinical Management

Editorial Board

Pain Research and Clinical Management

Volume 12

New Avenues for the Prevention of Chronic Musculoskeletal Pain and Disability

Edited by

Steven J. Linton

Department of Occupational and Environmental Medicine, Örebro Medical Center,
S-701 85 Örebro, Sweden

2002
ELSEVIER
AMSTERDAM • BOSTON • LONDON • NEW YORK • OXFORD • PARIS • SAN DIEGO •
SAN FRANCISCO • SINGAPORE • SYDNEY • TOKYO

ELSEVIER SCIENCE B.V.
Sara Burgerhartstraat 25
P.O. Box 211, 1000 AE Amsterdam, The Netherlands

First edition 2002

Library of Congress Cataloging in Publication Data
A catalog record of the Library of Congress has been applied for.

British Library Cataloguing in Publication Data
New avenues for the prevention of chronic musculoskeletal
   pain and disability. - (Pain research and clinical management ; v. 12)
   1. Chronic pain 2. Chronic pain - Prevention
   3. Musculoskeletal system - Diseases 4. Musculoskeletal system - Wounds and injuries
   J. Linton, Steven
   616'.0472

   ISBN 0444507329

ISBN: 0-444-50732-9 (hardbound)
ISBN: 0-444-50722-1 (paperback)
ISSN: 0921-3287 (series)

Dedication

to Ann-Charlotte

for 25 years of understanding that an ounce
of prevention is truly worth a pound of cure

List of Contributors

Benjamin H.K. Balderson
    Center for Health Studies, Group Health Cooperative, 1730 Minor Avenue, Suite 1600,
    Seattle, WA 98101, USA
    E-mail: balderson.b@ghc.org

Gunnar Bergström
    Section of Personal Injury Prevention, Karolinska Institute, S-112 94 Stockholm, Sweden
    E-mail: gunnar.bergstrom@cns.ki.se

Katja Boersma
    Department of Occupational and Environmental Medicine, Örebro University Hospital,
    S-701 85 Örebro, Sweden
    E-mail: katja.boersma@orebroll.se

A. Kim Burton
    Spinal Research Unit, University of Huddersfield, Huddersfield HD1 2SP, UK
    E-mail: kim@spineresearch.org.uk

Zoë Clyde
    INPUT Pain Management Unit, Guys and St. Thomas' NHS Hospital Trust, London SE1
    7EH, UK
    E-mail: zoe.clyde@gstt.sthames.nhs.uk

Michael Feuerstein
    Department of Medical and Clinical Psychology and Department of Preventive Medicine
    and Biometrics, Uniformed Services University of the Health Sciences, 4301 Jones Bridge
    Road, Bethesda, MD 20814, USA
    E-mail: mfeuerst@mx3.usuhs.mil

Robert J. Gatchel
    Department of Psychiatry, University of Texas Southwestern Medical Center, 5323 Harry
    Hines Boulevard, Dallas, TX 75235-9044, USA
    E-mail: robert.gatchel@utsouthwestern.edu

Mariëlle E.J.B. Goossens
    Institute for Rehabilitation Research, P.O. Box 192, 6430 CC Hoensbroek, The Netherlands
    E-mail: m.goossens@irv.nl

Sheilah Hogg-Johnson
    Institute for Work and Health, 481 University Avenue, 8th Floor, Toronto, ON M5G 2E9,
    Canada
    E-mail: shogg-johnson@iwh.on.ca

Grant D. Huang

Department of Medical and Clinical Psychology, Department of Preventive Medicine and Biometrics, Uniformed Services University of the Health Sciences, 4301 Jones Bridge Road, Bethesda, MD, USA
E-mail: ghuang@usuhs.mil

Irene B. Jensen

Section of Personal Injury Prevention, Karolinska Institute, S-112 94 Stockholm, Sweden
E-mail: irene.jensen@cns.ki.se

Steven J. Linton

Department of Occupational and Environmental Medicine, Örebro University Hospital, S-701 85 Örebro, Sweden
E-mail: steven.linton@orebroll.se

Ulf Lundberg

Department of Psychology and Centre for Health Equity Studies (CHESS), Stockholm University, S-106 91 Stockholm, Sweden
E-mail: ul@psychology.su.se

Gary J. Macfarlane

Unit of Chronic Disease Epidemiology, School of Epidemiology and Health Sciences, Stopford Building, University of Manchester, Oxford Road, Manchester M13 9PT, UK
E-mail: gary@fs1.ser.man.ac.uk

Chris J. Main

Department of Behavioural Medicine, Hope Hospital, Eccles Old Road, Salford M6 8HD, UK
E-mail: cmain@fs1.ho.man.ac.uk

John McBeth

Arthritis Research Campaign Epidemiology Unit, School of Epidemiology and Health Sciences, Stopford Building, University of Manchester, Oxford Road, Manchester M13 9PT, UK
E-mail: mack@fs1.ser.man.ac.uk

Bo Melin

National Institute for Working Life, Stockholm, Sweden
E-mail: bo.melin@niwl.se

Stephen Morley

Academic Unit, Psychiatry and Behavioural Sciences, School of Medicine, University of Leeds, Leeds LS2 9JT, UK
E-mail: s.j.morley@leeds.ac.uk

Michael K. Nicholas

Pain Management and Research Centre, University of Sydney and Royal North Shore Hospital, St. Leonards, NSW 2065, Australia
E-mail: miken@med.usyd.edu.au

Tamar Pincus

Department of Psychology, Royal Holloway, University of London, Egham, TW20 0EX, UK
E-mail: t.pincus@rhul.ac.uk

Carla B. Pulliam

Department of Psychiatry, University of Texas Southwestern Medical Center, 5323 Harry Hines Boulevard, Dallas, TX 75235-8898, USA
E-mail: carla.pulliam@utsouthwestern.edu

William S. Shaw

Liberty Mutual Center for Disability Research, 71 Frankland Road, Hopkinton, MA 01748, USA
E-mail: william.shaw@libertymutual.com

Sandra J. Sinclair

Institute for Work and Health, 481 University Avenue, 8th Floor, Toronto, ON M5G 2E9, Canada
E-mail: ssinclair@iwh.on.ca

Johanna H.C. Van den Hout

Department of Medical, Clinical and Experimental Psychology, Maastricht University, 6200 MD, Maastricht, The Netherlands
E-mail: anja.vandenhout@dep.unimaas.nl

Johan W.S. Vlaeyen

Pain Management and Research Center, University Hospital Maastricht, P.O. Box 5800, 6201 AZ Maastricht, The Netherlands; and Department of Medical, Clinical and Experimental Psychology, Maastricht University, P.O. Box 616, 6200 MD Maastricht, The Netherlands
E-mail: j.vlaeyen@dep.unimaas.nl

Michael Von Korff

Center for Health Studies, Group Health Cooperative, 1730 Minor Avenue, Suite 1600, Seattle, WA 98101, USA

Gordon Waddell

Glasgow Nuffield Hospital, Glasgow, UK

Rolf H. Westgaard

Division of Industrial Economics and Technology Management, Norwegian University of Science and Technology, N-7491 Trondheim, Norway
E-mail: rolf.westgaard@iot.ntnu.no

Amanda C.deC. Williams

Division of Psychological Medicine, GKT School of Medicine, Dentistry and Biomedical Sciences, INPUT Pain Management Unit, Guys and St. Thomas' NHS Hospital Trust, London SE1 7EH, UK

Jørgen Winkel

National Institute for Working Life West, Box 8850, SE-402 72 Gothenburg, Sweden
E-mail: jorgen.winkel@niwl.se

Contents

Section III. Early Identification and Preventive Interventions

New Avenues for the Prevention of Chronic Musculoskeletal Pain and Disability
Pain Research and Clinical Management, Vol. 12
Edited by S.J. Linton

CHAPTER 1

New research provides new avenues for prevention

Steven J. Linton [*]

Department of Occupational and Environmental Medicine, Örebro University Hospital, S-701 85 Örebro, Sweden

Exciting new findings are unveiling the mysteries of persistent pain and disability. Although we are far from understanding the whole story, there has been a surge of research that has identified important links to the development of chronic musculoskeletal pain. Not only are the roles of medical, workplace, societal, and psychological factors being illuminated, but also the connections between these areas are being defined. Slowly the mechanisms by which acute pain develops into a chronic problem are being delineated. Certainly, the development of chronic pain is complex involving a multidimensional process. Yet, great inroads are being made.

The advances being made provide new avenues for the prevention of musculoskeletal pain and disability. Indeed, a major stumbling block to prevention has been our lack of understanding and focus. Most early attempts at prevention produced meager results when evaluated scientifically. However, by better understanding the problem new inroads have been made for preventive interventions, and many of these are quite promising as demonstrated in controlled trials.

1. Aim of the book

The purpose of this book is to provide readers with the current trends and evidence about the prevention of chronic musculoskeletal pain. Although a broad approach is taken, the book nevertheless focuses on what might be done in professional settings. At the end of the day, the main question usually centers on what can be done. As a result, this book aims to provide important background for understanding how effective programs might be developed. This includes understanding the peculiarities of musculoskeletal pain problems that require that prevention programs are fundamentally different than for many other medical problems. In addition, there is a need to appreciate the intricacies of how chronic pain develops so that this information might be incorporated into prevention programs. This books also aims to provide readers with concrete ideas and examples of preventive programs, many of which have produced startling results. Finally, this book is designed to stimulate action. We know so much and yet do so little to prevent these problems. Thus, the book may be used as a handbook by a variety of professionals to develop specific or comprehensive programs for prevention.

[*] Correspondence to: S.J. Linton, Department of Occupational and Environmental Medicine, Örebro University Hospital, S-701 85 Örebro, Sweden, Tel.: +46 (19) 602-2456, E-mail: steven.linton@orebroll.se

2. The problem demands prevention

Never before has the need for the prevention of chronic pain and disability been so clear. The urgency for prevention is born out by some straightforward facts. Every year a vast number of people develop long-term pain problems that cannot be cured medically. This persistent pain results in untold suffering, considerable health-care utilization, as well as functional problems and disability. Since at least 85% of the population will at some time suffer from back pain alone, the socio-economic consequences are staggering. And, although medical advances are continually being made, there is no current cure for chronic musculoskeletal pain. At worst, persistence in applying the traditional medical model to these problems seems to inadvertently contribute to their development. Clearly, treatment as usual has failed to deal sufficiently with the problem and a fresh, preventive approach is needed. There is good reason to believe that providing new forms of health care at an early time point might prevent a considerable amount of suffering and disability.

The definition of prevention deserves examination already at this early point in the book. There are distinct differences between prevention aimed at musculoskeletal problems and those aimed at traditional diseases. First, traditional diseases are often definable from a biological test. For example, if we are interested in preventing cancer, tissue samples may be obtained to ascertain whether a given person has cancer. Musculoskeletal pain on the other hand, is defined mainly by self-reports. Whether a given person 'has' this problem is to a large extent based on the person's own report. Second, prevention is often based on hindering the etiology of the problem. That is, a clear biological mechanism is isolated and the prevention stops the mechanism. However, musculoskeletal pain is not a disease. It is natural that most people will at some point experience neck or back pain. Moreover, the pain serves as a warning signal and thus not all musculoskeletal pain should be prevented. Taken together, this means that primary prevention aimed at hindering the occurrence of any musculoskeletal pain is questionable. However, 'secondary' prevention that focuses on limiting the development of a persistent problem might be feasible. In addition, the goal need not strictly be the experience of pain, but rather a broad range of outcome variables including function. After all, one of the main negative consequences of the pain is dysfunction.

One reason that prevention has been neglected in this area is the difficulty in understanding the mechanisms involved in the transition from acute to chronic pain and another has been developing effective preventive interventions. Historically, preventing musculoskeletal pain has been a frustrating business. However, this may well be related to the fact that most attempts have been either focused on a medical model or a strict ergonomic approach. These have failed to produce a preventive effect. Instead, a combination of approaches from a broad perspective is producing exciting results.

One key element involved is the question of what is to be prevented. Although many attempts have focused on the obvious variable of 'pain', there is an increasing awareness that even outcome is multidimensional. Therefore, function has become a clear goal for prevention. Other aims are oriented toward the socio-economic impact, such as reducing sick absenteeism and health-care costs.

Another theme is the strategy for achieving prevention. Typically, prevention programs for back pain have focused on a single factor, such as exercise, relaxation or ergonomics. It has become clear that single-dimension programs are inadequate for a multidimensional problem. Moreover, prevention programs have often been generated by a school of thought or theory, rather than on scientific evidence. Yet, as we shall see in Section II, a number of 'risk' factors have been delineated. A new advancement is the strategy of addressing these factors in the prevention program.

A third theme in prevention is tailoring the program to the individual and his or her needs. Often prevention programs for back pain have been devised and then applied to an entire sector e.g. workers, patients, or students. Although this approach offers simplicity, it misses an important opportunity for increasing effectiveness. Early identification through screening and subsequent assessment may provide important insights into which factors are generating the development of a chronic problem for a given individual. With this information in hand, it is possible to provide an intervention tailored specifically to the patient's needs. This has the advantage of only needing to provide the intervention for those truly in need, and of enhancing the impact of the interventions applied.

However, despite the rapid growth in our knowledge and ability to prevent persistent musculoskeletal pain problems, little resources are currently being directed to this end. Only a small fraction of the huge resources spent each year on back pain are actually allocated to preventive interventions (Nachemson and Jonsson, 2000). For example, less than 10% of the vast economic resources being spent on back pain, are allocated for treatment. Of the money provided for treatment, the majority in reality pays for expensive procedures at hospitals. Therefore, only a small fraction trickles down to preventive interventions.

The prevention of chronic musculoskeletal pain is an important challenge for the twenty-first century since these pain problems cause a surprising amount of problems for the individual, his or her family, the workplace, the health-care system, and society at large. Although chronic neck and back pain are not ordinarily life threatening, they do inflict untold suffering and disability. Acute musculoskeletal pain serves an important function as a 'warning signal' and it sets boundaries on our behavior. Thus, we find that most people at some time during their life do suffer from it. Yet, for some people, the pain problem becomes recurrent or develops into a chronic problem that causes suffering and seriously disrupts normal life. The size of the problem demonstrates that we cannot simply continue in the same path; the problem demands prevention.

3. Overview of the book

To meet the aim of providing an evidenced-based tabulation of current the developing knowledge and practice, the book is divided into three main sections.

The first section concentrates on background factors and the need for prevention. Here the latest scientific studies on the extent of the problem, costs, and consequences for society are presented in detail. In addition, the breadth of the problem is analyzed and some basic considerations are perused.

The second section delves into the mechanisms that operate in the chronification process. Some analyses offer an overview of this process and aim to integrate large bodies of scientific information. However, some chapters focus on a particularly interesting factor so that the subject can be examined in greater depth. Several chapters deal with psychological variables since these have been firmly associated with the development of persistent pain and disability. Indeed, if we are to go forward it seems that these variables will need to be utilized to truly provide 'new avenues for prevention'.

Section III delves into the all-important question of how we might actually prevent chronic musculoskeletal pain problems. Early identification of people 'at risk' is a typical strategy. This allows one to concentrate limited resources on those most in need. It also offers the promise of being able to tailor the intervention to the individual and his or her profile. Thus, several chapters bring up the issue of applying our knowledge about risk factors to identify early on those patients at risk of developing a persistent pain problem. Identification alone, however, does not seem to be sufficient for prevention. The remaining chapters present various programs for prevention. Surprisingly positive results have been reported in many of the scientific reports on prevention providing a strong ray of hope. Indeed, it is my hope that this book will provide encouragement to scientists and practitioners alike so that we together can truly pave new avenues for the prevention of musculoskeletal pain.

References

Nachemson, A. and Jonsson, E. (2000) Neck and Back Pain: The Scientific Evidence of Causes, Diagnosis, and Treatment. Lippincott, Williams and Wilkins, Philadelphia, PA, 495 pp.

Section I

The Need for Prevention

This section provides a background concerning the need for prevention from a health, socioeconomic and systems perspective.

Objectives are for the reader to:
- understand the prevalence and nature of musculoskeletal pain
- understand the consequences of persistent pain
- obtain an introduction to prevention

New Avenues for the Prevention of Chronic Musculoskeletal Pain and Disability
Pain Research and Clinical Management, Vol. 12
Edited by S.J. Linton

CHAPTER 2

The prevalence of regional and widespread musculoskeletal pain symptoms

John McBeth [1] and Gary J. Macfarlane [1,2,*]

[1] *Arthritis Research Campaign Epidemiology Unit, School of Epidemiology and Health Sciences, Stopford Building,*
University of Manchester, Oxford Road, Manchester M13 9PT, UK
[2] *Unit of Chronic Disease Epidemiology, School of Epidemiology and Health Sciences, Stopford Building, University of*
Manchester, Oxford Road, Manchester M13 9PT, UK

Abstract: The purpose of this chapter is to examine the prevalence of musculoskeletal pain symptoms. Clear definitions of pain syndromes are important as this greatly impacts on prevalence rates. Other factors influencing these rates are methodological pitfalls, and the association between the pain symptom and population factors, such as age, gender, and occupation. The data are examined with regard to low back pain, shoulder pain, wide spread pain and fibromyalgia. Musculoskeletal pain is found to be common in community samples. It is also common in primary care and accounts for a large proportion of consultations. Although it has been suggested that the prevalence of musculoskeletal pain is increasing, this has yet to be scientifically confirmed. However, the high rate of musculoskeletal pain underscores the need for appropriate and effective preventive interventions.

1. Introduction

Pain originating from the musculoskeletal system may occur at single or multiple sites. In this chapter, we have chosen to focus on three main sites: low back pain, shoulder pain and chronic widespread pain, the symptomatic presentation of the 'fibromyalgia syndrome'. Of the regional sites, pain occurring in the low back is an obvious choice since it is the most commonly reported site of pain. It has been estimated that up to 60–80% of the population will, at some point in their lives, experience back pain (Biering-Sorensen, 1983). Back pain is one of the most commonly cited causes of absence from work and is associated with considerable socio-economic (Maniadakis and Gray, 2000) and individual costs (Hazard et al., 1997). Shoulder pain is the second most commonly reported site of pain (Badley et al., 1994). Shoulder pain also represents a considerable burden to the community and to the individual with up to two-thirds of community subjects with current shoulder pain reporting some associated disability (Pope et al., 1997). Although prevalent in the general population, chronic widespread pain syndromes have been less extensively studied. Recently, with the renewed interest in the fibromyalgia syndrome the issues of measurement and assessment of diffuse pain syndromes have begun to be addressed and the extent of widespread symptoms in community subjects and clinic populations has become apparent.

---

* Correspondence to: G.J. Macfarlane, Arthritis Research Campaign Epidemiology Unit, School of Epidemiology and Health Sciences, Stopford Building, University of Manchester, Oxford Road, Manchester, M13 9PT, UK. E-mail: mack@gary.ser.man.ac.uk

2. Case definition

Throughout the literature, 'diagnostic criteria' and 'classification criteria' are used interchangeably when discussing case definition and this can often lead to some confusion. In epidemiological studies it is more appropriate to discuss regional pain syndromes such as low back pain and shoulder pain, and diffuse pain syndromes such as chronic widespread pain and fibromyalgia in terms of classification criteria, since this term implies the identification of a homogenous group of persons with regard to symptoms. Epidemiological studies which investigate disease prevalence using the same classification criteria can then be compared and contrasted. In this chapter, the term classification criteria will be used when discussing case definition.

2.1. Low back pain

There is no generally accepted classification criteria which outlines the low back area in which to identify an episode of low back pain. Indeed, the classification of an episode is itself an issue for debate. Pain occurring in the low back can be attributed to a number of anatomical structures including muscles, ligaments, facet joints, blood vessels and spinal nerve roots (Deyo, 1992). However, in common with many pain disorders, objective findings on investigation may not predict who will have pain. For example, the radiographic identification of degenerative displacement of lumbar vertebrae has been shown to poorly predict reports of low back pain (Kauppila et al., 1998). Indeed, research informs us that only a small proportion of cases of back pain (approximately 10%) can be attributed to an underlying cause (Croft and Raspe, 1995).

In the face of a lack of objective findings which are associated with the occurrence of back pain, most research has relied on self-reported symptoms and this has led, in turn, to a diverse range of classification criteria being employed (Dionne, 1999). Often, simple statements such as "Have you ever been troubled with pain in your back?" have been used while others have enquired about pain, aches or stiffness in the lower back (Svensson and Andersson, 1989). The problem with this approach is that the response, whether positive or negative, is entirely dependent on the individuals definition of the low back area. In epidemiological studies of musculo-skeletal pain, it is essential to define the anatomical region. Anderson (1977) suggested that the lower back be defined as lying between the lower costal margins and the gluteal folds. With this in mind, a manikin (Fig. 1a) has been developed which outlines this anatomical area and which has been commonly used in population based studies of low back pain occurrence (Papageorgiou et al., 1995).

2.2. Shoulder pain

The shoulder complex essentially comprises five functional joints (sternoclavicular, acromioclavicular, subacromial, glenohumeral and scapulo-thoracic) with each joint playing a specific role in every upper extremity function. Each joint has a complex array of attendant soft-tissue components including ligaments, tendons, muscle and bursae which assist in movement. Shoulder pain can originate from multiple sites and multiple structures, and has many causes. Shoulder pain can be associated with pain referred from an extrinsic region (Kessel, 1986) or, more commonly, may be related to intrinsic factors. Pain originating in the joint complex itself is considered rare (Kessel, 1986). The two most common causes of intrinsic joint-related pain arise from osteoarthritis, which can effect the shoulder due to age or occupational wear, and rheumatoid arthritis which may manifest in the shoulder complex as part of a wider disorder. Pain arising from the soft-tissue components of the shoulder complex are more common (Calliet, 1991).

Given the complexity of the shoulder joint, the numerous interactions between the shoulder and surrounding areas, the wide spectrum of conditions and disorders that can cause shoulder pain and the frequent occurrence of referred shoulder pain it is not surprising that there are difficulties in formulating clear classification criteria for defining the shoulder region when assessing pain in epidemiological sur-

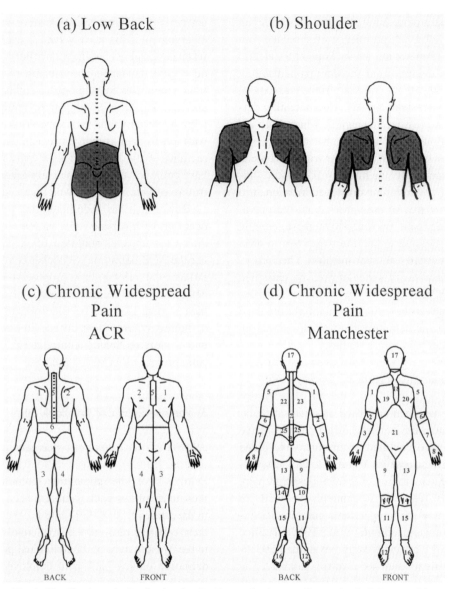

(a) Low Back

(b) Shoulder

(c) Chronic Widespread Pain ACR

(d) Chronic Widespread Pain Manchester

BACK   FRONT   BACK   FRONT

Fig. 1. Classification criteria of regional and widespread pain according to site shaded on manikin.

veys. Due to the potential for misclassification and the variability of diagnosis between studies, classifying individual conditions causing shoulder pain and assessing each in terms of occurrence and demographic spread is likely to be problematic. At present, there are no classification criteria suitable for use in population based studies and there is poor inter-clinician reliability (Bamji et al., 1996). Assessing the impact of shoulder pain in such a context would also underestimate the importance of a common musculoskeletal symptom which carries with it a substantial burden in terms of disability, absence from work and disability pensions. Conversely, employing an all-embracing definition of shoulder pain may also be problematic since short-lived transient episodes may be included and the prevalence of 'meaningful' shoulder pain overestimated.

What has been demonstrated is that, depending on the definition used, the prevalence of shoulder pain varies widely (Pope et al., 1997). Pope et al. (1997) employed four definitions of shoulder pain. The first definition was the direct question "Have you experienced pain in your shoulder(s)?". The remaining definitions used a pre-shaded manikin which outlined various definitions of the shoulder: the shoulder complex, the upper trunk, and the upper trunk and neck. Perhaps unsurprisingly, the findings of this study indicated that as the definition employed broadened to include a larger area of the upper trunk, the prevalence of shoulder pain was found to increase, ranging from 31% in response to the direct question to 48% using the upper trunk and neck manikin. The authors concluded that cases of shoulder pain be classified using an area restricted to the shoulder complex (Fig. 1b). However these findings highlight the need to be aware of the definition used when comparing rates of shoulder pain across studies.

2.3. Chronic widespread pain and fibromyalgia

Fibromyalgia has been described as a non-articular rheumatic syndrome whose cardinal features have traditionally been identified as chronic widespread pain in the presence of widespread tenderness. Focussing on the symptom of chronic widespread pain, the American College of Rheumatology (ACR) in a 16-centre study proposed criteria for the classification of fibromyalgia (Wolfe et al., 1990). Trained blinded assessors interviewed and examined 293 fibromyalgia patients and 265 control patients. The fibromyalgia patients were considered to have the disorder by the clinical diagnosis normally used by the investigator at the various centres. Age- and sex-matched patients with a variety of pain disorders including low back pain syndromes and trauma-related pain syndromes were used as controls. The presence of 11 of 18 tender points in the presence of widespread pain enabled fibromyalgia patients to be distinguished from controls with a sensitivity of 88.4% and a specificity of 81.1%.

The main problem with that criteria lies in the investigators a priori description of the defining characteristics of fibromyalgia, leading to a circularity of argument. This is, however, a common problem when developing classification criteria in the absence of a 'gold standard'. The strength of this classification criteria lies in enabling researchers to identify and investigate a homogenous group of subjects with the fibromyalgia syndrome. This criteria defines widespread pain as pain present in two contralateral sections of the body and axial pain (Fig. 1c), and have come to be the most widely used in prevalence studies of fibromyalgia.

However, it has been noted that patterns of pain distribution involving only a few local areas, as drawn by subjects, would qualify as widespread under the ACR definition (Schochat et al., 1994). Macfarlane et al. (1996a) have proposed a more stringent definition which identifies a group of subjects whose pain is more likely to be widespread (Fig. 1d). This definition requires more diffuse limb pain, present in two or more sections of contralateral limbs and axial pain, present for at least 3 months.

3. The prevalence of low back pain

3.1. Prevalence estimates in the general population

Estimates of the population cumulative lifetime prevalence of low back pain have been reported to lie in the range of 50–84% (Table I). The differences in these reported rates may be explained by differences in the age structure of the individual populations, the definition of low back pain employed and there is likely to be inaccurate recall when asking persons to recollect if they have ever experienced low back pain. Nevertheless, these studies do indicate that the cumulative lifetime prevalence is high, with over half of the general population reporting having ever experienced symptoms in their low back.

Studies examining more recent episodes can be categorised into those reporting period prevalence rates (symptoms in a defined period, usually the last 12 months) and those reporting point prevalence rates (symptoms on the day of contact) (Table II). The prevalence of current symptoms is generally lower

TABLE I

Population prevalence of low back pain (cumulative lifetime prevalence)

Setting	Age range (years)	Study population	Classification criteria	Prevalence (%)	Reference
Sweden	15–71	692	low back insufficiency, lumbago or sciatica	49	Hirsch et al., 1969
Netherlands	≥20	6584	low back pain	55	Valkenburg and Haanen, 1982
Sweden	40–47	940	pain, ache, stiffness or fatigue localised to lower back	61	Svensson and Andersson, 1982
Denmark	30–60	928	pain or other troubles in lower part of back	62	Biering-Sorensen, 1982
USA	18–55	1221	low back pain	70	Frymoyer et al., 1983
Sweden	38–64	1410	pain, ache, stiffness or fatigue localised to lower back	66	Svensson and Andersson, 1989
UK	20–59	2667	pain between 12th rib and gluteal folds, >24 h	58	Walsh et al., 1992
Belgium	≥15	4208	low back pain	59	Skovron et al., 1994
UK	25–64	3184	pain between 12th rib and gluteal folds, >24 h	59	Hillman et al., 1996
Canada	20–69	2184	low back pain	84	Cote et al., 1998

than the population cumulative lifetime prevalence. Nevertheless, depending on the definition used, between 20 and 60% of the general population report experiencing symptoms in the previous 12 months. Ascertaining symptoms by means of a telephone interview and using a broad definition of back pain, Sternbach (1986) reported the highest annual prevalence of 56%. When the definition was restricted to the low back region, the prevalence was slightly lower at 45% (Biering-Sorensen, 1982) while introducing a minimal time (pain present for more than 24 h) into the definition resulted in a slightly lower prevalence of 36% (Walsh et al., 1992). Similar rates were reported in a Swedish study which reported a prevalence of 50% amongst women and a slightly lower prevalence of 43% amongst men in one region of Sweden (Santos-Eggimann et al., 2000). An assessment of the prevalence of recurrent symptoms resulted in the lowest prevalence of 18% (Reisbord and Greenland, 1985) suggesting that a proportion of subjects with low back pain will have persistent symptoms over a 12-month period.

3.2. Prevalence estimates in primary care

Despite the high prevalence of low back pain in the general population, it has been estimated that in a 12-month period, fewer than 10% of those episodes will lead to a consultation with a health care practitioner (Papageorgiou et al., 1995). This finding is supported by studies which have conducted reviews of general practice records and have reported rates of consultation for low back pain of between 2 and 10% (Ward et al., 1968; Frymoyer et al., 1980). Amongst those consulting, it is often stated that 50% will have improved within 1 week while 90% will have improved within 1 month (Coste et al., 1994). However, the definition of low back pain in that study (acute low back pain lasting less than 72 h and without radiation below the gluteal folds) was restrictive and would represent only a small proportion of all those consulting with low back pain. Nevertheless, considering the population prevalence, this figure still indicates a sizeable number of persons who will go on to develop persistent symptoms for which they will continue to seek medical help. A recent study conducted in the UK (Croft et al., 1998) has examined the outcome of low back pain in general practice over 12 months. Of the 463 persons who consulted with a new episode of low back pain, 59% had a single consultation while 32% had consulted more than once but did not consult after 3 months following their initial consultation. These findings would appear to support the statement that

TABLE II

Population prevalence of low back pain (period and point prevalence)

Setting	Age range (years)	Study population	Classification criteria	Pain period	Prevalence (%)	Reference
Period prevalence						
USA	≥18	2,782	frequent pain in back	previous 12 months	18	Reisbord and Greenland, 1985
USA	≥18	1,254	backache on 1 or more days	previous 12 months	56	Sternbach, 1986
Denmark	30–60	928	pain or other symptoms in lower part of back	previous 12 months	45	Biering-Sorensen and Thomsen, 1986
USA	18–75	1,016	back pain, >24 h or several times	previous 6 months	41	Von Korff et al., 1988
UK	20–59	2,667	pain between 12th ribs and the gluteal folds	previous 12 months	41	Walsh et al., 1992
UK	18–75	4,501	low back ache or pain > 24 h	past month	39	Papageorgiou et al., 1995
UK	≥18	34,000	recurring backache	previous 12 months	24	Wright et al., 1995
UK	25–64	3,184	pain between 12th rib and gluteal folds, >24 h	past 12 months	59	Hillman et al., 1996
Canada	20–69	2,184	low back pain	previous 6 months	49	Cote et al., 1998
UK	20–59	10,363	low back pain	previous 12 months	49	Palmer et al., 2000
Sweden	25–74	1,718	low back pain on manikin > 7 days	past year	47	Santos-Eggimann et al., 2000
Point prevalence						
Netherlands	≥20	6,584	low back pain	day of interview	26	Valkenburg and Haanen, 1982
Sweden	40–47	940	pain, ache, stiffness or fatigue localised to lower back	day of interview	31	Svensson and Andersson, 1982
Sweden	18–84	827	pain in lower back	day of questionnaire	31	Brattberg et al., 1989
Sweden	38–64	1,410	pain, ache, stiffness or fatigue localised to lower back	day of interview	35	Svensson and Andersson, 1989

90% of episodes of low back pain would recover in 3 (not 1) months. However, the authors reported that when those persons were followed up at 3 months post-consultation only 21% had completely recovered in terms of pain and disability, while only 25% reported complete recovery at 12 months. These findings indicate that prevalence rates of persons who consult with low back pain symptoms do not necessarily reflect the true burden of low back pain in the general population.

3.3. Patterns in low back pain prevalence

It is often stated that the prevalence of low back pain increases with age and is more prevalent in women when compared to men. Indeed, studies of adult populations have tended to show an increase in the prevalence of low back pain until mid to late forties, with rates stabilising after that age until the mid sixties (Walsh et al., 1992; Skovron et al., 1994). In a population-based study of the prevalence of low back pain, Papageorgiou et al. (1995) reported a linear increase in pain prevalence in both men and women up until the sixth decade. The difference between the youngest age group (18–29 years) and those in the 45–59-year age group was more marked in women than in men (17% vs. 7.3%). Prevalence rates in the oldest, 60–75-year age group tended to drop for both men and women. Others have demonstrated that women are more likely to report low back pain than men (Skovron et al., 1994; Papageorgiou et al., 1995; Hurwitz and Morgenstern, 1997). However these findings are not consistent (Deyo and Tsui-Wu, 1987; Von Korff et al., 1988) and these basic assumptions of the relationship between pain prevalence, and age and gender have recently been questioned (LeResche, 1999). These relationships may be more complex and prevalence rates are likely to be subject to the influence of, amongst others, occupation, socio-economic status, ethnicity and lifestyle factors. For example, it has recently been reported that the prevalence of musculoskeletal pain is higher in ethnic minority groups (Allison et al., 2002) and varies by levels of social deprivation (Urwin et al., 1998).

3.4. Trends in the prevalence of low back pain

Several reports have highlighted the increasing costs associated with low back pain (Leboeuf-Yde et al., 1996; Croft, 2000; Palmer et al., 2000). It is unclear whether this is due to increasing health care costs, increasing sickness absences attributed to low back pain or to a real increase in the prevalence of back pain. Studies examining changes in the prevalence of back pain have reported conflicting results. A recent report examining self-reported chronic back pain from the General Household Survey (Symmons et al., 2002) found that prevalence rates were similar over the past decade. Similarly, a study of self-reported back pain in Finland concluded that there did not appear to be any change in prevalence over a 13-year period (Leino et al., 1994). These findings are in contrast to one of the most recent population-based studies which examined self-reported back pain in 2569 men and women aged between 20 and 59 years, from eight geographically diverse locations in the UK (Palmer et al., 2000). That study reported a 10-year increase in prevalence of just under 13%. This increase was reported to be consistent across age and gender groups, social class and geographical region. However, a study conducted in the Northwest of England reported a slight decrease in self-reported back pain of 3.5% over a 7-year period (Macfarlane et al., 2000). Further examination of prevalence rates in that study did not reveal any age- or gender-specific marked increase in symptom reporting. Both studies were conducted on large general population samples and used similar methods of ascertaining the presence of low back pain highlighting the discrepancies which can occur in prevalence rates when slight differences in study methodology are present.

4. The prevalence of shoulder pain

4.1. Prevalence estimates in the general population

Similar to those studies which have examined the prevalence of low back pain, those examining shoulder pain have employed different design methodolo-

TABLE III

Population prevalence of shoulder pain (period and point prevalence)

Setting	Age range (years)	Study population	Classification criteria	Pain period	Prevalence (%)	Reference
Period prevalence						
Finland	40–64	2,068	frequent pain in shoulder joint	past year	17	Takala et al., 1982
Sweden	79	129	pain in shoulder joint > 1 month	not stated	16	Bergstrom et al., 1985
Sweden	18–65	2,537	pain, tenderness, stiffness in shoulders	past year	6.1	Westerling and Jonsson, 1980
Sweden	52–62	574	shoulder pain	past month	14	Bergenudd et al., 1988
Sweden	50–70	445	subacromial shoulder pain > 6 weeks	past year	6.7	Jacobsson et al., 1989
UK	≥16	42,826	pain, swelling, stiffness in shoulder joint	not stated	6.9	Badley and Tennant, 1992
Sweden	25–74	1,806	pain manikin	not stated	20	Andersson et al., 1993
Norway	20–56	20,026	"how often do you have neck or shoulder pain?"	not stated	20.3	Hasvold and Johnsen, 1993
Sweden	18–59	637	pain manikin	past 6 months	37	Ekberg et al., 1995
UK	18–65	312	pain manikin	past month	34	Pope et al., 1997
Finland	30+	7,042	shoulder pain	past month	30	Mäkelä et al., 1999
Point prevalence						
USA	24–74	6,913	shoulder complaints	day of survey	6.7	Cunningham and Kelsey, 1984
Philippines	5–65	1,685	pain manikin	day of survey	2.3 [a]	Manahan et al., 1985
UK	>70	644	current shoulder pain	day of survey	2.6	Chard et al., 1991

[a] Subjects > 15 years.

gies in terms of the population studied, the definition of shoulder pain and the survey strategy used. There are only sparse data describing the cumulative lifetime prevalence of shoulder pain in the general population. In one available survey, which was conducted in a rural and urban population in South Africa (Meyers et al., 1982), 71% and 51%, respectively, of those examined reported shoulder pain. These data are likely to be a poor reflection of the actual cumulative lifetime population prevalence since the number of participants was extremely small (135 from the rural population, 35 subjects from the urban population). However, as shown in Table III, it is clear that whether we consider the period or point prevalence, shoulder pain is experienced by a considerable proportion of individuals in the community. Given the most stringent definition (adopted by Jacobsson et al., 1989 and based on a clinical diagnosis of subacromial shoulder pain experienced for at least 6 weeks) as many as 1 in 20 of a Swedish population aged 50–70 years were found to have shoulder pain in the past year. When shoulder pain is defined based on the subjective reporting of pain, the observed prevalence rates are considerably higher. For example, more than one-third of individuals of working age reported shoulder pain, indicated by the shading of symptoms in the shoulder complex on a pain drawing of the body, in both a Swedish population (pain experienced in the last 6 months; Ekberg et al., 1995) and a UK population (pain experienced in the past month; Pope et al., 1997). Population rates may not always be so high. Badley and Tennant (1992) reported a much smaller overall rate of 6.9% in a UK population. Although shoulder pain in the study was based on self-report, subjects were asked about pain at numerous sites and the shoulder area was not clearly defined. These small methodological differences may explain some of the discrepancies in reported rates.

4.2. Prevalence estimates in primary care

Rates of shoulder pain in primary care appear to be considerably lower than those in the general population. Recent reports have estimated the incidence of new cases of shoulder pain in general practice to be between 6.6 and 11.2 cases per 1000 registered patients per year (Van der Windt and Croft, 1999). This is perhaps unsurprising since it is known that the majority of episodes of shoulder pain will not be reported to health care providers (Chard et al., 1991), while those that are reported are more likely to be of longer duration or more severe in terms of pain, discomfort or disability (Chard and Hazleman, 1987; Croft et al., 1994). Nevertheless, after low back pain, shoulder pain has been estimated to be the second most frequent cause for musculoskeletal-related consultation in general practice (Croft et al., 1994). Data from the UK based 3rd National Morbidity Survey (OPCS, 1986) indicate that 2–4% of all general practice consultations, whether new or repeat consultations, concerned shoulder pain. Extrapolating these data, it has been estimated that a UK-based general practitioner will conduct approximately 100 consultations for shoulder pain per year. Prevalence rates based upon statistics which are derived from primary care sources are unlikely to reflect the burden of shoulder pain in the general population. However, they do indicate the clinical significance of a large proportion of cases. The importance of these consultations is further reflected in the fact that onward referrals from primary care account for a substantial number of new patients seen in rheumatology clinics (Symmons et al., 2002).

4.3. Patterns in shoulder pain prevalence

The prevalence of shoulder pain in men and women in the general population shows an inconsistent pattern of association. While most studies report an increase in women (Manahan et al., 1985; Jacobsson et al., 1989; Ekberg et al., 1995), others have reported that men are more likely to report symptoms (Allander, 1974) or have reported no differences (Takala et al., 1982). The pattern of increasing prevalence with age is somewhat clearer. A study conducted in the north of England (Badley and Tennant, 1992) reported a prevalence of self-reported shoulder pain of 0.7 in those aged 16–24 years which rose steadily to 15.9% in those aged 85 years and older. Others have reported that the prevalence tends to peak around 55–60 years and decreases thereafter (Allander, 1974; Andersson et al., 1993; Mäkelä et al., 1999). It has been suggested that degeneration of the rotor cuff as part of the ageing process is the most likely explanation of shoulder symptoms experienced by the elderly (Chard et al., 1991), although this is unlikely to explain symptoms in younger age groups. Again it is likely that other factors including socio-economic status, ethnic background, weight, occupation and individual lifestyle factors are all associated with prevalence rates of shoulder pain.

4.4. Trends in the prevalence of shoulder pain

It has been hypothesised that shoulder symptoms experienced in the general population are increasing in occurrence (Andersson et al., 1993). There are, however, no published data which have examined the increase in prevalence rates over time. Other sources of information are often cited to indicate that shoulder pain symptoms are increasing. For example, a study of a Swedish population assessed changes in sick leave for neck and shoulder pain between 1986 and 1994 and concluded that while sick leave for low back pain had steadily decreased over this period, sick leave for shoulder symptoms had increased towards the level of low back pain (Nygren et al., 1995). Many factors unrelated to musculoskeletal problems, such as increased awareness of shoulder pain as a disabling symptom, can influence insurance claims and ultimately reported prevalence rates based on those claims. Conclusions drawn from data based on insurance claims must therefore be treated with caution. Whether the prevalence of shoulder pain is increasing in community subjects is a question which requires further, rigorous study.

5. The prevalence of chronic widespread pain and fibromyalgia

5.1. Prevalence estimates in the general population

There are no studies of the cumulative lifetime prevalence of chronic widespread pain. However, it is clear that a significant proportion of cases persist (Macfarlane et al., 1996b; McBeth et al., 2001) and that symptoms are unlikely to respond to treatment (Leadingham et al., 1993). There are a limited number of studies which have specifically examined the prevalence of chronic widespread pain in the adult population (Table IV). Of those available, one was conducted in the USA (Wolfe et al., 1995), two in the UK (Croft et al., 1993; Hunt et al., 1999), one in Canada (White et al., 1999) and one in Sweden (Lindell et al., 2000). In a random sample of community based subjects Wolfe et al. (1995) reported a prevalence rate of chronic widespread pain using the ACR definition of 10.6%. The prevalence of chronic widespread pain was observed to increase by age in both men and women, and women were more likely to report symptoms when compared to men at all ages. This rate was similar to that reported in a survey of community subjects in the UK (Croft et al., 1993). In that study, of the 1340 subjects who responded to a postal questionnaire 13% (crude prevalence rate) reported having experienced pain symptoms which satisfied the ACR criteria for chronic widespread pain. When these rates were standardised to the population of England and Wales, the adjusted prevalence rate was 11.2%. Rates were 7% higher in women when compared to men (16% vs. 9%, respectively) with an overall tendency to increase with age in both sexes. Hunt et al. (1999) examined the prevalence of chronic widespread pain, defined using both the ACR criteria and the more stringent 'Manchester' criteria. The prevalence of ACR-defined chronic widespread pain of 12.9% was similar to that reported previously, while the prevalence using the Manchester definition was, as expected, lower at 4.7%. Lower rates of ACR-defined chronic widespread pain have been reported. In a telephone survey conducted in Ontario, White et al. (1999) reported a prevalence of chronic widespread pain of 7.3%, while an even lower rate of 4.2% has been reported in a Swedish population (Lindell et al., 2000).

There have been a number of studies which have assessed the prevalence of fibromyalgia in the general population (Table IV) with rates ranging from

TABLE IV

Prevalence of chronic widespread pain and fibromyalgia

Setting	Age range (years)	Study population	Classification criteria	Pain period	Prevalence (%)	Reference
Population studies						
Period prevalence						
Sweden	50–70	876	Yunus	past 12 months	1	Jacobsson et al., 1989
Norway	20–49	2038	ACR	past 12 months	10.5	Forseth and Gran, 1992
UK	18–85	1340	ACR	past month	11.2[a]	Croft et al., 1993
Denmark	18–79	1219	ACR	past 12 months	0.66	Prescott et al., 1993
Sweden	25–74	1609	chronic pain with multiple location	past 3 months	10.7	Andersson et al., 1996
Canada	≥18	3395	ACR	past 3 months	7.3[a]; 3.3	White et al., 1999
UK	18–65	1953	ACR and Manchester	past month	ACR, 12.9[a]; Manchester, 4.7[a]	Hunt et al., 1999
Point prevalence						
Finland	≥30	7217	Yunus	day of survey	0.75	Mäkelä and Heliövaara, 1991
US	≥18	3006	ACR	day of survey	10.6[a]; 2	Wolfe et al., 1995

Setting	Age range (years)	Study population	Disease definition	Prevalence (%)	Reference
Clinical studies					
Rheumatology	unclear	1473	diffuse aching, ≥7 tender points	14.6	Wolfe and Cathey, 1983
General medical	17–84	596	questionnaire and physical exam	5.7	Campbell et al., 1983
Rheumatology	unclear	280	diffuse aching, multiple tender points	13.6	Wolfe et al., 1984
Rheumatology	mean: 50	2781	diffuse aching, ≥7 tender points	4.6	Greenfield et al., 1992
SLE	mean: 38	102	ACR	22	Middleton et al., 1994
Spine	19–88	125	pain scale, 11/18 tender points	12	Borenstein, 1995
Rheumatology	14–61	100	diffuse aching, ≥4 tender points	20	Yunus et al., 1981
Family practice	20–70	692	various	9–39[b]	Hartz and Kirchdoerfer, 1987
Bowel disease	15+	521	ACR	3.5	Palm et al., 2001

[a] Chronic widespread pain.
[b] Depending on criteria.

approximately 1 to 11%. Overall, the population prevalence is estimated to be 2% (Lawrence et al., 1998). Two of the earliest studies (Jacobsson et al., 1989; Mäkelä and Heliövaara, 1991) reported rates of around 1% using a definition of fibromyalgia described by Yunus et al. (1989) which requires the presence of additional symptoms, such as morning and evening stiffness. A greater number of studies have used the ACR criteria. Wolfe et al. (1995) reported an overall prevalence of 2% with higher rates in women and an increase with age. Standardising these data to the population of the United States, the prevalence of fibromyalgia has been estimated to be 34 per 1000 women and 5 per 1000 men across all age groups (Lawrence et al., 1998). A slightly higher rate was reported in a population study of adults residing in Canada conducted by White et al. (1999). As described above, subjects in that study were contacted by telephone. Of 4674 subjects contacted, 3395 responded (response rate 73%). Of the 248 (7.3%) who reported widespread pain and who were invited to participate in a physical examination, 176 (71%) participated. The adjusted (for non-participation in examination and weighted by the number of adults in each household) rate of fibromyalgia was reported to be 3.3% with a higher rate in women (4.9%) when compared to men (1.6%). One recent study has examined the prevalence of fibromyalgia in the northern region of Pakistan (Farooqi and Gibson, 1998) although the classification criteria used was unclear. Overall the prevalence rate was found to be 2.1% with a male to female ratio of 1 : 13. Interestingly, there was a significant discrepancy in the prevalence rate between those persons who lived in an urban area and were poor (3.2%) and those who lived in the same area, but were classified as affluent (1.1%).

5.2. Prevalence estimates in primary care

There are no prevalence estimates of chronic widespread pain in primary care. There is only one estimate available of the prevalence of fibromyalgia in primary care (Hartz and Kirchdoerfer, 1987). Of 692 subjects examined, 2.1% satisfied the investiga-

tors classification criteria for fibromyalgia defined as unexplained diffuse musculoskeletal aching present for 3 months or more and having 4 or more tender points. Other investigators have examined the prevalence of fibromyalgia in a diverse range of specialist clinics which have included patients attending rheumatology, spine and systemic lupus erythematosus clinics (Table IV). These studies have reported rates of fibromyalgia ranging from 2 to 22%. However, they most certainly will not reflect the true prevalence in primary care since these rates are likely to be elevated due to differences in referral procedures and other factors associated with consultation at specialist clinics.

5.3. Patterns in chronic widespread pain and fibromyalgia prevalence

In persons with chronic widespread pain and fibromyalgia, the influence of age and gender on prevalence rates is much clearer. Women are consistently more likely to report chronic widespread pain and, on examination, to satisfy criteria for fibromyalgia (Croft et al., 1993; Wolfe et al., 1995). Croft et al. (1993) in a population survey of 2034 adults in the north west of England demonstrated that women were more likely to report ACR-defined chronic widespread pain when compared to men (15.6% vs. 9.4%, respectively) and this excess in reporting was maintained at all ages. For both women and men, self-reported widespread pain symptoms tended to increase with age. In a study conducted in the USA, Wolfe et al. (1995) found similar patterns for both age and gender-specific rates of ACR-defined chronic widespread pain in community subjects as those found in the UK study. The only difference being that in the latter study, the prevalence started to decrease in those aged 70 years and over, although this discrepancy may be accounted for by the small number of subjects in the upper age ranges in both studies (LeResche, 1999). Using the more stringent 'Manchester' criteria, similar patterns have been reported (Hunt et al., 1999). In a survey of 3004 men and women randomly selected from the general population, an overall point prevalence rate of 4.7%

was reported. Women were more likely to report Manchester-defined chronic widespread pain when compared to men (5.3% vs. 3.7%, respectively), although this difference was not statistically significant. Significant linear trends in pain prevalence by age were observed for both men and women. In women, the prevalence in the youngest age group (18–30 years) was 1.6% and rose to 10.6% in the oldest age group (51–65 years). The prevalence in men aged 18–30 years was 0.6% rising to 6.6% in those aged 51–65 years.

5.4. Trends in chronic widespread pain and fibromyalgia

Whether chronic widespread pain symptoms and fibromyalgia are increasing in prevalence is unknown. General population estimates do seem to be stable at around 10–13% between populations. Whether these rates are increasing within populations remains to be examined. A study conducted in Sweden reported an increase in pain-related consultations to primary care and that these consultations were primarily related to fibromyalgia (Andersson et al., 1999). However, that study was unable to determine whether this change was due to an increase in morbidity or an increase in care-seeking amongst that group. Two population-based studies have found that although a large proportion of subjects changed pain category over a 1-year (McBeth et al., 2001) and 2-year follow-up (Macfarlane et al., 1996a,b), movement between categories resulted in the prevalence of chronic widespread pain remaining stable.

6. Summary

Pain which originates from the musculoskeletal system is common in community subjects. Reported prevalence rates of musculoskeletal disorders are affected by numerous factors, including those inherent methodological difficulties associated with epidemiological research, and population factors which are associated with pain occurrence including age, gender, ethnicity, socio-economic status, occupation,

and so on. Low back pain, shoulder pain and chronic widespread pain are amongst the most common symptoms and are associated with considerable economic burden to both the individual and the health care system, and with considerable disability. It is clear that these symptoms account for a large proportion of consultations to primary care givers and contribute significantly to the new case loads of specialist clinics. It has been hypothesised that the prevalence of these pain symptoms is increasing although this has not been established. Nevertheless, the prevalence of musculoskeletal symptoms in the general population and primary care highlights the need for appropriate interventions to be developed.

References

Allander, E. (1974) Prevalence, incidence and remission rates of some common rheumatic disease or syndromes. Scand. J. Rheumatol., 3: 145–153.

Allison, T.R., Symmons, D.P.M., Brammah, T., Haynes, P., Rogers, A., Roxby, M. and Urwin, M. (2002) Musculoskeletal pain is more generalised among people from ethnic minorities than among whites in Greater Manchester. Ann. Rheum. Dis. Ann. Rheum. Dis., 61: 151–156.

Anderson, J.A. (1977) Problems of classification of low-back pain. Rheumatol. Rehabil., 16: 34–36.

Andersson, H.I., Ejlertsson, G., Leden, I. and Rosenberg, C. (1993) Chronic pain in a geographically defined general population: studies of differences in age, gender, social class, and pain localization. Clin. J. Pain, 9: 174–182.

Andersson, H.I., Ejlertsson, G., Leden, I. and Rosenberg, C. (1996) Characteristics of subjects with chronic pain, in relation to local and widespread pain report. Scand. J. Rheumatol., 25: 146–154.

Andersson, H.I., Ejlertsson, G., Leden, I. and Schertsen, B. (1999) Musculoskeletal pain in general practice. Studies of health care utilisation in comparison with pain prevalence. Scand. J. Prim. Health Care, 17: 87–92.

Badley, E.M. and Tennant, A. (1992) Changing profile of joint disorders with age: findings from a postal survey of the population of Calderdale, West Yorkshire, United Kingdom. Ann. Rheum. Dis., 51: 366–371.

Badley, E.M., Raooly, I. and Webster, G.K. (1994) Relative importance of musculoskeletal disorders as a cause of chronic health problems, disability, and health care utilization: findings from the 1990 Ontario Health Survey. J. Rheumatol., 21: 505–514.

Bamji, A.N., Erhardt, C.C., Price, T.R. and Williams, P.L. (1996) The painful shoulder: can consultants agree? Br. J. Rheumatol., 35: 1172–1174.

Bergenudd, H., Lindgärde, F., Nilsson, B. and Petersson, C.J. (1988) Shoulder pain in middle age. A study of prevalence and relation to occupational work load and psychosocial factors. Clin. Orthop., 231: 234–238.

Bergstrom, G., Bjelle, A., Sorensen, L.B., Sundh, V. and Svanborg, A. (1985) Prevalence of symptoms and signs of joint impairment at age 79. Scand. J. Rehab. Med., 17: 173–182.

Biering-Sorensen, F. (1982) Low back trouble in a general population of 30-, 40-, 50-, and 60-year-old men and women. Dan. Med. Bull., 29: 289–299.

Biering-Sorensen, F. (1983) A prospective study of low back pain in a general population. 3. Medical service — work consequences. Scand. J. Rehabil. Med., 15: 89–96.

Biering-Sorensen, F. and Thomsen, C. (1986) Medical, social and occupational history as risk indicators for low-back trouble in a general population. Spine, 11: 720–725.

Borenstein, D. (1995) Prevalence and treatment outcome of primary and secondary fibromyalgia in patients with spinal pain. Spine, 20: 796–800.

Brattberg, G., Thorslund, M. and Wilkman, A. (1989) The prevalence of pain in a general population. The results of a postal survey in a county of Sweden. Pain, 37: 215–222.

Calliet, R. (1991) Soft Tissue Pain and Disability, 2nd edn. Churchill Livingstone, New York, NY.

Campbell, S.M., Clark, S., Tindall, E.A., Forehand, M.E. and Bennett, R.M. (1983) Clinical characteristics of fibrositis I. A 'blinded' controlled study of symptoms and tender points. Arthritis Rheum., 26: 817–824.

Chard, M.D. and Hazleman, B.L. (1987) Shoulder disorders in the elderly (a hospital study). Ann. Rheum. Dis., 46: 684–687.

Chard, M.D., Hazleman, R., Hazleman, B.L., King, R.H. and Reiss, B.B. (1991) Shoulder disorders in the elderly: a community survey. Arthritis Rheum., 34: 766–769.

Coste, J., Delecoeuillerie, G., Cohen de Lara, A., Le Parc, J.M. and Paolaggi, J.B. (1994) Clinical course and prognostic factors in acute low back pain: an inception cohort study in primary care practice. Br. Med. J., 308: 577–580.

Cote, P., Cassidy, D. and Carroll, L. (1998) The Saskatchewan Health and Back Pain Survey: The prevalence of neck pain and related disability in Saskatchewan adults. Spine, 23: 1689–1698.

Croft, P., Rigby, A.S., Boswell, R., Schollum, J. and Silman, A. (1993) The prevalence of chronic widespread pain in the general population. J. Rheumatol., 20: 710–713.

Croft, P., Pope, D., Zonca, M., O'Neill, T. and Silman, A. (1994) Measurement of shoulder related disability: results of a validation study. Ann. Rheum. Dis., 53: 525–528.

Croft, P. and Raspe, H. (1995) Back Pain. Bailliere's Clin. Rheumatol., 9: 565–583.

Croft, P.R., Macfarlane, G.J., Papageorgiou, A.C., Thomas, E. and Silman, A.J. (1998) Outcome of low back pain in general practice: a prospective study. Br. Med. J., 316: 1356–1359.

Croft, P. (2000) Is life becoming more of a pain? People may be getting more willing to report pain. Br. Med. J., 320: 1552–1553.

Cunningham, L.S. and Kelsey, J.L. (1984) Epidemiology of musculoskeletal impairments and associated disability. Am. J. Public Health, 74: 574–579.

Deyo, R.A. (1992) What can history and physical examination tell us about low-back pain. J. Am. Med. Assoc., 286: 760–765.

Deyo, R.A. and Tsui-Wu, Y.H. (1987) Descriptive epidemiology of low-back pain and its related medical care in the United States. Spine, 12: 264–268.

Dionne, C.E. (1999) Low Back Pain. In: I.K. Crombie (Ed.), Epidemiology of Pain. IASP Press, Seattle, WA, 1999.

Ekberg, K., Karlsson, M. and Axelson, O. (1995) Cross-sectional study of risk factors for symptoms in the neck and shoulder area. Ergonomics, 38: 971–980.

Farooqi, A. and Gibson, T. (1998) Prevalence of the major rheumatic disorders in the adult population of North Pakistan. Br. J. Rheumatol., 37: 491–495.

Forseth, K.O. and Gran, J.T. (1992) The prevalence of fibromyalgia among women aged 20–49 years in Adrenal, Norway. Scand. J. Rheumatol., 21: 74–78.

Frymoyer, J.W., Pope, M.H., Costanza, M.C., Rosen, J.C., Goggin, J.E. and Wilder, D.G. (1980) Epidemiologic studies of low back pain. Spine, 5: 419–423.

Frymoyer, J.W., Pope, M.H., Clements, J.H., Wilder, D.G., MacPherson, B. and Ashikaga, T. (1983) Risk factors in low back pain. J. Bone Joint Surg., 65A: 213–218.

Greenfield, S., Fitzcharles, M. and Esdaile, J.M. (1992) Reactive fibromyalgia syndrome. Arthritis Rheum., 35: 678–681.

Hartz, A. and Kirchdoerfer, E. (1987) Undetected fibrositis in primary care practice. J. Fam. Pract., 25: 365–369.

Hasvold, T. and Johnsen, R. (1993) Headache and neck or shoulder pain-frequent and disabling complaints in the general population. Scand. J. Prim. Health Care, 11: 219–224.

Hazard, R.G., Haugh, L.D., Reid, S., McFarlane, G. and MacDonald, L. (1997) Early physician notification of patient disability risk and clinical guidelines after low back injury. A randomized, controlled trial. Spine, 22: 2951–2958.

Hillman, M., Wright, A., Rajaratnam, G., Tennant, A. and Chamberlain, M.A. (1996) Prevalence of low back pain in the community: implications for service provision in Bradford, UK. J. Epidemiol. Community Health, 50: 347–352.

Hirsch, C., Jonsson, B. and Lewin, T. (1969) Low back symptoms in a Swedish female population. Clin. Orthopaed., 63: 171–176.

Hunt, I.M., Silman, A.J., Benjamin, S., McBeth, J. and Macfarlane, G.J. (1999) The prevalence and associated features of chronic widespread pain in the community using the 'Manchester' definition of chronic widespread pain. Rheumatology, 38: 275–279.

Hurwitz, E.L. and Morgenstern, H. (1997) Correlates of back problems and back related disability in the United States. J. Clin. Epidemiol., 50: 669–681.

Jacobsson, L., Lindgärde, F. and Manthorpe, R. (1989) The commonest rheumatic complaints of over six weeks' duration in a twelve-month period in a defined Swedish population. Prevalences and relationships. Scand. J. Rheumatol., 18: 353–360.

Kauppila, L.I., Eustace, S., Kiel, D.P., Felson, D.T. and Wright,

A.M. (1998) Degenerative displacement of lumbar vertebrae. A 25 year follow up study in Framingham. Spine, 23: 1868–1873.

Kessel, L. (1986) Clinical Disorders of the Shoulder, 2nd edn. Churchill Livingstone, New York.

Lawrence, R.C., Helmick, C.G., Arnett, F.C., Deyo, R.A., Felson, D.T., Giannini, E.H., Heyse, S.P., Hirsch, R., Hochberg, M.C., Hunder, G.G., Liang, M.H., Pillemer, S.R., Steen, V.D. and Wolfe, F. (1998) Estimates of the prevalence of arthritis and selected musculoskeletal disorders in the United States. Arthritis Rheum., 41: 778–799.

Leadingham, J., Doherty, S. and Doherty, M. (1993) Primary fibromyalgia syndrome: an outcome study. Br. J. Rheumatol., 32: 139–142.

Leboeuf-Yde, C., Klougart, N. and Lauritzen, T. (1996) How common is low back pain in the Nordic population? Data from a recent study on a middle-aged Danish population and four surveys previously conducted in the Nordic countries. Spine, 21: 1518–1525.

Leino, P., Berg, M.A. and Puska, P. (1994) Is back pain increasing? Results from national surveys in Finland during 1978/1979–1992. Scand. J. Rheumatol., 23: 269–276.

LeResche, L. (1999) Gender considerations in the epidemiology of chronic pain. In: I.K. Crombie (Ed.), Epidemiology of Pain. IASP Press, Seattle, WA, pp. 43–52.

Lindell, L., Bergman, S., Peterson, I.F., Jacobsson, L.T. and Herrstrom, P. (2000) Prevalence of fibromyalgia and chronic widespread pain. Scand. J. Prim. Health Care, 18: 149–153.

Macfarlane, G.J., Croft, P.R., Schollum, J. and Silman, A.J. (1996a) Widespread pain: is an improved classification possible. J. Rheumatol., 23: 1628–1632.

Macfarlane, G.J., Thomas, E., Papageorgiou, A.C., Schollum, J., Croft, P.R. and Silman, A.J. (1996b) The natural history of chronic pain in the community: a better prognosis than in the clinic. J. Rheumatol., 23: 1617–1620.

Macfarlane, G.J., McBeth, J., Garrow, A. and Silman, A.J. (2000) Life is much a pain as it ever was. Br. Med. J., 321: 897.

Mäkelä, M. and Heliövaara, M. (1991) Prevalence of primary fibromyalgia in the Finnish population. Br. Med. J., 303: 216–219.

Mäkelä, M., Heliövaara, M., Sainio, P. and Knekt, P. (1999) Impivaara, O. and Aromaa. A. (1999) Shoulder joint impairment among Finns aged 30 years or over: prevalence, risk factors and co-morbidity. Rheumatology, 38: 656–662.

Manahan, L., Caragay, R., Muirden, K.D., Allander, E., Valkenburg, H.A. and Wigley, R.D. (1985) Rheumatic pain in a Philippine village. A WHO-ILAR Copcord study. Rheumatol. Int., 5: 149–153.

Maniadakis, N. and Gray, A. (2000) The economic burden of back pain in the UK. Pain, 84: 95–103.

McBeth, J., Macfarlane, G.J., Hunt, I.M. and Silman, A.J. (2001) Risk factors for persistent chronic widespread pain: a community-based study. Rheumatology, 40: 95–101.

Meyers, O.L., Jessop, S. and Klemp, P. (1982) The epidemiology of rheumatic disease in a rural and urban population over the age of 65 years. S. Afr. Med. J., 62: 403–405.

Middleton, G.D., McFarlin, J.E. and Lipsky, P.E. (1994) The

prevalence and clinical impact of fibromyalgia in systemic lupus erythematosus. Arthritis Rheum., 8: 1181–1188.

Nygren, A., Berglund, A. and von Koch, M. (1995) Neck-and-shoulder pain, an increasing problem. Strategies for using insurance material to follow trends. Scand. J. Rehabil. Med., 32: 107–112.

Office of Population Census and Surveys (OPCS) (1986) Royal College of General Practitioners, Department of Health and Social Security. Morbidity Statistics from General Practice 1981–1982 — Third National Study. HMSO, London.

Palm, O., Moum, B., Jahnsen, J. and Gran, J.T. (2001) Fibromyalgia and chronic widespread pain in patients with inflammatory bowel disease: a cross sectional population survey. J. Rheumatol., 28: 590–594.

Palmer, K.T., Walsh, K., Bendall, H., Cooper, C. and Coggon, D. (2000) Back pain in Britain: comparison of two prevalence surveys at an interval of 10 years. Br. Med. J., 320: 1577–1578.

Papageorgiou, A.C., Croft, P.R., Ferry, S., Jayson, M.I.V. and Silman, A.J. (1995) Estimating the prevalence of low back pain in the general population. Evidence from the South Manchester Back Pain Survey. Spine, 20: 1889–1894.

Pope, D.P., Croft, P.R., Pritchard, C.M. and Silman, A.J. (1997) Prevalence of shoulder pain in the community: the influence of case definition. Ann. Rheum. Dis., 56: 308–312.

Prescott, E., Kjoller, M., Jacobsen, S., Bulow, P.M., Danneskiold-Samsoe, B. and Kamper-Jorgensen, F. (1993) Fibromyalgia in the adult Danish population: 1. A prevalence study. Scand. J. Rheumatol., 22: 233–237.

Reisbord, L.S. and Greenland, S. (1985) Factors associated with self-reported back-pain prevalence: a population-based study. J. Chronic Dis., 38: 691–702.

Rohrer, M.H., Santos-Eggimann, B., Paccaud, F. and Haller-Maslov, E. (1994) Epidemiologic study of low back pain in 1398 Swiss conscripts between 1985 and 1992. Eur. Spine J., 3: 2–7.

Santos-Eggimann, B., Wiertlisbach, W., Rickenbach, M., Paccaud, F. and Gutzwiller, F. (2000) One-year prevalence of low back pain in two Swiss regions: estimates from the population participating in the 1992–1993 MONICA project. Spine, 25: 2473–2479.

Schochat, T., Croft, P. and Raspe, H. (1994) The epidemiology of fibromyalgia. Br. J. Rheumatol., 33: 783–786.

Skovron, M.L., Szpalski, M., Nordin, M., Melot, C. and Cukier, D. (1994) Sociocultural factors and back pain. Spine, 19: 129–137.

Sternbach, R.A. (1986) Pain and 'hassles' in the United States: findings of the Nuprin pain report. Pain, 27: 69–80.

Svensson, H.-O. and Andersson, G.B.J. (1982) Low back pain in forty to forty seven year old men. 1. Frequency of occurrence and impact on medical services. Scand. J. Rehabil. Med., 14: 47–53.

Svensson, H.-O. and Andersson, G.B.J. (1989) The relationship of low back pain, work history, work environment and stress. Spine, 14: 517–522.

Symmons, D., Asten, P., McNally, R. and Webb, R. (2002) Healthcare Needs Assessment for Musculoskeletal Diseases:

The First Step – Estimating the Number of Incident and Prevalent Cases. 2nd edn. Arthritis Research Campaign, Chesterfield, in press.

Takala, J., Sievers, K. and Klaukka, T. (1982) Rheumatic symptoms in the middle-aged population in Southwestern Finland. Scand. J. Rheumatol., 47: 15–29.

Urwin, M., Symmons, D., Allison, T., Brammah, T., Busby, H., Roxby, M., Simmons, A. and Williams, G. (1998) Estimating the burden of musculoskeletal disorders in the community: the comparative prevalence of symptoms at different anatomical sites, and the relation to social deprivation. Ann. Rheum. Dis., 57: 649–655.

Valkenburg, H.A. and Haanen, H.C.M. (1982) The epidemiology of low back pain. In: A.A. White and S.L. Gordon (Eds.), Symposiums on Idiopathic Low Back Pain. CV Mosby, St Louis, MO, pp. 9–22.

Van der Windt, D. and Croft, P.R. (1999) Shoulder Pain. In: I.K. Crombie (Ed.), Epidemiology of Pain. IASP, Seattle, WA, pp. 257–278.

Von Korff, M., Dworkin, S.F., LeResche, L. and Kruger, A. (1988) An epidemiologic comparison of pain complaints. Pain, 32: 173–183.

Walsh, K., Cruddas, M. and Coggon, D. (1992) Risk of low back pain in people admitted to hospital for traffic accidents and falls. J. Epidemiol. Community Health, 46: 231–233.

Ward, T., Knowelden, J. and Sharrard, W.J.W. (1968) Low back pain. J. R. Coll. Gen. Pract., 15: 128–136.

Westerling, D. and Jonsson, B.G. (1980) Pain from the neck–shoulder region and sick leave. Scand. J. Soc. Med., 8: 131–136.

White, K.P., Speechley, M., Harth, M. and Ostbye, T. (1999) The London fibromyalgia epidemiology study: the prevalence of fibromyalgia syndrome in London, Ontario. J. Rheumatol., 26: 1570–1576.

Wolfe, F. and Cathey, M.A. (1983) Prevalence of primary and secondary fibrositis. J. Rheumatol., 10: 965–968.

Wolfe, F., Cathey, M.A. and Kleinheksel, S.M. (1984) Fibrositis (fibromyalgia) in rheumatoid arthritis. J. Rheumatol., 11: 814–818.

Wolfe, F., Smythe, H.A., Yunus, M.B., Bennett, R., Bombardier, C., Goldenberg, D.L., Tugwell, P., Campbell, S.M., Abeles, M., Clark, P., Fam, A.G., Farber, S.J., Fiechtner, J.J., Franklin, C.M., Gatter, R.A., Hamaty, D., Lessard, J., Lichtbroun, A.S., Masi, A.T., McCain, G.A., Reynolds, W.J., Romano, T.J., Russell, I.J. and Sheon, R.P. (1990) The American College of Rheumatology 1990 Criteria for the Classification of fibromyalgia. Arthritis Rheum., 33: 160–172.

Wolfe, F., Ross, K., Anderson, J., Russell, I.J. and Hebert, L. (1995) The prevalence and characteristics of fibromyalgia in the general population. Arthritis Rheum., 38: 19–28.

Wright, D., Barrow, S., Fisher, A.D., Horsley, S.D. and Jayson, M.I. (1995) Influence of physical, psychological and behavioural factors on consultations for back pain. Br. J. Rheumatol., 34: 156–161.

Yunus, M.B., Masi, A.T., Calabro, J.J., Miller, K.A. and Feigenbaum, S.L. (1981) Primary fibromyalgia (fibrositis): clinical study of 50 patients with matched normal controls. Semin. Arthritis Rheum., 11: 151–171.

Yunus, M.B., Masi, A.T. and Aldag, J.C. (1989) Preliminary criteria for primary fibromyalgia syndrome (PFS): multivariate analysis of a consecutive series of PFS, other pain patients, and normal subjects. Clin. Exp. Rheumatol., 7: 63–69.

New Avenues for the Prevention of Chronic Musculoskeletal Pain and Disability
Pain Research and Clinical Management, Vol. 12
Edited by S.J. Linton

CHAPTER 3

Economic aspects of chronic musculoskeletal pain

Mariëlle E.J.B. Goossens [*]

Institute for Rehabilitation Research, P.O. Box 192, 6430 CC Hoensbroek, The Netherlands

Abstract: Musculoskeletal pain constitutes one of the most common and expensive disorders in the Western countries. Since the incidence and costs of musculoskeletal pain are large and the socio-economic implications due to disability are growing rapidly, it is becoming important to examine how much of the burden and costs can be avoided by effective therapies and at what costs. The aim of this chapter is to give insight into important economic consequences, economic characteristics of musculoskeletal problems and trends in costs. The chapter summarizes the available economic impact studies of various countries which have reported on the costs of musculoskeletal pain, from a societal perspective. Comparisons between calculations of costs of illness are difficult to make, because of differences in several aspects. Nevertheless these studies indicate similarities in the structure and characteristics of the costs between these countries, which needs to be taken into account when planning new health care interventions. The characteristics of costs indicate that preventing the musculoskeletal problem for a small group of people could produce considerable economic savings. Insight into the cost-effectiveness of new and existing treatment modalities will allow one to consider the relative priority of different needs for chronic musculoskeletal pain.

1. Introduction and background

Musculoskeletal pain has a major impact on society in most western countries. The incidence and prevalence of musculoskeletal complaints are large. Payments for health care as well as for sick leave and work disability are enormous. The consequences of musculoskeletal complaints are not restricted to the patient, but are also felt by many other parties, such as the family, the health care providers, the employers and society as a whole. Therefore, when the economic consequences of musculoskeletal pain are to be considered, usually the societal perspective is taken into account. This means that those costs are taken into account which are important for the society as a whole.

This chapter gives an overview of the most important economic consequences of musculoskeletal problems considered from a societal perspective. The second part of this chapter gives a description of the most relevant economic definitions. The second part furthermore gives an overview of available international cost-of-illness data. The third part shows characteristics of costs of musculoskeletal pain and future trends in costs. Finally, the last part explains the need for economic evaluation in the health care planning process and shows the results of a systematic review in this area.

---
[*] Correspondence to: M.E.J.B. Goossens, Institute for Rehabilitation Research, P.O. Box 192, 6430 CC Hoensbroek, The Netherlands. Tel.: +31 (45) 523-7578; Fax: +31 (45) 523-1550; E-mail: m.goossens@irv.nl

2. Cost of illness

The economic burden of a particular disease on society is measurable in terms of direct costs and indirect costs. Direct costs include health care utilization (primary care, outpatient care, inpatient care, institutional care and medications) and patients' and family costs, such as out-of-pocket costs, paid and unpaid help and travel costs. Indirect costs refer to the value of production lost to society due to illness-related absence from (paid and unpaid) work and days of inactivity.

Musculoskeletal disorders appear to be one of the most expensive disease categories. Total costs of back pain, which accounts for more than half of all musculoskeletal incapacity, are estimated at 1–2% of the GNP (Norlund and Waddell, 2000). In western countries, back and neck pain are leading causes of sick leave compensation and early retirement expenditures (Waddell, 1998). In the Netherlands, in 1994, musculoskeletal disorders are ranked as the fourth most expensive disease category regarding health care costs and together with mental disorders they constitute the most expensive disease category in terms of absenteeism and disability (Meerding et al., 1998). Half of the direct medical cost was related to hospital care, 1% to medical specialist care, 6% to visits in primary care and 36% to paramedical care (Van Tulder et al., 1995). In the UK, statistics from the Department of Social Security (1994) showed that musculoskeletal disorders are now the most common cause of chronic incapacity (Waddell, 1998). The total costs are estimated to put musculoskeletal diseases among the most expensive illnesses in society, together with cardiovascular diseases and psychiatric illnesses. In Sweden, the group of back disorders and other diseases in the musculoskeletal organs were responsible for the major part of the cost of sick leave. Problems in the musculoskeletal system accounted for 48% of the newly granted early retirement pensions. Back diagnoses were mainly responsible for early retirement pensions (Jonsson and Husberg, 2000).

These estimates indicate that the economic burden of musculoskeletal pain is significant. To present accurate cost figures, however, we have to be cautious. Several countries, like the US, UK, Sweden, Canada, Australia, Germany and the Netherlands, have attempted to estimate the economics of back pain. From epidemiological studies we have learned that comparisons between these studies and across countries are difficult for several reasons, such as differences in methodology, differences in study population, differences in diagnosis and classification of (musculoskeletal) pain. When comparing the economic aspects, it is crucial to take these factors into consideration, since they may have caused changes in costs in time or differences in costs between countries. Furthermore, when comparing economic consequences, we also deal with the large number of (apparent and less apparent) cost components, differences in definitions and differences in measurement and valuation techniques. Furthermore, differences in health care and insurance systems, legislation, socio-economic aspects, wealth, and in the perception of musculoskeletal pain are important to bear in mind. One other major factor that can lead to different cost estimates is the perspective from which the economic consequences have been considered. As indicated earlier, cost-of-illness studies should preferably be performed from a societal perspective, which means that all relevant costs should be included in the estimates. Most US estimates, however, have not been calculated from a societal perspective. In these studies, workers' compensation rather than wages has been used as the indicator of productivity losses. Moreover, US studies have mainly been updates from two original reports estimating the total costs of back pain disorders between 1972 and 1978 at US $16 billion a year and in 1986 at US $11.1 billion a year. A few European countries used the societal perspective to estimate the economic consequences of back pain: the UK for 1991–1992, the Netherlands for 1991, and Sweden for 1995. Table I shows that the total costs per inhabitant of illness caused by back pain seemed to fall within approximately the same range for the studies in the Netherlands and in Sweden (Norlund and Waddell, 2000). For the UK, costs were lower, but using the same method for calculating losses of productivity

TABLE I

Cost of back pain in US dollars in the United Kingdom, Sweden and The Netherlands [a]

Cost categories	United Kingdom		Sweden		The Netherlands	
	Cost in million US $ (% of total)	Cost per inhabitant	Cost in million US $ (% of total)	Cost per inhabitant	Cost in million US $ (% of total)	Costs per inhabitant
Direct costs	385 (11.5)	7	213 (8)	24	368 (7.4)	24
Indirect costs	2948 (88.5)	113	2262 (92)	266	4600 (92.6)	299
Total costs	3333 (100)	120	2475 (100)	290	4968 (100)	323

[a] The costs estimated by each study were converted to US $ for the same base year, i.e. 1991, by using OECD currency and divided per inhabitant according to demographic statistics from the OECD (OECD, 1996).

as was used for Sweden and for the Netherlands, i.e. average wage plus costs for societal security, the cost per inhabitant for the UK could be calculated as about 80% of that for the Netherlands.

Although the studies cited above do not provide a complete overview of the economic impact of musculoskeletal pain, they indicate that the economic burden is significant. Nevertheless, it is valuable not only to focus on the final cost figures, but also to analyze the different cost components qualitatively, so as to identify particular features of the costs of musculoskeletal pain.

3. Characteristics of costs of musculoskeletal pain

A tentative analysis of the studies incorporating the costs of musculoskeletal pain indicated that the costs have several important characteristics that need to be taken into account when planning new health care interventions.

A first important feature concerns the structure of the total costs of musculoskeletal pain. For diseases in general, 70% of the costs are direct and 30% are indirect. For musculoskeletal pain, it is the other way around; although the health care costs are considerable, they contribute to less than 30% of the total costs, whereas the indirect costs are responsible for more than 70% of the total costs of musculoskeletal pain (Coyle and Richardson, 1994; Meerding et al., 1998; Jonsson and Husberg, 2000). As can be seen from Table I, this structure is similar in the different countries. An important observation in this respect

is that a large share in sick leave and compensation does not automatically indicate large medical costs. It is also surprising that most of the health care costs arise from hospital visits, physical therapy and diagnostic examinations, rather than from early rehabilitation, secondary prevention and pain management, in order to stop the further escalation of the indirect costs.

Second, the estimates of the direct costs of musculoskeletal pain fail to include important cost components, which may have led to an underestimation of the total direct costs. None of the studies calculating the economic burden took into consideration direct non-medical costs, such as personal expenses, expenses for informal care, non-reimbursed medical costs (alternative medicine and over-the-counter medication) and other out-of-pocket expenses. Especially for the chronic group of patients, the disorder is generally believed to have an enormous social and economic impact on the individual and family. Patients undertake a lot in order to feel in better (physical and mental) shape, such as alternative medicine, over-the-counter medication, Yoga, and other health care expenses. The impact is even more striking considering that expenditures due to pain increase, whereas income due to disability decreases. Two studies evaluating cognitive behavioral rehabilitation for fibromyalgia and chronic back pain assessed the economic impact on the individual patient, using a cost diary. One year after treatment, direct non-health care costs (such as informal care, transportation and out-of-pocket expenses) accounted for 66% and 71% of the fibromyalgia and chronic low back pain patient's total health care expenditures respectively, as compared to 34% and 29% for direct health care costs (such as doctor visits and hospitalizations) (Goossens et al., 1996, 1998). These data indicate that, although difficult to measure, estimates related to the economic impact of chronic musculoskeletal pain should, whenever possible, also assess the financial burdens imposed on the patient and the family. Since several of these cost components cannot be measured by ordinal data bases (such as those from the health care institutions and insurance companies), effort should be made to measure these costs from the patients themselves by use of diaries (Goossens et al., 2000).

In the same context, the available cost-of-illness studies did not include unpaid labor, lower productivity at the workplace and costs of (work)replacements in the calculations of the indirect costs. It has been shown that despite high ratings of pain, less than one-quarter of the sufferers said they had called in sick at their work (Linton and Ryberg, 2000). It is very plausible that respondents who stay at work in spite of the pain are less productive in their usual activities. Previous studies on the economic consequences of migraine has shown that on average work losses related to reduced productivity are higher than those related to work absence (Van Roijen et al., 1995; Ferrari, 1998). Furthermore, there may be an underestimation of the reporting of sick leave, due to the variability in duration of sick leave and type of employment, which is estimated at about 10% (Moens, 2001). Failure to include these aspects in the calculations of the indirect costs may lead to substantial underestimation. Effort thus has to be made to estimate these costs.

A third, more frequently publicized observation shows that the total costs of musculoskeletal pain are not normally distributed. Between 10 and 25% of the patients, account for more than 75% of the costs (Cats-Baril and Frymoyer, 1991; Moffet et al., 1995). This small group generally comprises chronic patients who suffer from musculoskeletal complaints recurrently or for a longer period (usually longer than 3 months). Watson et al. (1998) showed that (in Jersey, UK) half of the days of absenteeism were ac-

counted for by 15% of the employees with back pain who were on sick-leave for more than 1 month. The Dutch MORGEN project showed that about 32% of the respondents with chronic back pain had been on sick-leave in the last 12 months, compared with 15% of the respondents with acute back complaints. With regard to the direct medical costs, about 60% of the respondents with chronic complaints had used some kind of health care in the last 12 months, compared with 25% of the respondents with acute back pain (Picavet et al., 1999). Linton and Ryberg (2000) showed that 6% of the neck and back sufferers in their study accounted for 50% of the health care costs.

It is also remarkable that within this tiny group of chronic patients the costs are skewed as well. Goossens et al. (1998) showed a large discrepancy between the mean and median direct health care costs of chronic low back pain patients. About 20% of the patients turned out to be responsible for 56% of the total direct health care costs.

Special attention should be paid to explain the medical shopping behavior of this tiny group and how we can prevent these patients becoming chronic and finally disabled.

The characteristics highlight the fact that the high share of the indirect costs may be interpreted to mean that treatments and interventions available at the moment are not effective or are not being used effectively enough. The imbalance between direct and indirect costs highlights the need for new treatment methods.

Preventing the musculoskeletal problem for a small group of people could produce considerable economic savings (Reid et al., 1997). In that case, it is important to look beyond the results of the cost-of-illness studies. Cost-of-illness studies add little to the creation of an efficient health care system (Byford et al., 2000). Current research efforts should rather be focused on undertaking economic evaluations, such as cost-effectiveness analysis, which involve assessing both the costs and the outcomes. This will provide insight into what treatment ingredients will work for which subgroups of patients and which subgroups of patients run the risk of becoming chronic and as a consequence will cause the largest costs.

Better early and tailored interventions might reduce the suffering and as a consequence reduce the health care costs and costs of disability.

3.1. Trends in costs

The complexity of musculoskeletal pain makes it very difficult to give a reliable prognosis for a possible trend in its economic burden. Fordyce (1995) and Waddell (1998) conclude that we are dealing with a paradox: "the so-called pain-disability paradox"; on the one hand there are no indications that the incidence and prevalence of back pain has changed in the past 40 years. The large amount of scientific research in this area and the increase in knowledge about the mechanism of pain and effective treatments have not led to a change in the prevalence of back pain. All the evidence is that back pain is no more common, no different and not more severe than it always has been (Waddell, 1998). On the other hand, however, there has been a major increase in the societal and economic consequences of musculoskeletal pain. In all western countries, the number of persons who became legally categorized as disabled as a result of low back pain has increased enormously (Einerhand et al., 1995; Waddell, 1998) (Fig. 1).

The number of persons who are on sick-leave because of musculoskeletal complaints and the number of days benefit paid for musculoskeletal incapacities have increased enormously. According to experts, this increase in number of sickness and invalidity benefits may be explained by social, economic and demographic factors, rather than because of the back pain itself (Waddell, 1998). In many western countries, there has been a gradual shift in the concept of disability and conditions to which it applies. The concept of disability has broadened to include matters difficult to assess and that has gone well beyond the original intent of what constitutes a compensable disability (Fordyce, 1995). What is remarkable too is the fact that the increase in benefits claims is not, as it has been for years, only a male problem. Recently there has been an increase in claims from women, which probably reflects a social trend towards sexual equality. A second important demographic factor is the increasing risk of chronic musculoskeletal complaints with age (Rossignol et al., 1988; Van Doorn, 1995; Andersson, 1999). The prevalence of back pain increases with age till 65 years. In the MORGEN project, it was concluded that the reporting of chronic complaints in the Netherlands increased from 12% between the ages 20 and 29 years to 27% between 50 and 59 years (Picavet et al., 1999).

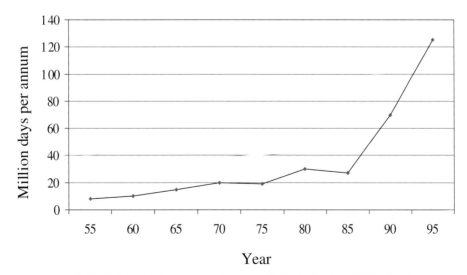

Fig. 1. Trends in UK sickness and invalidity benefits for back pain (Waddell, 1998).

Prospective studies should investigate the natural course of musculoskeletal complaints and factors influencing the development of chronic musculoskeletal complaints, such as physical, social and psychosocial factors. Undoubtedly, future shifts in the (economic) burden of musculoskeletal pain should be sought in changes in these social-economic and demographic factors, in the increasing role of psychosocial factors, and as a consequence in the shift in treatment.

4. Need for economic evaluation

Cost-effectiveness analysis has taken on an increasingly larger role in health care policy debates about interventions for chronic musculoskeletal pain. Cost-of-illness studies give valuable information, but add little to the creation of a more efficient health care system. One step in that direction is evidence-based research. In recent years, many systematic reviews of the effectiveness of treatment of musculoskeletal pain have been performed. The results of these reviews are without a doubt partly responsible for the current shift in treatment focus towards more active and behavioral interventions.

However, nowadays, decision-makers are striving for efficiency and looking for more evidence than only the effectiveness of interventions. Insight into the cost-effectiveness of treatments allows one to consider the relative priority of different needs and allows the implementation of successful and efficient interventions in the health care system.

More and more studies in the field of chronic musculoskeletal pain incorporate cost issues in their analysis. A MEDLINE-search with key-words 'musculoskeletal disorders/back pain/spine' and 'cost-and-cost-analysis' shows both an absolute and a relative increase of the number of chronic musculoskeletal pain studies that include economic aspects (see Fig. 2) (Goossens et al., 1999).

This does not indicate whether the results of all these studies can ultimately be used for decision making. Government, insurers and other payers will be willing to implement a certain intervention only when its effectiveness and cost-effectiveness are clearly established and compared to other treatments. The field of study in which both the costs and outcomes of alternative interventions are weighed against each other is called 'economic evaluation'. Drummond et al., 1997). Three recent reviews of economic evaluation of interventions for musculoskeletal pain syndromes showed that among the already small number of studies included in the reviews (not more than 30), the number of studies which actually demonstrated a good quality economic evaluation was a lot smaller (Ferraz et al., 1997; Maetzel et al., 1998; Goossens and Evers, 2000). The most recent review included a wide range of interventions. Four of the studies dealt with injury prevention programs, 10 with post-incidence management and secondary prevention programs and 16 studies with different kinds of pain remedies and clinical treatment, such as manipulation and physical therapy. The injury prevention program (except for back school programs) and post-incidence management and secondary prevention programs appear to produce cost savings due to reduced absenteeism generally for (acute) musculoskeletal pain in the workplace. Economic evaluations of chronic musculoskeletal pain interventions and other types of pain management seem to be lacking. This is remarkable, given the considerable (societal) costs related to musculoskeletal pain. Furthermore, the quality of the evaluation studies included in the review was low. A sound economic evaluation study should compare the costs and the consequences of two or more alternative interventions. Several studies included in the review evaluated only one single treatment or included only the costs of the intervention without mentioning the process of cost measurement and cost valuation. Then, little attention was paid to the measurement of patient-related costs (as mentioned in the previous section) and health-related quality of life. This is also remarkable, since the acceptance of quality of life measures as valid indicators of whether or not a therapy is beneficial has grown in recent decades, especially in pain-related disorders. Moreover, the review showed that from the studies included, it was impossible to draw definite con-

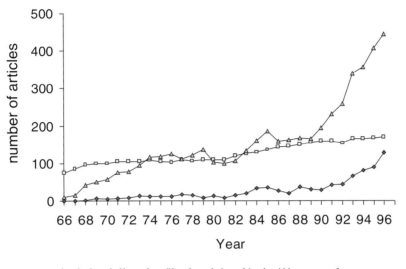

Fig. 2. Number of studies in the field of musculoskeletal pain incorporating cost issues (Goossens et al., 1999).

clusions on the cost-effectiveness of each treatment category. The small number of comparable treatments, the large differences in and low quality of the costing methodology and the large differences between the study population, limited the comparisons between the estimates in the studies reviewed. It should be borne in mind, however, that in some studies reviewed, the main purpose was not the economic evaluation of the treatment, but the assessment of the effect of the treatment instead. As a result, the methodology of performing an economic evaluation was backgrounded. Differences in cost-effectiveness then possibly reflect the characteristics of the programs evaluated and the differences between methods, rather than the differences between costs and effects. The review concluded that, due to the small number of comparable treatments and the large differences in costing methodology, it was impossible to draw conclusions in favor of any type of program, and to interpret the results with regard to policy decisions. This again demonstrates the need to perform good quality cost-effectiveness studies.

5. Conclusions

Growing health care costs and productivity losses, disappointing treatment results and changing beliefs in health and pain have led to an increase in concern about the amount of money spent on chronic musculoskeletal pain. Musculoskeletal disorders seem to be one of the most expensive disease categories in most western countries. Although the incidence and prevalence seem to have stabilized in recent years, the costs resulting from disability pensions and absenteeism have increased enormously. These so-called 'indirect costs' contribute to more than 70% of the total costs of musculoskeletal pain. It is important to realize that only a small group of patients, the so-called 'chronic patients' are responsible for the largest part of the costs. Nevertheless, the total costs of this small subgroup of musculoskeletal pain patients are expected to be underestimated, since important cost components are lacking in the calculation. The indirect costs fail to include unpaid labor and lower productivity at the workplace, which can be expected to be enormous in (chronic) musculoskeletal pain. The direct costs fail to include direct non-medical costs, such as personal expenses, expenses for informal care, non-reimbursed medical costs and other out-of-pocket costs.

The imbalance between direct and indirect costs seems to indicate that the majority of the existing treatments are not getting to the root of the problem and are not addressing the correct issues for certain subgroups of patients, especially for chronic patients. Insight into the cost-effectiveness of new and existing treatment modalities will allow one to consider the relative priority of different needs for chronic musculoskeletal pain. Special attention needs to be paid to prevent a subgroup of patients becoming chronic and finally disabled This could produce considerable economic savings. Furthermore, secondary prevention of chronic musculoskeletal complaints, (chronic) disuse, sick-leave and absenteeism may contribute to the desirable easing of this enormous medical, economic and social problem.

References

Andersson, G.B. (1999) Epidemiological features of chronic low-back pain. Lancet, 354(9178): 581–585.

Byford, S., Torgerson, D. and Raftery, J. (2000) Cost of illness studies. Br. Med. J., 320: 1335.

Cats-Baril, W. and Frymoyer, J. (1991) The Economics of Spinal Disorders, The Adult Spine. Raven press, New York.

Coyle, D. and Richardson, G. (1994) The Cost of Back Pain. HSMO, London.

Drummond, M.F., O'Brien, B., Stoddard, G.L. and Torrance G.W. (1997) Methods for the Economic Evaluation of Health Care Programmes. Oxford University press, Oxford.

Einerhand, M., Knol, G., Prins, R. and Veerman, T. (1995) Sickness and Invalidity Arrangements. Facts and Figures from Six European Countries. Vuga, Den Haag.

Ferrari, M.D. (1998) The economic burden of migraine to society. Pharmacoeconomics, 13(6): 667–676.

Ferraz, M.B., Maetzel, A. and Bombardier, C. (1997) A summary of economic evaluations published in the field of rheumatology and related disciplines. Arthritis Rheum., 40(9): 1587–1593.

Fordyce, W. (1995) Back Pain in the Workplace: Management of Disability in Nonspecific Conditions. IASP Press, Seattle, WA.

Goossens, M. and Evers, S. (2000) Cost-effectiveness of Treatment for Neck and Low Back Pain. Lippincott, Williams and Wilkins, Philadelphia, PA.

Goossens, M.E., Rutten van Molken, M.P., Leidl, R.M., Bos, S.G., Vlaeyen, J.W. and Teeken Gruben, N.J. (1996) Cognitive-educational treatment of fibromyalgia: a randomized clinical trial. II. Economic evaluation. J. Rheumatol., 23(7): 1246–1254.

Goossens, M.E., Rutten Van Molken, M.P., Kole Snijders, A.M., Vlaeyen, J.W., Van Breukelen, G. and Leidl, R. (1998) Health economic assessment of behavioural rehabilitation in chronic low back pain: a randomised clinical trial. Health Econ., 7(1): 39–51.

Goossens, M.E., Evers, S.M., Vlaeyen, J.W., Rutten van Molken, M.P. and van der Linden, S.M. (1999) Principles of economic evaluation for interventions of chronic musculoskeletal pain. Eur. J. Pain, 3(4): 343–353.

Goossens, M.E., Evers, S.M., Vlaeyen, J.W., Rutten van Molken, M.P. and van der Linden, S.M. (2000) The cost diary: a method to measure direct and indirect costs in cost-effectiveness research. J. Clin. Epidemiol., 53: 688–695.

Jonsson, D. and Husberg, M. (2000) Socioeconomic costs of rheumatic diseases. Implications for technology assessment. Int. J. Technol. Assess. Health Care, 16(4): 1193–1200.

Linton, S.J. and Ryberg, M. (2000) Do epidemiological results replicate? The prevalence and health-economic consequences of neck and back pain in the general population. Eur. J. Pain, 4(4): 347–354.

Maetzel, A., Ferraz, M.B. and Bombardier, C. (1998) A review of cost-effectiveness analyses in rheumatology and related disciplines. Curr. Opin. Rheumatol., 10(2): 136–140.

Meerding, W., Bonneux, L., Polder, J., Koopmanschap, M. and van der Maas, P. (1998) Demographic and epidemiological determinants of health care costs in the Netherlands: cost of illness study. Br. Med. J., 317: 111–115.

Moens, G. (2001) Socio-economic Aspects of Low Back Pain. Multidisciplinary Treatment of Chronic Pain. Belgian Pain Society.

Moffet, J., Richardson, G., Sheldon, T. and Maynard, A. (1995) Back Pain: Its Management and Costs to Society (Discussion paper 129). University of York, York.

Norlund, A. and Waddell, G. (2000) Cost of back pain in some OECD countries. In: A. Nachemson and E. Jonsson (Eds.), Neck and Back Pain: The Scientific Evidence of Causes, Diagnosis and Treatment. Lippincott, Williams and Wilkins, Philadelphia, PA, pp. 421–425.

OECD (1996) Historical Statistics 1960–1994, Paris.

Picavet, H.S., Schouten, J.S. and Smit, H.A. (1999) Prevalence and consequences of low back problems in The Netherlands, working vs. non-working population, the MORGEN-Study. Monitoring Project on Risk Factors for Chronic Disease. Public Health, 113(2): 73–77.

Read , S., Haugh, L.D., Hazard, R.G. and Tripathi, M. (1997) Occupational low back pain: recovery curves and factors associated with disability. J. Ooccup. Rehabil., 7: 1–14.

Rossignol, M., Suissa, S. and Abenhaim, L. (1988) Working disability due to occupational back pain: three-year follow-up of 2,300 compensated workers in Quebec. J. Occup. Med., 30(6): 502–505.

Van Doorn, J.W. (1995) Low back disability among self-employed dentists, veterinarians, physicians and physical therapists in The Netherlands. A retrospective study over a 13-year period ($N = 1,119$) and an early intervention program with 1-year follow-up ($N = 134$). Acta Orthop. Scand. Suppl., 263: 1–64.

Van Roijen, L., Essink-Bot, M.L., Koopmanschap, M.A., Michel, B.C. and Rutten, F.F. (1995) Societal perspective on the burden of migraine in The Netherlands. Pharmacoeconomics, 7(2): 170–179.

Van Tulder, M.W., Koes, B.W. and Bouter, L.M. (1995) A cost-of-illness study of back pain in The Netherlands. Pain, 62(2): 233–240.

Waddell, G. (1998) The Back Pain Revolution. Churchill Livingstone, Edinburgh.

Watson, P.J., Main, C.J., Waddell, G., Gales, T.F. and Purcell-Jones, G. (1998) Medically certified work loss, recurrence and costs of wage compensation for back pain: a follow-up study of the working population of Jersey. Br. J. Rheumatol., 37(1): 82–86.

New Avenues for the Prevention of Chronic Musculoskeletal Pain and Disability
Pain Research and Clinical Management, Vol. 12
Edited by S.J. Linton
© 2002 Elsevier Science B.V. All rights reserved

Reducing disability in injured workers: the importance of collaborative management

Michael K. Nicholas [*]

Pain Management and Research Centre, University of Sydney and Royal North Shore Hospital, St. Leonards, NSW 2065, Australia

Abstract: There is a great deal of knowledge available to explain why so many apparently minimally injured workers become long-term disability cases with poor return to work outcomes and associated high costs. A number of studies have demonstrated that particular interventions, at the individual injured worker level, at the clinical and workplace management levels and even changes to compensation systems can have an impact on the levels and persistence of injury-related disability and associated costs. However, rarely are these effects uniform across studies, suggesting that there is unlikely to be a single solution to the problem of growing levels of disability associated with musculoskeletal conditions. Thus, simply funding evidence-based treatments alone is unlikely to be sufficient if the rest of the injured worker's environment does not assist the rehabilitation process. This chapter attempts to outline some of the contributing factors to long-term disability cases as well as possible options for their improved management and even prevention in the first place. There is already good evidence available for many of these options. It is argued that ways of developing comprehensive and collaborative interventions, incorporating (at least) the injured worker, his/her health-care providers, the workplace, the funding bodies (and the system under which they operate) need to be found if improved overall outcomes are to be achieved and sustained.

1. Introduction

In most cases, workers with mild musculoskeletal work injuries (commonly referred to as 'strains and sprains') recover and return to work within days. By 2 weeks after such injuries, 70–80% of workers have returned to work. By 3 months, this figure is close to 80–90% back at work. After this period, there seems to be little improvement. These figures can be found in Australian statistics (WorkCover New South Wales, 1997) and similar data are available from Europe and North America (e.g. Deyo, 1993; Waddell, 1994). Those who successfully return to work are not all pain-free, but most remain at work, in many cases with modified duties (Von Korff and Saunders, 1996; Miedema et al., 1998; Carey et al., 2000; Cohen et al., 2000). Those who do not return to work after 3 months commonly report persisting pain and disability. They also continue to consume health-care resources in the form of multiple investigations and treatments, often to no avail (Engel et al., 1996; Williams et al., 1998; Cohen et al., 2000).

[*] Correspondence to: M.K. Nicholas, Pain Management and Research Centre, University of Sydney and Royal North Shore Hospital, St. Leonards, NSW 2065, Australia. Tel.: +61 (2) 9926-7318; Fax: +61 (2) 9926-6548; E-mail: miken@med.usyd.edu.au

Indeed, once such pain becomes chronic (after 3–6 months or so) and no treatable pathology is identified, there are no real cures available at present (Nachemson, 1992; Loeser, 1996). Over time, they resemble the long-term unemployed and they represent a cost — to the employer and the community — that is out of proportion with their relatively small numbers (Frymoyer, 1992; Engel et al., 1996). Australian data (WorkCover New South Wales, 1997), for example, indicate that those with back complaints lasting more than 26 weeks (10% of cases) accounted for around 42% of total costs for back problems. Similar findings have been reported elsewhere (e.g. Engel et al., 1996). Furthermore, there is good international evidence that the level of disability attributed to complaints like back pain has been rising despite reported advances in medical care and evidence that the incidence of back pain, at least in Western countries, has barely changed (Waddell, 1994; Grellman, 1997).

At least two questions confront us: (1) why are people with seemingly little wrong with them becoming so disabled; and (2) what can be done to prevent it?

2. Why is it that most injured workers with so-called 'strains and sprains' are able to return to work, while some do not?

There are a number of elements to this answer and their weight may vary from case to case.

2.1. The injured workers' responses

There is now good evidence that while medical/physical factors do play a role, psychological and environmental factors play a more important role (see chapters in Section II of this book for more detailed analyses). A recent review (Linton, 2000) of 39 prospective studies on back and neck/arm pain revealed that psychological factors such as fear, anger, depression as well as beliefs that pain equals damage (and thus the belief that activities which aggravate pain must be avoided) are strongly predic-tive of greater disability. Those with similar medical conditions who do not respond in these ways do not suffer as much, nor are they so disabled (Burton et al., 1995; Cohen et al., 2000).

2.2. The treatment provider

Evidence that commonly practised medical (somatic) treatments for persisting pain conditions are effective in terms of health outcomes and work restoration is quite limited. A recent large six-country prospective study with people sick-listed due to low back pain, for example, concluded that "almost none of the commonly occurring and frequently practiced medical (including physiotherapy and chiropractic) interventions . . . had any positive effects on either recorded health measures or work resumption" (Hansson and Hansson, 2000, p. 3055).

Medications (such as, analgesics and anti-inflammatory agents) may ease chronic musculo-skeletal pain but they will not cure it, and of course, they will have side effects which many find unpleasant and are unwilling to tolerate (see Deyo, 1996 for a review of evidence for drug therapies). It is worth noting that systematic reviews have often used pain reductions of 50%, rather than 100%, as a sort of benchmark of treatment effectiveness (e.g. McQuay et al., 1997). Somewhat surprisingly, the amount of pain reduction, even with opioid drugs, is often quite modest. Studies using controlled designs have indicated that typical pain reductions with opioid analgesics are not much better than 2/10, on a 0–10 scale (Stein, 2000). At the same time, Stein (2000) pointed out there is little evidence available to suggest that such agents reliably achieve improvements in disability or distressed mood and these have to be balanced against the high rates of side effects and withdrawal from treatment. Certainly, by themselves there seems little reason to utilise these agents.

Relative to advice on resuming normal daily activities and assistance in achieving that, there is no good evidence to support ongoing use of passive physical treatments, such as manipulation, ultrasound, interferential, massage, and hydrotherapy, especially in relation to rehabilitation outcomes in people with non-specific low back pain (Von Korff et al., 1994; Waddell and Burton, 2000). Very few of such patients require surgery (Loeser, 1996). Some surgical procedures (e.g. radiofrequency lesions) may provide pain relief for varying periods in a small group of selected patients, but they do not last and usually need to be repeated (Lord et al., 1997). Some procedures that show promise in uncontrolled trials have not fared so well under randomised, placebo-controlled conditions (e.g. Barendse et al., 2001). Thus, there are few real curative options with ongoing physical or medical treatments in the vast majority of workers with chronic musculoskeletal pain. In the main, such people will have to learn to live with their pain and to minimise its impact on their lives. The epidemiological evidence is that while many do this with little outside help, some do need help (Engel et al., 1996). Unfortunately, many seem to get too much ineffective help (Engel et al., 1996; Williams et al., 1998; Cohen et al., 2000).

In addition to the limited effectiveness of ongoing passive treatments, there is a real risk of such treatments actually causing disability — ongoing, ineffective treatments should not be assumed to be benign (e.g. Loeser, 1996; Fordyce, 1997). Such ongoing treatments risk perpetuating beliefs held by the patient that they are helpless and must wait for their doctor or physical therapist to come up with solutions. If the focus of intervention is on pain relief before activation, the therapist may inadvertently be reinforcing avoidance of pain. This approach could actually risk maintaining the patient's focus on pain and other symptoms (e.g. Hadler, 1998; Crombez et al., 1999). As a result, passivity and dependence (on others) can be promoted, leading ultimately to more disability (e.g. Von Korff et al., 1994; Kouyanu et al., 1997).

A recent study by Cohen et al. (2000) on a sample of Australian workers with back or neck/arm work injuries, revealed that those who had not returned to work within 2 years after injury received twice the amount of (passive) treatment than those who had return to work, even though there was no major medical difference between the two groups. It was also notable that those who had not returned to work displayed many more psychological problems (than those with persisting pain who had returned to work), yet these were attended to in only a minority of cases. The members of this group were also much more disabled than those who had returned to work (even though their medical conditions were similar). Thus, the additional treatment would seem to have had no effect on functional outcomes. Similar findings were observed in a large US study (Williams et al., 1998) where, despite the readily available evidence (in the literature) that psychosocial factors play a significant role in the development of disability, the health-care providers attended to such factors in only 0.5% of injured workers who had not returned to work within 6 months. In both the US and Australian studies the treatment providers seemed to have no obvious management plan for these cases, other than to persist with pain or symptom focussed treatments which had not helped and were unlikely to help.

2.3. The workplace

There is evidence that job dissatisfaction is a significant predictor of workers reporting injuries and of developing disabling chronic pain following an episode of acute pain as well (e.g. Bigos et al., 1992; Thomas et al., 1999). There is also evidence that those injured workers who remain at work tend to have better outcomes than those who lose their jobs (not just in terms of financial costs but also in clinical terms) (e.g. Sanderson et al., 1995). Equally there is evidence that employers with proactive policies that facilitate return to work (e.g. find alternative duties) tend to have fewer work days lost due to injury (Hunt and Harbeck, 1993)

Thus, it appears that return to work as soon as possible after injury is important in preventing the development of disability, even when pain persists. This action is now routinely recommended in clinical guidelines (e.g. Carter and Birrell, 2000). When that does not happen due to the employer's inaction or lack of assistance, the employer could be effectively contributing to the problem of long-term disability cases. Recent reports from New Zealand's Accident

Compensation Corporation scheme have provided graphic illustrations of the importance of this issue, with one abattoir company employing 5500 workers reported having 1500 injury claims in the last year but no long-term injury cases off work (Stevens, 2000). Stevens attributed this to their having found ways to keep the injured workers at work and to coordinate their medical management and rehabilitation with the workplace. This report would seem to be consistent with findings reported by Sanderson et al. (1995) who concluded that whether or not injured workers were at work was a more potent determinant of disability than compensation status alone.

2.4. The compensation system

There is less evidence for the role of the actual compensation system, partly because it is difficult to study, with many layers of interacting factors in each country. But the compensation system in any country does set the contingencies under which all parties — injured workers, health care providers, employers and insurance companies — operate. For example, most compensation systems require the injured person to repeatedly report symptoms in order to be compensated. Thus, it can be expected to be making some contribution to the outcomes achieved. Certainly, a number of concerns have been expressed about compensation systems and some evidence for these concerns is available.

Some of these concerns are discussed below.

2.4.1. Delayed recovery for those with compensation claims

There is a widely held belief (and some evidence) that those with injury compensation claims take longer to recover or regain normal function than those who are similarly injured but without a claim (e.g. Greenough and Fraser, 1989; Filan, 1996). Cassidy et al. (2000), for example, reported on the effects of changes in the third-party accident compensation scheme in a province of Canada. The changes included a shift from a 'fault' to a 'no-fault' scheme, whereby injured people did not have to prove someone else was 'at fault' in order to receive benefits. This also meant that injured people could not sue for pain and suffering, although treatments were funded and income benefits were increased. Cassidy et al. examined those with whiplash injuries and noted a 28% drop in number of claims in the first year of the new system compared to the last 6 months of the old system. Also, the median duration of claims dropped by over 200 days (i.e. between date of injury and closure of the claims file by the insurer). Cassidy et al. concluded that elimination of compensation for pain and suffering was associated with both decreased incidence and improved prognosis of whiplash injury. In a similar vein, a recent US study (Atlas et al., 2000) concluded that patients covered by workers compensation were less likely to report relief from symptoms and improved quality of life than those not receiving compensation at long-term follow-up. However, both groups had similar return to work outcomes, suggesting that good health outcomes per se, do not automatically predict return to work.

However, there are also studies which have found no real difference between patients with and without compensation claims (Mendelson, 1984; Mayou, 1996), suggesting that this aspect is not the only factor involved in prolonged disability. It also needs to be remembered that most injured workers actually recover and return to work quite quickly, despite their eligibility for compensation.

2.4.2. The adversarial nature of the system

Hadler (1995) has noted that "anyone who has to prove he or she is ill cannot get better... they will only get more disabled, any other option will compromise their veracity" (p. 646). In other words, where a compensation system takes an adversarial stance, there is a risk of effectively promoting the focus of attention on pain, symptoms, disability and suffering, rather than rehabilitation and functioning, which is often what is observed in injury claimants (Filan, 1996; Turk and Okifuji, 1996; Rainville et al., 1997; Cohen et al., 2000).

As an alternative, Hadler (1997) suggested that workplaces need to be comfortable when we are well and accommodating when we are ill. In other words, the focus should be on finding ways to help people stay at work while their rehabilitation proceeds. It may be argued that the Cassidy et al. (2000) findings of the effects of moving to a no-fault compensation scheme would tend to support this concern about adversarial systems. However, even no-fault schemes can be associated with prolonged disability as McNaughton et al. (2000) showed in New Zealand (which has a no-fault scheme). In that case, income replacement was thought to be a contributing factor.

2.4.3. The lawyers

As part of an adversarial system, the lawyers are frequently criticised for appearing to encourage injured workers to maximise their disabilities. For their part, the lawyers usually say that it is their ethical responsibility to get as much financial compensation for their clients as possible. Anecdotal accounts from injured workers have supported some of these impressions, but objective evidence is lacking, and no doubt difficult to obtain. It should be noted that since the mid-1970s New Zealand has largely done away with the use of lawyers in their accident compensation scheme, but that by itself was not enough to avoid increased disability rates through the 1990s (McNaughton et al., 2000). So it seems likely that lawyers cannot be held responsible for all the problems of long-term cases, though it seems reasonable to expect they make some contribution along with others in an adversarial system.

2.4.4. The insurance companies

There are numerous complaints by injured workers about the behaviour of insurance companies in dealing with their claim. These often relate to issues such as the use of covert (and not so covert) surveillance to check the veracity of their claims, delays in approvals for treatment or funding of expenses, refusal to fund recommended treatments, or simply what is perceived as rudeness. Whether accurate or not (or whether these are even totally avoidable) it is not difficult to see that such perceptions held by injured workers can provide ready grist for their anger and risk noncompliance and tardiness in rehabilitation (e.g. Mayou, 1996). Again, objective evidence is dif-

ficult to obtain, but from the writer's own experience there are some facets of insurance company behaviour that clearly do go against generally accepted principles of effective rehabilitation.

These include:

Failure to review cases that become long-term and to develop strategies to deal with them as early as possible. This was evident in the research conducted for the paper by Cohen et al. (2000) where actual insurance company files were examined by the researchers.

Delays in approval for recommended treatments. This can take many forms, from referring the injured worker to independent reviewers (who often seem to be people who do not agree with the treating doctors, but cannot suggest anything else) to repeated telephone calls (at the author's clinic it is estimated that each approval by an insurance company for admission to our pain management program takes an average of 10 phone calls between the clinic and the insurance company and often this results in delays of 2 months or longer — the worst case being 45 calls over 12 months).

Approval for treatments of unproven value or no value (but often cheaper than more effective treatments which are denied approval). This is always hard to understand, apart from obvious short-term monetary considerations and the possibility (hope) that the person will get better or withdraw their claim. This flies in the face of available evidence with long-term cases. For example, a systematic review of published randomised controlled trials of multidisciplinary rehabilitation programs by Guzman et al. (2001) demonstrated that with disabled chronic back pain patients, more intensive (and usually more expensive) interventions are more effective than similar but briefer interventions. Williams et al. (1998, 1999) demonstrated a similar effect in a heterogeneous sample of disabled chronic pain patients.

In practice, repeated sessions of passive physiotherapy may be approved ($40–45 per session in Australia) or repeated injections of steroids or nerve blocks for back pain may be approved (for $300–400 per occasion, depending upon country), but funding for an intensive multidisciplinary cognitive–behavioural pain management program (about $8000 in Australia or £4000 in the UK) with better evidence of effectiveness may be denied 'because it is too expensive'. Turk (1996) pointed to an apparent bias in evidence-based criteria for funding approval by third party payers in the US, with single modality physical treatments for low back pain requiring lower standards of evidence of effectiveness than multidisciplinary pain centre interventions.

A recent example at the author's clinic involved an insurance company denying approval for a long-term injured worker with disabling, persisting pain to attend our intensive 3-week pain management program (which has a record of good outcomes, consistent with the international literature on such programs). Despite our multidisciplinary assessment (by very experienced staff) and the patient's general practitioner's support for this intervention, the patient had been reviewed by an 'independent' psychologist (who had no formal clinical qualifications and no qualifications in pain management, but in Australia can still be registered as a psychologist) at the request of the insurance company. This psychologist concluded that the patient did not require the pain management program at all, but rather thought some individual sessions with him, as it happened, would suffice (for a smaller fee than that of the program). No mention was made of the fact that the proposed individual treatment had no good supporting evidence in the scientific literature. The patient felt uncertain about her options, but said she did not wish to antagonise the insurance company by going against their recommendation that she attend the psychologist for individual 'pain management'. Such machinations are not uncommon and it is hard to see that they assist in improving outcomes.

2.5. Summary

There are a number of possible contributors to the development of long-term disability cases following work injuries. The important point is that we know that many of them are psychological and environmental (health, employment and compensation systems), rather than underlying physical pathology. One implication of this finding is that these psychological and environmental factors ought to be amenable to change. In addition to doing more research on the factors contributing to disability and their identification in individual cases (e.g. Linton and Hallden, 1998; Vlaeyen and Linton, 2000), we need to find ways of implementing existing knowledge. The second section concerns what can be done about the identified psychological and environmental problems, based on available evidence, to prevent persisting painful musculoskeletal conditions from becoming chronically disabling.

3. Preventing musculoskeletal injuries from becoming chronic disabling conditions

There is unlikely to be one simple solution for every case, but it is likely that attending to only one of the problem areas outlined above will be insufficient to achieve substantial general reductions in disability in the injured worker population. Thus, simply improving the quality of treatments (providing evidence-based treatments only, for example) could well founder in a system which effectively reinforces attention on pain and disability and does not adequately support rehabilitation. A number of principles can be enunciated to act as a guide in this process. Wherever possible, these principles should be based on reasonable evidence. Each contributor identified above will be addressed in turn.

3.1. The injured workers

Given that, in the absence of serious pathology, the main obstacles to their rehabilitation are likely to be psychological and environmental, these issues must be addressed. They will not go away by wishful thinking. Fortunately, we now have good quality evidence that these obstacles can be effectively resolved, providing the injured worker adheres to the treatment (Nicholas, 1995).

In the first instance, the work of Indahl et al. (1995) from Norway have shown that providing these injured workers (around 8–12 weeks after onset of back pain) are given a comprehensive musculoskeletal assessment by an appropriate physician (to exclude signs of major pathology) then a large proportion of these cases who are worried about their pain and other symptoms can be reassured and encouraged to resume normal activities in a graduated manner. Lindstrom et al. (1992) from Sweden have also shown that providing such people with a structured exercise program utilising behavioural principles to facilitate performance and adherence (to the exercises) can also help restore function.

However, not all cases respond to reassurance and encouragement to resume normal activities. For example, Indahl et al. (1995) reported that about 30% of cases did not respond to this approach in the first 6 months. This figure is actually worse than that achieved in the current, much criticised, New South Wales (Australia) workers compensation system (Grellman, 1997), which suggests that differences in compensation schemes between Norway and Australia may be contributing to the outcomes achieved. In addition, it could be argued that those who are particularly worried or distressed or fearful do not respond to simple reassurance (e.g. Salkovskis and Warwick, 1986); they need something more.

Recently, Linton and colleagues (e.g. Linton and Andersson, 2000; Linton and Ryberg, 2001) from Sweden have shown that such cases can respond to a brief, structured cognitive–behavioural treatment program aimed at teaching them ways of coping and adjusting to persisting pain. In the Linton and Anderson study with a large group of injured workers with back pain (around 6 months after onset of symptoms), those who received this intervention (six 2-h group sessions with a clinical psychologist) on top of normal rehabilitation had a 9-fold improvement in days lost from work (in the following year) compared to two other groups who got the same rehabilitation input as the first group, but differing amounts of information on back care. The cognitive–behavioural group also had significantly less use of both medical and physiotherapy services in the 1-year follow-up period compared to the rehabilitation-only groups.

More recently, Linton and Ryberg (2001) found that a similar brief cognitive–behavioural program strongly prevented the development of disability in a large group of workers with persisting, but only mildly disabling neck or back pain. Significantly, at 1-year follow-up, days lost from work due to pain were substantially reduced in this group compared to those who received 'treatment as usual' from their general practitioner, physiotherapist or chiropractor.

Thus, there is now good evidence that if these (largely psychological) factors (beliefs, coping strategies, fears, etc.) can be tackled early (ideally within 6 months of onset) there is a good chance of preventing longer-term disability much more cheaply, and effectively, than is likely to be the case when extensive and repeated physical modalities have been tried and failed for 2–3 years (which is when many such cases are finally referred for cognitive–behavioural pain management).

It is also possible to tackle these problems several years later, as more intensive programs have shown (Guzman et al., 2001), but it is much more difficult, more expensive and less effective than when a similar (but less intensive) approach is employed earlier — and the injured worker still has a job to return to (as Linton and Andersen have shown). Williams et al. (1999), for example, demonstrated that more disabled, long-term cases with persisting pain will respond to such an approach, but they require a more intensive versus less intensive cognitive–behavioural pain management program. A study by Marhold et al. (2001) illustrates this point from another perspective. In this study, recently injured workers versus those with longer-standing problems (and longer-term absences from work) revealed that a brief cognitive–behavioural intervention (training in pain management and problem-solving strategies) was significantly more effective with the recent-onset cases compared to the long-term cases. Taken together, these studies suggest that while recent-onset cases can respond well to brief, targeted cognitive–behavioural interventions, not surprisingly the more disabled, longer-term cases require more intensive versions of the same approach.

3.2. The treating doctors

The doctors, whether they be general practitioners or specialists, are in an important but difficult position. On the one hand, they are expected (by the patients, the community and themselves) to treat. However, they have few evidence-based treatments for this population of patients, and if they provide ongoing treatments with little evidence of effectiveness they risk promoting passivity and disability in their patients (e.g. Loeser, 1996). On the other hand, expert advice from people like Indahl and various international panels (e.g. Fordyce, 1995; CSAG, 1994; Carter and Birrell, 2000), recommend more of a 'hands off' approach (after initial examination) with an emphasis on reassurance and encouragement to resume normal activities and to avoid bed-rest and other passive modalities. Not all doctors are comfortable with this role and many seem to feel that they must 'do something' (Australasian Faculty of Occupational Medicine, 2001). Further training for these doctors has been recommended, but it remains to be shown that more training for doctors will help or that they actually want it (e.g. Waddell and Burton, 2000).

Some have suggested that preventing chronic disability in relatively mildly injured workers is akin to dealing with an emergency and should require specialised multidisciplinary teams be established to deal with them (as such care may be beyond the capacity of most individual doctors or therapists) (Australasian Faculty of Occupational Medicine, 2001). This model would be based on the current use of specialised emergency centres for critically injured patients where additional but limited resources are required. Given the possible impact of long-term disability on a person's life this model would seem to have enough validity to be worth exploring, especially once a milestone like 3-months post-injury is reached without discernable progress, especially where so-called 'yellow' psychosocial flags (Kendall et al., 1997) are identified. To the best of the author's knowledge, such an approach has not been done yet.

A less dramatic proposition has been put forward by Von Korff (1997). Von Korff suggested that

doctors should be encouraged to work in a more collaborative way with their patients. Von Korff (1997) pointed out, in the case of chronic illnesses, medical care was seldom effective in the absence of adequate self-care (by the patient). Thus, just as in the case of people with diabetes or asthma, people in persisting pain need to play an active role in the management of their pain rather than simply passively waiting for the doctor to do things to them.

Von Korff (1997) proposed the physician should employ a typical behavioural approach in his/her management plan, that would be characterised by the physician and the patient firstly negotiating their respective roles, responsibilities and expectations. In this case, they would act like equal members of a team with the doctor playing more of a trainer's role and the patient being an active participant, taking responsibility for showing initiative and implementation of the agreed 'game plan'. Von Korff emphasised the importance of both parties negotiating agreed goals for the treatment plan as well. Clearly, unless the goals were those sought by the patient, the patient's active participation is unlikely. A similar theme was explored by Weinstein (2000) in his call for more shared decision making between the doctor and patient, rather than leaving it all up to the doctor to make the decisions on what was 'best' for the patient.

By extension, the same approach could be employed by the treating doctor including any others involved in helping the same patient/injured worker, such as other health-care/rehabilitation providers and workplace representatives, in a coordinated collaborative plan (e.g. Nordin, 2001). There is already some evidence that this is possible and can achieve improved functional outcomes (Rossignol et al., 2000; Waddell and Burton, 2000).

Theoretically, basic behavioural principles of reinforcement would support the importance of all those professionally involved with the patient actively collaborating on their interventions to ensure that these interventions are consistent (giving the same messages), and coordinated in their demands and expectations. Thus, one provider should not be advising rest and 'being careful' when another is advising the opposite. Equally, if the physician involved is prescribing medication, the use of this should be clearly related to the rehabilitation or re-activation plan. Waiting until the pain is sufficiently relieved before commencing rehabilitation is likely to promote the problems identified earlier. Rather, the patient should be encouraged to employ self-management strategies (whether or not they are taking an analgesic drug). Nor should a patient be encouraged to use an analgesic, say, to enable him/her to do activities they could not otherwise do without the drug (e.g. Nicholas and Wright, 2001). This approach is unlikely to be sustainable.

Unfortunately, it may be salutary to consider the extent to which the different health-care provider professions have been trained to work collaboratively with providers from other professions, such as physicians working with psychologists, or psychologists working with physical therapists. In many countries, and Australia is one, professional training often seems to occur in what might be termed a 'silo-like' approach, with each profession training itself with little attention paid to the activities of others or issues involved in working with others, even using what amounts to different languages (e.g. terms) at times (e.g. Miller and Swartz, 1990). As a result, one might be justified in having little confidence that effective cooperation is likely to be achieved in a general way between health-care professions, although the review by Waddell and Burton (2000) did indicate that some have managed it. However, when system issues, like differential funding for certain interventions rather than others (e.g. greater support for passive, unimodal medical procedures than active multidisciplinary programs, seemingly regardless of outcome evidence — see Turk, 1996, Williams, 1998 and Chapman, 2000 for discussions), are considered, there is even more reason for doubt about the feasibility of collaborative, evidence-based health care.

A recently published (WorkCover New South Wales, 2000) handbook for medical practitioners on injury management and the Workers Compensation System is a case in point here. Although injured workers frequently receive treatment from a range of non-medical providers, such as physiotherapists

and in some cases psychologists, there is no mention in this handbook of how the medical practitioner could or should collaborate with them in the care of the same patients. Given that the more doctors and other health-care providers that people see the more opinions they are likely to receive (e.g. Cohen et al., 2000), it is remarkable that so little attention was paid to this issue. Rehabilitation providers were mentioned in the handbook and it would be a major step forward if they were better able to work closely with the treating doctors, but many medical practitioners still seem uncertain (and in some cases unwilling) as to how to achieve this.

It is possible that arrangements like health maintenance organisations might offer a possible mechanism for a more collaborative system (e.g. Saper, 1996; Klein et al., 2000), but these are largely confined to the US and even there their acceptance is not total. As would be expected, issues of power and control over decision making remain hotly contested (e.g. Saper, 1996; Klein et al., 2000; McCarberg and Lande, 2000).

In sum, there is good evidence and sound, considered advice available for treating doctors to follow as a means of preventing excessive disability in injured workers but to date there is limited evidence of general acceptance of this advice within the profession. Waddell and Burton (2000) concluded that the impact of guidelines on actual clinical practice still remains to be demonstrated and Davies et al. (1993) have already pointed to documented evidence of medical practitioners persisting with ineffective treatments despite the evidence against their use.

3.3. The workplace

As mentioned earlier, there is evidence that certain measures when adopted by employers can greatly improve return to work outcomes for injured workers (see the Michigan Disability Prevention Study by Hunt and Harbeck, 1993). This study is also reviewed in the report by the IASP's 'Backpain in the Workplace' (Fordyce, 1995), which also makes a number of considered recommendations for employers. Not surprisingly, Hunt and Harbeck reported that those employers with pro-active return to work policies had better return to work outcomes than those who did not have such policies.

The recent New Zealand initiatives in this area mentioned earlier report impressive outcomes achieved by individual employers. However, some reviewers (e.g. Volinn, 1999) have cautioned against ready acceptance of outcomes from workplace studies due to concerns about methodological and research design issues, especially the common lack of suitable control groups and appropriate randomisation of subjects. Nevertheless, in the absence of better studies, we have to consider the evidence that is available. In this context, it should be remembered that given the complexities of this area, no single intervention in isolation is likely to be sufficient and mixed results are inevitable across studies in different settings (e.g. Greenwood et al., 1990; Loisel et al., 1997). Even so, Carter and Birrell (2000) concluded there was moderate evidence available to assert that a combination of optimum clinical management, a rehabilitation programme, and organisational interventions arranged to facilitate return to work in a worker with low back pain was effective.

At the more pragmatic level, the usual question raised about workplace interventions is the likely difficulty that small employers can have in finding alternative duties for injured employees, compared to large employers who usually have more options. The answer to this possibly lies within the workers compensation system to provide assistance in this regard to employers with small numbers of staff.

3.4. The compensation system

While it is beyond the focus of this paper to address every issue, it is also the case that improved injury management cannot occur without attention being paid to the overall system in which it operates. Many models have been tried (e.g. from those where fault is relevant to those where it is not) and all systems have their opponents and proponents. In this context, the comments of Hadler (1995) comments (referred to earlier) about shifting the focus of attention from proving something is wrong with the injured worker

to finding ways of helping that person return to work and other normal roles would seem to be a reasonable general framework. However, given the evident political realities of vested interests in maintaining the status quo, there will always be constraints on what is likely to be achieved. Nevertheless, it may be possible to address some of the other issues identified earlier. For example, the results of the Cassidy et al. (2000) study would seem to indicate that providing appropriate treatment for pain and suffering was funded, providing compensation for pain and suffering per se could be withdrawn as part of an inducement to focus efforts on recovery and rehabilitation.

3.4.1. Reducing delays in the system

This would appear critical if the first 3-months post-injury seems to be a defining period in the development of long-term disability.

In addition to current requirements for early reporting of injury or suspected injury and the speedy development of rehabilitation and return to work plans (in consultation between treating doctor, rehabilitation provider and workplace), there is a strong case for a comprehensive medical and psychological review of all injured workers who are not back at work within 3 months of injury (e.g. Linton, 2000). By this stage, they are already unusual (for those with back, neck/arm or strain/sprain conditions), and given that most others with similar physical problems are already back at work urgent, attention is required to determine why these people have not done so.

Given the evidence that psychological and environmental issues are very likely to be involved, these should be assessed by properly qualified and experienced people (mainly clinical psychologists and psychiatrists with relevant experience). In the author's experience, it should not be assumed that all psychologists and psychiatrists are equal in this task — even those with recognised clinical qualifications may have no direct experience or training in assessing injured workers in pain. A survey of practising Australian psychiatrists, for example, indicated that while 78% of those surveyed felt that specialised training was required for those psychiatrists wishing to work with this population, 54% of those completing their training felt they were incompetent to deal with this patient group (Harris, 1997). Undoubtedly, finding suitably qualified and trained psychiatrists or clinical psychologists may not be possible in under-resourced rural areas, but patients can still travel for appropriate expert assessments and consultations. The less specialised local practitioners could then work in a consultative way with their more specialised colleagues to provide a reasonable local service.

The results of these psychological assessments must be incorporated into a specific treatment plan for each patient. That means close collaboration between clinical psychologist or psychiatrist and treating doctor. Expertise by that doctor in musculoskeletal and pain medicine should also be expected or at least a doctor with such expertise should be involved in the review and development of a treatment plan. In some cases, such patients might be assessed at one centre, like a multidisciplinary pain centre, but others would be assessed at different sites (providing those involved are able to liaise cooperatively and often in their management planning and treatment implementation).

Where the injured worker continues to be concerned that "something might have been missed" in his/her assessment, scans like CT or MRI may be recommended as part of the assessment process and negative findings (i.e. no signs of major pathology) interpreted as 'positive' to reframe this aspect of the problem (e.g. Indahl et al., 1995). This can help to resolve this concern and as those cases which involve litigation will tend to get one anyway at some stage, delay may only prolong the uncertainty and interfere with the patient's willingness to commit to a re-activation program. Alternatively, such concerns can also be addressed within a cognitive–behavioural framework by an appropriate health-care provider (e.g. Linton and Andersson, 2000).

In addition, the insurance company or funding authority would need to play a role here to expedite the approval decision process or to come up with a better one if they do not agree with what the treating clinicians have advised. Using doctors, psychologists and others who do not have appropriate qualifications and expertise in injury management and/or pain management for independent opinions on the management of these cases should be strongly discouraged.

Finally, there needs to be a system in place for regular reviews of progress (towards expected and specified goals) with any treatment/rehabilitation plan, as well as a means of addressing any identified obstacles or difficulties.

3.4.2. Emphasis on treatments with good evidence early: avoiding a trial-and-error approach

Once the injured worker has reached the 3-month point (post injury) and is not back at work, it is critical that appropriate treatments be instituted as soon as possible. This would mean funding preferentially those treatments which have demonstrable evidence that they are likely to achieve the stated goals (ideally increased function and reduced use of health-care services) so that return to work can be facilitated (in conjunction with the rehabilitation provider and employer). In addition, this would mean addressing the issues identified in the 3-month comprehensive review that are proving obstacles to improvement. This should be done in a planned way with all steps and expectations explained to the injured worker (who must be an informed participant in the process). All those health-care providers involved in the case would need to commit themselves to the plan as well. Thus, proposed changes to the plan would need to be negotiated between the key participants (including the injured worker).

In suitable cases (where pain or concerns about pain interfering with function are a factor), a structured cognitive–behavioural pain management program like that described by Linton and Andersson (2000) should be instituted at least within 3–6 months of injury (when no curative medical treatments are likely). That would involve something like five to ten 1-h individual sessions or six 2-h group sessions. Such an approach may be combined with an exercise program supervised by a physiotherapist skilled in that form of treatment, providing it was coordinated with the cognitive–behavioural intervention and targeted at appropriate return to work and other functional goals (e.g. Lindstrom et al., 1992; Frost et al., 1995). Such interventions should not, of course, be long-term and must be reviewed regularly to ensure that progress is being made. If that is not happening then the reasons for that must be identified and addressed.

3.5. Conclusion

There is a great deal of knowledge and expertise available to help identify the reasons why so many apparently minimally injured workers become long-term disability cases with poor return to work outcomes and associated high costs. Attempts are being made by various funding authorities and various clinical and professional groups to improve the lot of those already in the long-term basket and to prevent others becoming unnecessarily disabled. However, it should be accepted that there is unlikely to be a single solution to the problem of growing levels of disability associated with musculoskeletal conditions — the history of the treatment of back pain should at least tell us that. Thus, simply funding evidence-based treatments alone is unlikely to be sufficient if the rest of the injured worker's environment does not assist the rehabilitation process. This paper has attempted to identify some of the contributing factors to long-term cases as well as possible options for preventing their development in the future. There is already good evidence available for many of these options. What is still required is a comprehensive and concerted attempt to implement them in a coherent manner.

References

Atlas, S.J., Chang, Y., Kammann, E., Keller, R.B., Deyo, R.A. and Singer, D.E. (2000) Long-term disability and return to work among patients who have a herniated lumbar disc: the effect of disability compensation. J. Bone Joint Surg. Am., 82A: 4–15.

Australasian Faculty of Occupational Medicine (2001) Compensable injuries and health outcomes. The Royal Australasian College of Physicians, Sydney.

Barendse, G.A.M., van den Berg, S.G.M., Kessels, A.H.F., Weber, W.E.J. and van Kleef, M. (2001) Randomized controlled trial of percutaneous intradiscal radiofrequency thermocoagulation for chronic discogenic back pain. Spine, 26: 287–292.

Bigos, S.J., Battie, M.C., Spengler, D.M., Fisher, L.D., Fordyce, W.E., Hansson, T., Nachemson, A.L. and Zeh, J. (1992) A longitudinal prospective study of industrial back injury reporting. Clin. Orthop., 279: 21–34.

Burton, A.K., Tillotson, K.M., Main, C.J. and Hollis, S. (1995) Psychosocial predictors of outcome in acute and subacute low back trouble. Spine, 20: 722–728.

Carey, T.S., Garrett, J.M. and Jackman, A.M. (2000) Beyond the good prognosis: examination of an inception cohort of patients with chronic low back pain. Spine, 25: 115–120.

Carter, J.T. and Birrell, L.N. (Eds.) (2000) Occupational Health Guidelines for the Management of Low Back Pain at Work. London, Faculty of Occupational Medicine.

Cassidy, D.J., Carroll, L.J. and Cote, P. (2000) Effect of eliminating compensation for pain and suffering on the outcome of insurance claims for whiplash injury. New Engl. J. Med., 342: 1179–1186.

Chapman, S.L. (2000) Chronic pain rehabilitation: lost in a sea of drugs and procedures? APS Bull., 10: 1.

Cohen, M., Nicholas, M. and Blanch, A. (2000) Medical assessment and management of work-related low back or neck/arm pain. J. Occupat. Health Safety-Aust. N.Z., 16: 307–317.

Crombez, G., Eccleston, C., Baeyens, F., van Houdenhove, B. and van den Broeck, A. (1999) Attention to chronic pain is dependent upon pain-related fear. J. Psychosom. Res., 47: 403–410.

CSAG (Clinical Standards Advisory Group), back Pain: Report of a CSAG Committee on Back Pain, HMSO, London, 1994.

Davies, H.T.O., Crombie, I.K. and Macrae, W.A. (1993) Polarised views on treating neurogenic pain. Pain, 54: 341–346.

Deyo, R.A. (1993) Practice variations, treatment fads, rising disability. Do we need a new clinical research paradigm? Spine, 18: 2153–2162.

Deyo, R.A. (1996) Drug therapy for back pain: which drugs help which patients? Spine, 21: 2840–2849.

Engel, C.C., Von Jorff, M. and Katon, W.J. (1996) Back pain in primary care: predictors of high health-care costs. Pain, 65: 197–204.

Filan, S.J. (1996) The effect of worker's or third-party compensation on return to work after hand surgery. Med. J. Aust., 165: 80–82.

Fordyce, W.E. (Ed.) (1995) Back Pain in the Workplace. IASP, Seattle, WA, 1995.

Fordyce, W.E. (1997) On the nature of illness and disability. Clin. Orthop. Relat. Res., 336: 47–51.

Frost, H., Klaber Moffett, J., Moser, J. and Fairbank, J. (1995) Evaluation of a fitness programme for patients with chronic low back pain. Br. Med. J., 310: 151–154.

Frymoyer, J.W. (1992) Predicting disability from low back pain. Clin. Orthop., 279: 101–109.

Greenough, C.G. and Fraser, R.D. (1989) The effects of compensation on recovery from low-back injury. Spine, 14: 947–955.

Greenwood, J.G., Harvey, H.J., Pearson, J.C., Woon, C.L., Posey, P. and Main, C.F. (1990) Early intervention in low back disability among coal miners in West Virginia: negative findings. J. Occup. Med., 32: 1047–1052.

Grellman, R.J. (1997) Inquiry into Workers' Compensation System in NSW (Final report). Department of the NSW Attorney-General and Minister for Industrial Relations.

Guzman, J., Esmail, R., Karjaleinan, K., Malmivaara, A., Irvin, E. and Bombardier, C. (2001) Multidisciplinary rehabilitation for chronic low back pain: systematic review. Br. Med. J., 322: 1511–1515.

Hadler, N.M. (1995) The disabling backache: an international perspective. Spine, 20: 640–649.

Hadler, N.M. (1996) If you have to prove you are ill, you cannot get well: the object lesson of fibromyalgia. Spine, 21: 2397–2400.

Hadler, N.M. (1997) Back pain in the workplace. What you lift or how you lift matters far less than whether you lift or when. Spine, 22: 935–940.

Hadler, N.M. (1998) Coping with arm pain in the workplace. Clin. Orthop. Relat. Res., 351: 57–62.

Hansson, T.H. and Hansson, E.K. (2000) The effects of common medical interventions on pain, back function, and work resumption in patients with chronic low back pain. Spine, 25: 3055–3064.

Harris, N.L. (1997) The role of psychiatrists in the assessment and management of chronic (non-malignant) pain syndromes in NSW. Unpublished Masters of Medicine (Pain Management) Treatise, University of Sydney.

Hunt, A. and Harbeck, R. (1993) The Michigan Disability Prevention Study. WE Upjohn Institute for Employment Research, Kalamazoo, MI.

Indahl, A., Velund, L. and Reikeraas, O. (1995) Good prognosis for low back pain when left untampered: a randomized clinical trial. Spine, 20: 473–477.

Kendall, N.A.S., Linton, S.J. and Main, C.J. (1997) Guide to assessing psychosocial yellow flags in acute low back pain: risk factors for long-term disability and work loss. Accident Rehabilitation and Compensation Insurance Corporation of New Zealand and the National Health Committee. Wellington, New Zealand.

Klein, B.J., Radecki, R.T., Foris, M.P., Feil, E.I. and Hickey, M.E. (2000) Bridging the gap between science and practice in managing low back pain. Spine, 25: 738–740.

Kouyanu, K., Pither, C.E. and Wesley, S. (1997) Iatrogenic factors and chronic pain. Psychosom. Med., 59: 597–604.

Lindstrom, I., Ohland, C., Eek, C., Wallin, L., Peterson, L.E. and Nachemson, A. (1992) Mobility, strength, and fitness after a graded activity program for patients with subacute low back pain. A randomized prospective clinical study with a behavioral therapy approach. Spine, 17: 641–649.

Linton, S.J. (1991) A behavioral workshop for training immediate supervisors: the key to neck and back injuries? Percept. Motor Skills, 73: 1159–1170.

Linton, S.J. (2000) A review of psychological risk factors in back and neck pain. Spine, 25: 1148–1156.

Linton, S.J. and Andersson, T. (2000) Can chronic disability be prevented? A randomized trial of a cognitive–behavioral intervention and two forms of information for spional pain patients. Spine, 25: 2825–2831.

Linton, S.J. and Hallden, X. (1998) Can we screen for problematic back pain? A screening questionnaire for predicting outcome in acute and subacute back pain. Clin. J. Pain, 14: 209–215.

Linton, S.J. and Ryberg, M. (2001) A cognitive–behavioral group intervention as prevention for persistent neck and back pain in a non-patient population: a randomized trial. Pain, 90: 83–90.

Loeser, J.D. (1996) Mitigating the dangers of pursuing cure. In: M.J.M. Cohen and J.N. Campbell (Eds.), Pain Treatment Centres at a Crossroads: a Practical and Conceptual Reappraisal, Progress in Pain Research and Management, Vol. 7. IASP Press, Seattle, WA, pp. 101–108.

Loisel, P., Abenhaim, L., Durand, P., Esdaile, J.M., Suissa, S., Gosselin, L., Simard, R., Turcotte, J. and Lemaire, J. (1997) A population-based, randomized clinical trial on back pain management. Spine, 22: 2911–2918.

Lord, S., Barnsley, L., Wallis, B.J. and Bogduk, N. (1997) Percutaneous radiofrequency neurotomy for chronic cervical zygapophyseal joint pain. N. Engl. J. Med., 335: 1721–1726.

Marhold, C., Linton, S.J. and Melin, L. (2001) A cognitive–behavioral return-to-work program: effects on pain patients with a history of long-term versus short-term sick leave. Pain, 91: 155–163.

Mayou, R. (1996) Accident neurosis revisited. Br. J. Psychiatry, 168: 399–403.

McCarberg, B. and Lande, S.D. (Eds.) (2000) APS Managed Care Forum on Pain. APS Bull. 10: 10–14.

McNaughton, H.K., Sims, A. and Taylor, W.J. (2000) Prognosis for people with back pain under a no-fault 24-hour cover compensation scheme. Spine, 25: 1254–1258.

McQuay, H.J., Moore, R.A., Eccleston, C., Morley, S. and Williams, A.C.deC. (1997) Systematic review of outpatient services for chronic pain control. Health Technol. Assess. 1(6): 11–12.

Mendelson, G. (1984) Compensation, pain complaints, and psychological disturbance. Pain, 20: 169–177.

Miedema, H.S., Chorus, A.M.J., Wevers, C.W.J. and van der Linden, S. (1998) Chronicity of back problems during working life. Spine, 23: 2021–2029.

Miller, T. and Swartz, L. (1990) Clinical psychology in general hospital settings: issues in interprofessional relationships. Prof. Psychol. Res. Pract., 21: 48–53.

Nachemson, A. (1992) Newest knowledge of low back pain: a critical look. Clin. Orthop., 279: 8–20.

Nordin, M. (2001) Backs to work: some reflections. Spine, 26: 851–856.

Nicholas, M.K. (1995) Compliance: a barrier to occupational rehabilitation? J. Occup. Rehab., 5: 271–282.

Nicholas, M.K. and Wright, M. (2001) Management of acute and chronic pain. In: J. Milgrom and G.D. Burrows (Eds.),

Psychiatry and Psychology: Integrating Medical Practice. John Wiley and Sons, Chichester, pp. 127–154.

Rainville, J., Sobel, J.B., Hartigan, C. and Wright, A. (1997) The effect of compensation involvement on the reporting of pain and disability by patients referred for rehabilitation of chronic low back pain. Spine, 22: 2016–2024.

Rossignol, M., Abenhaim, L., Seguin, P., Neveu, A., Collet, J.-P., Ducruet, T. and Shapiro, S. (2000) Coordination of primary health care for back pain: a randomized controlled trial. Spine, 25: 251–259.

Salkovskis, P.M. and Warwick, H.M.C. (1986) Morbid pre-occupations, health anxiety and reassurance: a cognitive–behavioural approach to hypochondriasis. Behav. Res. Ther., 24: 597–602.

Sanderson, P.L., Todd, B.D., Holt, G.R. and Getty, C.J. (1995) Compensation, work status, and disability in low back pain patients. Spine, 20: 554–556.

Saper, J.R. (1996) Health care reform and access to pain treatment: a challenge to managed care concepts. In M.J.M. Cohen and J.N. Campbell (Eds.), Pain Treatment Centres at a Crossroads: a Practical and Conceptual Reappraisal, Progress in Pain Research and Management, Vol. 7. IASP Press, Seattle, WA, pp. 275–286.

Sinclair, S.J., Hogg-Johnson, S., Murdoch, M.V. and Shields, S.A. (1997) The effectiveness of an early active intervention program for workers with soft-tissue injuries. Spine, 22: 2919–2931.

Stein, C. (2000) What's wrong with opioids in chronic pain? Curr. Opin. Anaesthesiol., 13: 557–559.

Stevens, K. (2000) Industrial case management. Paper presented at Spine in Action 2000 Conference: Managing Low Back Pain in the Workplace. ACC Injury Prevention and Christchurch School of Medicine. Wellington, New Zealand.

Thomas, E. et al. (1999) Predicting who develops chronic low back pain in primary care: a prospective study. Br. Med. J., 318: 1662–1667.

Turk, D.C. (1996) Efficacy of multidisciplinary pain centres in the treatment of chronic pain. In: M.J.M. Cohen and J.N. Campbell (Eds.), Pain Treatment Centres at a Crossroads: a Practical and Conceptual Reappraisal, Progress in Pain Research and Management, Vol. 7. IASP Press, Seattle, WA, pp. 257–274.

Turk, D.C. and Okifuji, A. (1996) Perception of traumatic onset, compensation status and physical findings: impact on pain severity, emotional distress, and disability in chronic pain patients. J. Behav. Med., 19: 435–453.

Vlaeyen, J. and Crombez, G. (1999) Fear of movement/(re)injury, avoidance and pain disability in chronic low back pain patients. Man. Ther., 4: 187–195.

Vlaeyen, J. and Linton, S.J. (2000) Fear-avoidance and its consequences in chronic musculoskeletal pain: a state of the art. Pain, 85: 317–332.

Volinn, E. (1999) Do workplace interventions prevent low-back disorders? If so, why?: a methodologic commentary. Ergonomics, 42: 258–272.

Von Korff, M. (1994) Studying the natural history of back pain. Spine, 19: 2041S–2046S.

Von Korff, M. (1997) Collaborative Care. Ann Intern. Med., 127: 1097–1102.

Von Korff, M., Barlow, W., Cherkin, D. and Deyo, R.A. (1994) Effects of practice style in managing back pain. Ann. Intern. Med., 121: 187–195.

Von Korff, M. and Saunders, K. (1996) The course of back pain in primary care. Spine, 21: 2833–2839.

Waddell, G. (1994) The epidemiology and cost of back pain. Annex to the Clinical Advisory Group (CSAG) report on back Pain, HMSO, London, pp. 1–64.

Waddell, G. and Burton, K. (2000) Evidence review. In: J.T. Carter and L.N. Birrell (Eds.), Occupational Health Guidelines for the Management of Low Back Pain at Work — Principal Recommendations. Faculty of Occupational Medicine, London.

Weinstein, J.N. (2000) The missing piece: embracing shared decision making to reform health care. Spine, 25: 1–4.

Williams, A.C.deC. (1998) Evidence-based health care: applying fine words to one's fingertips. Pain Forum, 7: 55–57.

Williams, D.A., Feurstein, M., Durbin, D. and Pezzello, J. (1998) Health care and indemnity costs across the natural history of disability in occupational low back pain. Spine, 23: 2329–2336.

Williams, A.C.deC., Nicholas, M.K., Richardson, P.H., Pither, C.E. and Fernandes, J. (1999) Generalizing from a controlled trial: the effects of patient preference versus randomization on the outcome of inpatient versus outpatient chronic pain management. Pain, 83: 57–65.

Williams, A.C.deC., Richardson, P.H., Nicholas, M.K., Pither, C.E., Harding, V.R., Ralphs, J.A., Ridout, K.L., Richardson, I.H., Justins, D.M. and Chamberlain, J.H. (1996) Inpatient versus outpatient pain management: results of a randomised controlled trial. Pain, 66: 13–22.

WorkCover New South Wales, Back injuries statistical profile 1995/6. New South Wales Workers Compensation Statistics. ISSN 1039–1487. Statistics Branch, Sydney, WorkCover Authority, 1997.

WorkCover New South Wales, Injury Management and Workers Compensation System: A Medical Practitioner's Handbook. Sydney, 2000.

New Avenues for the Prevention of Chronic Musculoskeletal Pain and Disability
Pain Research and Clinical Management, Vol. 12
Edited by S.J. Linton

CHAPTER 5

Concepts of treatment and prevention in musculoskeletal disorders

Chris J. Main [*]

Department of Behavioural Medicine, Hope Hospital, Eccles Old Road, Salford M6 8HD, UK

Abstract: This chapter focuses on basic concepts concerning the prevention of musculoskeletal pain and disability. First, we examine the idea of whether pain can and should be prevented. Then a historical overview provides background for how we might view the prevention of pain and disability. Various concepts of treatment and prevention in relation to musculoskeletal disorders, using non-specific low back pain (LBP) as an example are therefore examined. We find that there is a need to move from ideas about preventing pain to preventing disability. In particular, occupational aspects appear to be relevant. This includes occupational risk factors, but also organizational factors. It is argued that there is a clear need to develop better clinical–occupational interfaces. Moreover, there is a call to move beyond traditional pathology-based concepts of sickness and disability. Health care and social systems are slow to change and the power of underling models of illness in directing the focus of attention needs to be recognized. To develop effective prevention, we must then reconsider our fundamental assumptions, not only regarding the objectives for intervention, but also the type of interventions. The concept of prevention, within the field of musculoskeletal disorders has developed mainly from a clinical perspective. We need to expand our role in terms of a 'systems' perspective. We may need to expand our clinically derived concepts of prevention; broaden our skills and develop closer and more effective liaison with other agencies. This must, however, be carried out within an evidence-based framework.

1. Introduction

Since the advent of public health medicine, concepts of prevention have been a cornerstone of medicine. Indeed, it could be argued that the success of prevention for diseases such as polio has fuelled unrealistic and unachievable targets for prevention. Even within the category of clearly identified disease, problems such as malaria can re-emerge as nature finds ways of combating prevention by the development of drug-resistant organisms. The optimism borne of early success established an expectation that modern medicine was powerful enough to tackle the most intransigent of diseases such as cancer; an achievement not as yet realized despite the advent of high tech medicine and a colossal research program underpinned by the pharmaceutical industry. What then of pain? Eighty percent of people will suffer from significant pain problems and pain is the most common presenting symptom in hospitals. Can we prevent pain? How should we view prevention? In this chapter, I shall attempt to review concepts

---
[*] Correspondence to: C.J. Main, Department of Behavioural Medicine, Hope Hospital, Eccles Old Road, Salford M6 8HD, UK. E-mail: cmain@fs1.ho.man.ac.uk

of treatment and prevention in relation to musculo-skeletal disorders, using non-specific low back pain (LBP) as an example. (Evidence-based appraisal of our success in 'prevention' is the subject of later chapters.)

2. A historical perspective on treatment and prevention

Early approaches to the treatment of LBP were dom-inated by a search for structural abnormality. Ac-cording to Waddell (1998), after Mixter and Barr (1934) first described 'disc prolapse' as a cause of sciatica, disc rupture was postulated as a possible cause for back pain, the notion of back pain as an 'injury' became established and orthopedic surgery was established as a major focus of treatment. Mean-while, a range of manual therapies had also devel-oped. Orthopedic medicine incorporated manipula-tion for spinal fractures and dislocations, but the treatment of musculoskeletal symptoms by manual therapy was taken up unorthodox practitioners, orig-inally 'bone-setters' and developed within a much more holistic frame of reference. Osteopathy (Still, 1899) and Chiropractic (Palmer, 1910) developed as distinct professions. Although both claim to offer a more holistic approach o treatment than orthodox medicine, to the 'uncommitted' they seem very sim-ilar in application in that they rely principally on a type of physical readjustment to the spine; and are 'holistic' only in terms of their stated philosophies of healing. Neither seem to require much in the way of patient perception or engagement.

Within the orthodox tradition, however, there was also a move to promote manual therapy, now mainly the province of physiotherapists. More recently, a number of 'schools' of physiotherapy, such as Cyriax (1969) have developed; each of which have their 'disciples', but in general the approaches can be considered in terms of 'hands-on' techniques, such as massage and manipulation; or more 'hands-off' techniques with a primary emphasis on exercise and re-activation. In traditional physiotherapy, although education of the patient may play a part, back pain

is viewed principally as a physical abnormality and managed as such. To the extent that there is a focus on prevention, it has a postural and biomechanical focus.

The accompanying widely promulgated tenet "Let pain be your guide", the precise origin of which is uncertain, arguably has been responsible for an approach to prevention which has led to much unnecessary fear and pain-associated limitations.

It would certainly appear to be the case that, treat-ments focused on surgery, manipulative adjustment (with or without associated pharmacological inter-vention) have failed to prevent the progressive rise in pain-associated dysfunction during the latter third of the 20th Century.

2.1. Prevention of pain as the primary focus of treatment

The use of anesthetics for the relief of pain in the context of surgery represents perhaps the most dramatic success in the prevention of pain. Unfor-tunately, from the strict perspective of pain control, it had an unacceptably high cost in rendering the patient unconscious. The success of postoperative analgesia, however, illustrated that pain prevention was possible in the context of significant tissue dam-age. Peripherally and centrally acting drugs were developed to disrupt the nociceptive pathways link-ing peripheral tissue damage with activation of pain centers in the brain (and the experience of pain it-self). The principle of prevention was extended with the development of chemical, electrical and surgi-cal approaches to 'interruption' of pain pathways. Unfortunately, the exclusive focus on the nocicep-tive component was not always successful, either in the relief of pain, in the relief of suffering, or in the prevention of chronic pain-associated incapacity. Analgesics vary in potency. Weaker analgesics seem to be effective only for transitory painful episodes of relatively mild intensity. Stronger analgesics are sometimes associated with troublesome side effects and patients may build up tolerance to them. Sci-entific research has not supported long-term efficacy of most specific modality treatments of back pain, over and above the simple passage of time. More specifically, there was some evidence for efficacy of manipulation within the first 6 weeks of a new episode of LBP, there was no evidence for the efficacy of most physical modalities, only weak evidence for back exercises, or back schools, while bed rest, extended use of narcotics or benxiodiazipines was positively contraindicated (RCGP, 1996). Similarly, in the more recent Occupational Health Guidelines for the management of low back pain at work stated:

> Do not recommend lumbar belts and supports or traditional biomedical education as methods of preventing LBP. There is insufficient evidence to advocate general exercise or physical fitness programmes.

It seems clear that our assumptions about the nature of prevention require re-examination. As a precursor, it is necessary to re-examine our assumptions about the nature of pain.

3. New understandings about the nature of pain: from Descartes to GCT

During the first half of the last century, the primary focus of clinical endeavor in the treatment of LBP was on the *cure* of pain. Only more recently has the emphasis shifted from pain relief to pain management with a parallel shift from a specific focus on pain to pain-associated dysfunction. Nonetheless, much of our current understanding of pain is still based on earlier perspectives. Pain has puzzled man for centuries, but modern theories of pain have their origins in the writings of Descartes (1664), and his Cartesian view of the world. In understanding pain mechanisms specifically, there have been two major assumptions which have been inherited from Descartes; firstly that of a one-to-one relationship between amount of damage (or nociception) and the pain experiences; and secondly the separation of mind and body. Descartes never resolved satisfactorily the relationship between mind and body, but the assumption of a direct correspondence between the two was established.

This model of a one-to-one relationship between the amount of tissue damage and the amount of pain experienced has attractiveness, in that it seems to be consistent with the everyday experience of acute pain, but the inherent 'dualism' led to a concept of prevention in which interaction between mind and body was not addressed and that in addressing pain relief all that was required was to address the nociceptive component.

The advent of Melzack and Wall's theory was of critical importance in changing our understanding of pain and in offering new opportunities for prevention. According to the Gate-Control Theory or GCT (Melzack and Wall, 1965) and its later derivatives (Melzack and Casey, 1968), pain perception depends on complex neural interactions in the nervous system where impulses generated by tissue damage are modified both by ascending pathways to the brain and by descending pain suppressing systems activated by various environmental and psychological factors. Pain thus is *not* merely the end product of a passive transmission of nociceptive impulses from receptor organ to an area of interpretation. It is the result of a dynamic process of perception and interpretation of a wide range of incoming stimuli, some of which are associated with actual or potential harm and some which are benign but interpreted and described in terms of damage.

The GCT opened up new opportunities for both physiological and psychological enquiry, but it has a particular importance from the point of view of prevention. Simply put, to the extent that psychological factors had an influence on the experience of pain, new possible targets for prevention become available.

4. The genesis of psychological approaches to treatment and management

A key to understanding how chronic pain was viewed can be gleaned from the disease model of illness of Virchow (1858) in which symptoms were viewed as secondary to physical signs, and to be understood almost exclusively in terms of their relationship to the physical signs. A range of 'equivalence' or symptom–sign mapping was assumed. Where the mismatch, however, fell without this range, the symptoms were viewed with suspicion, either in terms of their nature, or in terms of their legitimacy. As aforementioned, pain which persisted required explanation. Over-reliance on orthopedically based concepts of injury, and rheumatological concepts of 'tissue-healing time' led to attempts to explain the persistence of pain on *psychological* grounds. However, many such psychological formulations effectively were 'diagnoses by exclusion'. There were, however, attempts to explain the persistence of pain in terms of positive psychological features. Until the advent of more systematic cognitive and behavioral perspectives on pain, chronic pain was viewed as a manifestation of psychiatric illness, and treated as such, with little attention directed specifically at the perception of pain or psychological adjustment to its effects. The 'mental illness model', had appeal, not only because of the similarity in symptom presentation between chronic pain patients and depressed patients, but also because the symptoms could be explained in terms of a disease model (albeit 'mental' rather than 'physical'. Thus articles feature in the early 1980s where pain is conceptualized as a 'depressive equivalent'. The treatment of pain exclusively as a symptom of depression was at times resented by pain patients who felt (correctly) that the nature and effects of their pain was not being given sufficient attention. It is easy to be somewhat dismissive of early psychiatric perspectives, until it is realized that many of the early studies into the psychiatric concomitants of pain were carried out on *psychiatric* patients who reported pain, rather than on chronic pain patients manifesting distress in medical or surgical clinics. Arguably, without such studies, the psychological concomitants of pain might not have been so fully investigated. In fact, only relatively recently have epidemiologically grounded prospective studies been able to offer evidence on the strength of the causal link between chronic pain and depression (Magni et al., 1994). It would seem that while a history of depression gives an increased risk of developing a chronic pain problem in the

future, persistence of pain is a much higher risk for depression. Construing depression as primarily *reactive* rather than *causative*, however, has important therapeutic implications for the management of chronic pain patients. Pain-associated depression is perhaps viewed as a type of 'learned helplessness', with its cognitive, emotional and behavioral components. The level of depression seems to be associated not so much with the severity of pain as such, but with the extent to which it interferes with quality of life and function (Rudy et al., 1988). In a minority of chronic pain patients demonstrating marked clinical depression, primary psychiatric treatment is the treatment of choice, but in most patients, the best way of alleviating 'depression' is pain management (i.e. enabling patients to regain some control over their pain and pain-associated limitations). Viewed from the perspective of *prevention* therefore, addressing pain.

4.1. The advent of cognitive and behavioral perspectives

Experimental investigations into animal behavior demonstrated scientifically that behavior could be learned and change in behavior could be produced by the experimental manipulation of the antecedents and consequence of the behaviors in question. behavior therapy was developed as an effective treatment initially for specific psychiatric disorders, such as phobias and obsessive–compulsive disorders, but gradually other anxiety-related problems were targeted. A key ingredient of the approach was a careful analysis of the circumstances in which the behavior was occurring. This offered a radically different approach to treatment from both organic psychiatry and psychodynamic psychotherapy, and offered new opportunities for the investigation and treatment of pain. Behavioral medicine, the forerunner of modern clinical health psychology, offered an alternative to the traditional 'pathology-based' medical model. The 'behavioral perspective' was not confined simply to traditional psychosomatic disorders, but shown to be of relevance in the understanding and management of all sorts of disease. This development was not just a disguised version of psychosomatic medicine. Clinical researchers demonstrated the powerful influence of psychological factors not only on the development of disease, but also on response to treatment and adjustment to disease-associated incapacity. Medical sociologists such as Mechanic (1968) had brought the term 'illness behavior' to the medical and scientific communities. This construct has had a profound impact on the management of pain (Pilowsky and Katsikitis, 1994).

Fordyce (1976) first clearly articulated the behavioral management of pain; although the approach had been a cornerstone of the earlier North American pain management programs. In one of the first RCTs of the behavioral approach, Fordyce et al. (1986) demonstrated the superiority of behavioral management to traditional medical management for acute LBP. The early fairly radical behaviorist perspective which to the uncommitted appeared to pay insufficient attention to the role of thoughts and feelings, was later integrated with cognitive perspectives, such as those of Beck (1976) into cognitive–behavioral therapy, which has become the dominant paradigm within psychologically oriented pain management (Turk et al., 1983).

The development of the cognitive–behavioral perspective heralded an entirely new approach to prevention with a shift from a primary focus on the prevention of *pain* per se to an new focus on *adjustment* and prevention of unnecessary pain-associated disability.

5. Cognitive and behavioral approaches to treatment and management

The cognitive perspective differs from psychodynamic psychotherapy in that it is based on a detailed investigation and systematization of patients explicit beliefs and attributions. This approach had been shown to be particularly important in the treatment of depression in which the important role of 'cognitive distortion' was identified.

Similar cognitive 'distortions' were identified among chronic pain patients and the development of cognitive approaches to the treatment of pain was a logical consequence (Turk et al., 1983). The specific focus on understanding of pain, perception of symptoms and expectations of outcome became key components of cognitive approaches to pain management, whether in terms of individual psychological therapy, or whether part of a broader therapeutic approach, such as cognitive–behavioral therapy (CBT), which blends behavioral and cognitive approaches into a powerful therapeutic approach involving a combination of 'patient-centeredness' and specification of clear outcomes for treatment. CBT (and variants of it) has become the dominant therapeutic approach to the management of non-specific pain. It has been shown to be effective (Morley et al., 1999) and has the further advantage of lending itself to evaluation in terms of specific outcome measures.

5.1. Importance for prevention

The development of behavioral and cognitive perspectives changed clinicians views about the nature of clinical intervention in three important ways. Firstly, a focus on psychological effects, on adjustment and on enhancement of positive or adaptive coping strategies allowed a wider range of therapeutic targets than simply pain itself. Secondly, a shift from the concept of cure to optimal adjustment not only offered a much more honest and realistic outcome for many patients with established pain problems, but also introduced the notion that certain aspects of pain-associated dysfunction might be preventable. Thirdly, since CBT is predicated on planned and systematic change, involving the 'deconstruction' of disability, the role of the patient's understanding and active engagement becomes paramount.

6. The move from pain to disability: further development of the biopsychosocial perspective

Many theoreticians and several different research groups have developed models of disability. Although some of the models are labeled as 'pain models', they are perhaps more appropriately understood as 'disability' or 'illness models'. A historical perspective on the development of models of pain associated disability is offered elsewhere (Main and Spanswick, 2000). These models were important in the context of prevention since they offered empirical support for the multifactorial nature of disability. Thus although the original biopsychosocial model of disability (Waddell et al., 1984) was cross-sectional in nature, it demonstrated that psychological (behavioral and emotional) factors could not only be distinguished, but that they made an independent contribution to the understanding of disability. The later development of tools for the assessment of cognitive factors provided a more comprehensive biopsychological perspective on disability; stimulating the development of multi-faceted pain management. The success of the pain-management approach, although essentially rehabilitative demonstrated that if was possible to reduce disability and increase function; with a concomitant improvement in the psychological parameters. Prevention of unnecessary (or recoverable) disability became a key focus for pain management.

6.1. Development of psychologically oriented pain management

During the 1970s and 1980s individualized cognitive and behavioral therapy became an established part of the pain clinic repertoire, although many pain services 'contracted in' psychological therapy on an out-patient basis. Cognitive therapies might focus on the abolition of pain using distraction techniques; or adopt more psychophysiological approaches directed at reduction of muscle tension or generalized emotional arousal. The precise focus of intervention, whether on cognition, emotional reaction or behavioral adjustment was not always clear. There is some evidence that pain tolerance mostly associated with the affective rather than the sensory component of pain. Some therapeutic activity therefore can be seen as the prevention of suffering, and focus specifically on the emotional component catered for in psychological support, re-establishment of confidence; reduction of fear. behavioral approaches were more specifically directed at remediation of behavioral dysfunction, such as excessive medication use or 'down time', leading to necessary disability. It is clearly unwise, however, to completely distinguish cognitive, behavioral and emotional components since they interact. With less chronic and less disabling pain, individualized psychologically oriented pain management may be helpful, but for more significant problems, the multidimensional aspects of pain and disability require a multidisciplinary approach, as is offered in multi- and inter-disciplinary Pain Management Programs (Main and Spanswick, 2000).

6.2. Pain management: implications for prevention

Outcome data from PMPs consistently demonstrated positive change in a range of clinical parameters, although there is little evidence that they prevented pain as such. While the importance from a rehabilitation perspective of demonstrating that psychologically oriented pain management could go some way to improving function should not be underestimated, there is little evidence of their efficacy specifically in prevention of reduction of sick leave, increased rate of return to work or improvement in sub-optimal work functioning. In summary, in terms of chronic disability, while PMPs appear to be effective in the treatment of certain facets of pain-associated disability, they are best viewed in the context of partial restoration of function rather than prevention as such.

7. Occupational concepts of prevention

Many patients seek professional help when their pain becomes disabling to the point of compromising their work and threatening their livelihood. Funding of clinical services, however, is becoming conditional increasingly on demonstration of satisfactory outcome. Traditionally, outcome of clinical programs has been appraised in terms of improvement in clinical parameters such as reduction in pain, self-reported disability or health-care usage.

Although there have always been programs funded principally in terms of work rehabilitation, in most clinical programs, impact on work is seldom appraised, and there frequently is little in the way of specific occupational focus in design of treatment. Identification of the increasing costs of pain-associated disability, however, is driving new initiatives designed to extend rehabilitation into work. It is important, therefore, to consider prevention from an occupational perspective.

7.1. Biomechanical and ergonomic perspectives

In many countries, there is now workplace legislation designed to regulate working practices and prevent injury. Much of the emphasis on primary prevention of injury has relied on epidemiological studies which have addressed principally anthropomorphic and physical risks factors, with a heavy biomechanical and ergonomic emphasis.

Burton (1997) has highlighted an apparent contraction in the way in which occupational injury is viewed and managed. "On the one hand, ergonomists and biomechanists strive to reduce physical stress in the work place with the intent of lowering the risk of musculoskeletal problems, while clinical scientists and psychologists are suggesting not only that psychological factors are important, but that rehabilitation of the back-injured worker should involve physical challenges to the musculoskeletal system" (Burton, 1997, p. 2575.

This dilemma illustrates not only a management problem, as Burton asserts, but also illustrates a fundamental conflict in models of injury. At the heart of the debate lies the nature of mechanisms of chronicity.

The basic 'injury/damage' model is based on the commonly held view that physically demanding work is detrimental to the back in the sense that it can cause injury through sudden or cumulative trauma, and the injury in turn leads to pain and disability. Much clinical and non-clinical scientific research has been directed at the nature of injury and the possible underlying mechanisms. There are have been many variants on the basic themes, but in the field

of occupational injury, the primary focus has been on biomechanical analysis of the physical stresses sustained during various movements or postures under various conditions of load. It might appear that there ought to be a direct relationship between the physical demands of work and the occurrence of injury, but in fact there are significant inconsistencies in the scientific literature (Burton and Main, 2000a). Certainly there is evidence of increased risk of work-related disorders affecting the back, neck and upper limbs with certain types of work, but not all workers become injured, and certainly do not all become significantly disabled. Marras et al. (1993) found that risk of musculoskeletal symptoms could be predicted from a combination of five risk trunk motion and workplace factors, but since not all jobs with high injury rates require the same physical abilities (Halpern, 1992), the relationship between these risk factors and actual injury is not straight-forward.

7.2. How successful is this approach to occupational prevention?

There have been energetic attempts to improve the working environment, with ergonomic redesign, to reduce the risk of injury. Most ergonomic interventions focus on strategies to reduce spinal loading, but the only intervention which has been formally evaluated has been worker training in manual handling techniques. Occupational guidelines for manual handling designed to constrain task performance to within safety limits of lifting and handling, have been produced. It appears that while lifting techniques can be improved, it has not been possible to demonstrate a corresponding reduction of injury rates (Smedley and Coggan, 1994). The explanation for the lack of success in preventing injury is perhaps not all that surprising. According to Burton (1997), although epidemiological studies can link the occurrence of initial back pain with certain physical stressors (such as spinal loading and physical usage), there is little evidence that the symptoms are due to irreversible damage to spinal structures. Furthermore, there is increasing evidence that recurrence and disability are mediated by psychosocial phenomena, such as the perception of comfort and the ability to cope.

This specific focus on primary prevention has perhaps hindered proper analysis of the mechanisms of recovery from injury, many of which seem to be psychosocial rather than biomechanical or ergonomic. Recognition, particularly in North America of the increasing costs of long-term disability led to investigations into its predictors and a number of researchers examined a wide range of presenting characteristics in an effort to find predictors of chronicity. Early reviews of risk factors in industrial low back pain, Bigos et al., 1990; Cats-Baril and Frymoyer, 1991) had implicated not only clinical history, and work characteristics, but also perceptions of work as risk factors for the development of disability, although the studies were later criticized on methodological grounds. "The population of patients who have already incurred two weeks of off-work time secondary to low back trouble probably are anticipating long-term disability, and, perhaps more importantly, so are their health care providers, employers, and insurers. These expectations may trigger illness behaviors that help establish long-term disability" (Lehmann et al., 1993, p. 1110).

The evidence seems to show that the back can certainly be injured in various ways (whether at work or leisure), but the 'injury model' is not able to explain the wide variation in resultant disability. Nonetheless, many workers *perceive* their musculoskeletal symptoms to be work-related. In a recent UK survey (Jones et al., 1998), of individuals reporting musculoskeletal symptoms, nearly 80% identified a work task, or set of tasks, as leading to their complaint, but in considering prevention, psychosocial factors seems to have been largely ignored.

In a recent review of the available evidence, Burton et al. (1998) concluded: "The possible role of ergonomics for reducing recurrence rates seems at best equivocal, but there is no convincing evidence that continuation of work is detrimental in respect of disability. It is likely that much back pain is only work-related in as much that people of working age get painful backs. It is becoming clear that reduc-

ing spinal loads or awkward postures is likely to have only a small impact on the overall pattern of back pain. Non-biomechanical approaches (organisational and social) seemingly are more effective in maintaining ability to work" (p. 1134).

In considering the design of prevention, therefore, it is important to consider what is known in terms of psychosocial aspects of work, and how these features might be incorporated into effective prevention.

8. Psychosocial perspectives on work

8.1. Stress and work

The nature of work stress has been a major focus of research. It can be viewed in terms of characteristics of the working environment, in terms of physiological stress or as a consequence of interaction between the individual and their environment. According to Cox (1993): "The experience of stress is therefore defined, first, by the realisation that they are having difficulties in coping with demands and threats to their well being and, second, that coping is important and the difficulty in coping depresses or worries them" (p. 17).

However, such general definitions are of limited utility since psychosocial factors are multiple and diverse, as illustrated by Carayon and Lim (1999) in Table I.

They stress that such factors need to be understood in the context of societal changes in the economic, social, technological, legal and physical environments.

However, stress affects people differently. Whether or not they become ill appears to depend to a considerable extent on what they think about the stressor and how they cope with it. Researchers have studied individual differences both in the way stressors are perceived and also the extent to which these appraisals might moderate the relationship between stress and health (Payne, 1988). Griffiths (1998) identifies a large number of work organizational factors associated with poor health and well-being, but unfortunately much of the research

TABLE I

Selected psychosocial work factors and their facets

1. Job demands
    Quantitative workload
    Variance in workload
    Work pressure
    Cognitive demands

2. Job content
    Repetitiveness
    Challenge
    Utilization and development of skills

3. Job control
    Task/instrumental control
    Decision/organizational control
    Control over the physical environment
    Resource control
    Control over workplace: machine-pacing

4. Social interactions
    Social support from supervisor and colleagues
    Supervisor complaint, praise, monitoring
    Dealing with (difficult) clients/customers

5. Role factors
    Role ambiguity
    Role conflict

6. Job future and career issues
    Job future ambiguity
    Fear of job loss

7. Technology issues
    Computer-related problems
    Electronic performance monitoring

8. Organizational and management issues
    Participation
    Management style

After Table 15.2 in Carayon and Lim (1999), p. 278.

into specific work organizational characteristics is of poor quality.

They are frequently confounded with physical work load (Bongers et al., 1993; Vingard and Nachemson, 2000; Davis and Heaney, 2000), and most studies to date have been unable to quantify either their individual importance or specific interactions. Nevertheless, the available evidence provides most support for influence of the factors shown in Table II (Bongers et al., 1993; Vingard and Nachem-

TABLE II

Work organizational factors most clearly associated with occupational stress/musculoskeletal disorders

High demand and low control
Time pressure/monotonous work
Lack of job satisfaction
Unsupportive management style
Low social support from colleagues
High perceived workload

son, 2000), and it seems that workers' reactions to psychosocial aspects of work may be more important than the actual aspects themselves (Davis and Heaney, 2000), with stress acting as an intermediary (Bongers et al., 1993).

8.2. Conclusion: what lessons can be learned from the occupational stress literature?

The occupational stress literature has been important in the identification of adverse features of the working environment. Many different organizational characteristics have been associated with ill-health, sickness absence or impaired productivity. Certain characteristics of the working environment appear to constitute risk factors in their own right, but it seems that *perceptual* factors may be even more important than objective characteristics. Most jobs have irritating, difficult or stressing features which can be thought of as risk factors for sickness or ill-health. Individuals, however, vary in their reaction to difficult circumstances or adversities and the extent to which a specific individual copes with such risk factors will influence job satisfaction, morale and psychological well-being.

The principal lessons from the occupational stress literature are summarized in Table III.

In recovery from musculoskeletal injury, an adverse view of work may become an additional obstacle to return to work. In addressing issues of prevention of unnecessary work absence or work compromise, therefore, it would seem to be important to incorporate occupational characteristics, particularly perceptions of work, into the therapeutic strategy.

TABLE III

Lessons from the occupational stress literature

Aspects of work can have an adverse psychological impact in terms of stress
Work stress can adversely affect health and lead to sickness absence
A number of the key influences on health have been identified
Coping styles and strategies may mediate or moderate the relationship between work stress, ill-health and work absence
Perception of work may be more important than actual working conditions or characteristics
There has, however, been no systematic research into the relationship between occupational stress, musculoskeletal symptomatology and
  recovery from injury

The Occupational Health Guidelines state:

Advise employers that high job satisfaction and good industrial relations are the most important organisational characteristics associated with low disability and sickness absence rates attributed to LBP.

(Carter and Birrell, 2000)

8.3. Specific psychological factors predicting return to work

A historical perspective on the nature of psychological aspects of work is presented elsewhere (Main and Burton, 1998; Carayon and Lim, 1999). Specific psychological features have been investigated in more detail in a number of more recent studies. Carosella et al. (1994) found that patients with low return to work expectations, heightened perceived disability, pain and somatic focus had problems complying with an intensive work rehabilitation program. Haazen et al. (1994) have shown that change in distorted pain cognitions, worker's compensation status and use of medication were the most important predictors in behavioral rehabilitation of low back pain (They were, however, pessimistic about the overall level of prediction achieved.) The above studies, although tantalizing, do not identify the putative psychological factors with sufficient degree of accuracy to evaluate their specific importance.

Feuerstein et al. (1994) categorized variables predicting return to work by 1 year into five categories: medical history, demographics, physical findings, pain and psychological indices.

The specific psychological factors identified by them in different studies are shown in Table IV.

TABLE IV

Specific psychological factors predicting return to work

Lower pain severity
Pain drawing scores
Higher treatment satisfaction
Higher co-operativeness during treatment
Lower levels of hypochondriasis
Distrust/stubbornness
Depression
Premorbid pessimism

In addition to these clinical psychological variables, Feuerstein and Huang (1998), grouped the factors associated with delayed recovery into medical, ergonomic and psychosocial (although they did not sub-classify the latter specifically into clinical and occupational perceptions). Feuerstein and Zastowny (1999) did, however, recognize that in occupational rehabilitation the psychological problems specifically associated with job stress and work re-entry should be specific targets for psychological intervention (in addition to the usual clinical targets).

Finally, in two recent controlled studies, a large difference in prevalence of musculoskeletal disorders in Dutch and Belgian nurses, was explained not by workload, or attribution of work as a cause, but was explained by attitudes to work and depressive symptoms (Burton et al., 1997). In another study, Burton et al. (1996), in a comparison of musculoskeletal complaints among police in Northern Ireland and in Manchester (UK), found that the proportion of officers with persistent (chronic) back complaints did not depend on length of exposure to physical stressors, but to psychosocial factors, such as distress and blaming work. According to a relatively recent review: "Monotonous work, high perceived work load, and time pressure are related to musculoskeletal symptoms. The data also suggest that low control on the job and lack of support by colleagues are positively associated with musculoskeletal disease. Perceived stress may be an intermediary in the process" (Bongers et al., 1993, p. 297).

It would seem that there is now overwhelming evidence that psychosocial factors influence musculoskeletal symptomatology and effect on work. Studies have been carried out in a wide range of settings, with varying degrees of precision and differences in measurement tools. The studies have offered evidence in the form of statistical associations between a range of psychosocial variables, work performance and illness characteristics. In an attempt to integrate some of these findings, consideration will now be given specifically to the nature of obstacles to recovery.

9. The emergence of secondary prevention

It would seem that further success in primary prevention, whether in terms of education about lifting and posture, or in terms of ergonomic redesign of the physical demands of work is unlikely. Such initiatives may have decreased the likelihood specifically of workplace accidents, but they seem to have been unsuccessful in stemming the rise in back-associated disability. A clear focus on the psychological concomitants of pain and disability does appear, however, to have had some success with chronic pain patients (Morley et al., 1999). The logic of trying to prevent some of the 'recoverable' disability seems irresistible. As Linton and Van Tulder (2000) has pointed out, here are some ambiguities in the term 'secondary prevention' (discussed below), but it generally refers to prevention of chronic incapacity in patients who are not yet chronically incapacitated. There is also epidemiological and economic support for such an endeavor. Since back pain is both common and recurrent (Von Korff et al., 1988; Waddell, 1996), prevention of *disabling* back pain would appear to be a much more realistic target than primary prevention.

As aforementioned, identification of rapidly increasing costs of pain-associated disability (CSAG, 1994) has stimulated redirection of the primary focus of clinical activity from treatment to prevention. It has been shown that costs of subsequent episodes of low back pain are more costly than new episodes, and that the burden of work-associated sickness costs is a consequence of chronic sufferers (Watson et al., 1997).

Early intervention, however, requires a system for identification of those potentially at risk of chronicity. The term 'risk' is, however, used in a number of different ways, and so before consideration of possible targets for prevention, a degree of conceptual clarification is necessary.

10. Risks, flags and obstacles to recovery

10.1. Concepts of risk

Traditionally, primary prevention has been targeted at entire clinical (or preclinical) groups or at workforces. Initiatives in health education such as smoking cessation programs or occupationally based initiatives such as training programs in lifting and handling techniques are examples of this approach. Such population-based initiatives do not involve any selection or targeting of 'vulnerable' individuals, since they will be included. There are two major problems with such initiatives: firstly, they are expensive and inefficient (to the extent that they target not only those 'at risk', but also those not at risk. Secondly, there can be problems of compliance if the initiative is viewed as irrelevant. In many circumstances, this may not be a problem, but in targeting preventative interventions, disaffection with an initiative, as evident in non-compliance, may compromise other initiatives in the future, and there may be pressures to minimize costs. In secondary prevention, it is frequently necessary to focus and target resources and identification of those 'at risk' becomes important.

10.2. From risks to obstacles

Concepts of risk have usually been based on identification of factors associated with poor outcome, but there are different types of predictors of outcome, and not all are potential targets for intervention. *Epidemiological* studies are primarily descriptive, rather than explanatory and are population based. Statistically significant associations may serve as a foundation for major clinical initiatives (such as immunization) or social policy decisions involving the re-direction of resources, but such risk factors are usually not sufficiently powerful to be useful for decision making on an individual basis. The *clinical* perspective on risk tends to focus primarily on factors associated with health-care outcome. Although clinical studies are more narrowly focused than epidemiological investigations, and therefore provide a better basis for clinical intervention, the incorporation of demographic and educational factors, for example, may be helpful in targeting certain groups, they may not provide particular therapeutic targets or assist in the design of the preventative intervention. *Occupational* risk factors tend to be wide-ranging, may be very different from clinical risk factors, but equally may be of little help in the targeting or design of preventative interventions. It may be helpful to base prevention not on risk as such, but to refocus attention on *obstacles to recovery*.

10.3. The concept of 'red flags'

In the field of back pain, the concept of risk has been examined in terms of 'flags'. Waddell (1998) as part of an assessment strategy for patients presenting with back pain, recommends an initial diagnostic triage into simple back pain, nerve root pain or serious spinal pathology. The signs and symptoms considered indicative of possible spinal pathology or of the need for an urgent surgical evaluation became known as 'red flags'. These 'risk factors' for serious pathology or disease became incorporated into screening tools recommended for use in primary care by clinicians to identify those patients in whom an urgent specialist opinion was indicated. Assessment

of these risk factors were included within a several new sets of clinical guidelines for the management of acute low back pain (CSAG, 1994; AHCPR, 1994).

10.4. Yellow flags

The increasing costs of chronic incapacity, despite advances in technological medicine, stimulated the search for other solutions to the problem of low back disability. In New Zealand, increasing costs of chronic non-specific low back pain became an unmanageable burden. This fuelled a new initiative designed to complement a slightly modified set of acute back pain management guidelines with a psychosocial assessment system designed systematically to address the psychosocial risks factors which had been shown in the scientific literature to be predictive of chronicity (Kendall et al., 1997). The main categories of the yellow flags are shown in Table V.

They also included a number of specific guidelines for behavioral management which are shown in Table VI (Kendall et al., 1997).

It can be seen that there are clear *preventative components within the management guidelines*. It is important to note also that the yellow flags were developed not only from a clinical perspective, but also from an occupational perspective and consisted of both psychological and socio-occupational risk factors.

11. Occupational factors as obstacles to recovery: the blue flags and black flags

The occupational component of the original New Zealand yellow flags focused on the perception of work, but in terms of obstacles to recovery, it is necessary to make a distinction also between two types of occupational risk factors. They can be thought of as factors concerning the *perception* of work (blue flags) and objective work characteristics (black flags). The distinction is similar to the distinction between *intrinsic* and *extrinsic* factors by Herzberg (1974), but with a focus on obstacles to recovery, i.e. potential targets for a some sort of biopsychoso-

TABLE V

Yellow flags

Attitudes and beliefs about back pain
Behaviors
Compensation issues
Diagnostic and treatment issues
Emotions
Family
Work

TABLE VI

Behavioral management guidelines

1. Provide a *positive* expectation that the individual will return to work
2. Be directive in scheduling regular reviews of progress
3. Keep the individual active and at work
4. Acknowledge difficulties of daily living
5. Help maintain positive co-operation
6. Communicate that having more time off work reduces the likelihood of successful return
7. Beware or expectations of 'total cure' or expectation of simple 'techno-fixes'
8. Promote self-management and self-responsibility
9. Be prepared to say "I don't know"
10. Avoid confusing the report of symptoms with the presence of emotional distress
11. Discourage working at home
12. Encourage people to recognize that pain can be controlled
13. If barriers are too complex, arrange multidisciplinary referral

cial intervention. In tackling obstacles to recovery, whether from the perspective of actual clinical management or occupational rehabilitation, however, it seems necessary to distinguish concerns that the individual has about their personal well-being from specific concerns about work. It was decided, therefore, to subdivide the yellow flags into clinical yellow flags and occupationally focused blue flags (Main and Burton, 1998; Burton and Main, 2000b).

11.1. Blue flags

The blue flags have their origin in the stress literature, as reviewed above. They are perceived features of work which are generally associated with higher rates of symptoms, ill-health and work loss which in the context of injury may delay recovery, or constitute a major obstacle to it. They are characterized by features such as high demand/low control, unhelpful management style, poor social support from colleagues, perceived time pressure and lack of job satisfaction. Individual workers may differ in their perception of the same working environment. According to Bigos et al. (1990), perception may be more important than the objective characteristics since: "Once an individual is off work, perception about symptoms, about the *safety* of return to work, and about impact of return to work on one's personal life can affect recovery even in the most well-meaning worker" (Bigos et al., 1990, p. 184).

It should be emphasized that blue flags incorporate not only issues related to the perception of job characteristics, such as job demand, but also perception of social interactions (whether with management or fellow-workers).

11.2. Black flags

'Black flags' are *not* a matter of perception, and affect all workers equally. They include both nationally established policy concerning conditions of employment and sickness policy and working conditions specific to a particular organization. Some examples are shown in Table VII.

It is not always possible to make an absolute distinction between black and blue flags, Since here are also content-specific aspects of work which characterize certain types of job and which are associated with higher rates of illness, injury or work loss. They are shown in Table VIII.

These features of work, following injury, may require a higher level of working capacity for successful work retention. After certain types of injury, such jobs may be specifically contraindicated and therefore constitute an absolute obstacle to return to work. It might be hoped that many such risk factors could be 'designed' out of the working environment, but such factors certainly need to be evaluated in the context of work retention or rehabilitation. In

TABLE VII

Occupational black flags. I: Job context and working conditions

National
Rates of pay
Nationally negotiated entitlements
    Sick certification
Benefit system
Wage re-embursement rate

Local
Sickness policy
    Entitlements to sick leave
    Role of occupational health in 'signing off' (?) and 'signing on'
        Requirement for full fitness
    Possibility of sheltered work
        Restricted duties
Management style
Trade Union support/involvement
Organizational size and structure

TABLE VIII

Occupational black flags. II: Content-specific aspects of work

Ergonomic
Job heaviness
Lifting frequency
Postures
Sitting/standing postural requirements

Temporal characteristics
Number of working hours
Shift pattern

terms specifically of *prevention*, they are matter primarily for legislation, establishment of satisfactory job design, and adherence to recommended work practices; in negotiation, where appropriate, between employers and employee organizations.

11.3. Concluding comment

Despite the acknowledged methodological weaknesses in many of the studies, the general picture is clear. Certain working conditions and adverse work characteristics place an individual at increased risk of ill-health and associated absence from work. These occupational features, in the context of individual

vulnerabilities or additional external stressors, may lead to impaired performance and work absence. In the context of injury, they may delay recovery and return to work.

12. Concluding comment: need for a new perspective on prevention

12.1. New directions for prevention

There would seem to be a clear need to develop better clinical–occupational interfaces.

For example, in a recent predictive study, examining the transition from acute to chronic low back pain, Williams et al. (1998) evaluated the influence of job satisfaction, pain, disability and psychological distress at baseline with outcome 6 months later. They found that job satisfaction may protect against the development of chronic pain and disability, and conversely that dissatisfaction may heighten the risk.

In summary, with regard to prevention, there are several further stages beyond traditional pathology-based concepts of sickness and disability. These are shown in Table IX.

The advantages of an integrated approach was demonstrated in a study in the United Kingdom (Watson and Main, in preparation) in which a short occupationally oriented pain management program was designed for unemployed benefit claimants with back pain as the principal reason for unemployment. Despite the fact that the group had been out of work for an average of 44 months and had on average been symptomatic for more than 8 years, 43% were

TABLE IX

New directions for prevention

From pathology to biopsychosocial illness
From psychopathology to adjustment and optimal adaptation
From a clinical to a combined clinical and occupational focus
From sickness and disability management to optimization of function
From individualized to integrated individual and organizational perspectives

rehabilitated into work and 71% into useful function. Although it was not possible to design a RCT, as a feasibility of an integrated clinical and occupational initiative, the study offers a challenge, since previously the accepted wisdom (Waddell, 1998) for such a group was that less than 2% would be likely to return to work.

Finally it should be noted that return to work was achieved despite a residual level of disability such that they would be considered appropriate for further treatment.

12.2. Beyond sickness and disability

The most important conceptual shift needed in relationship to prevention is to move beyond the traditional concepts of sickness and disability. Pain and disability are more than a health-care issue. Indeed they are more than a social policy or political issue. We need to move beyond our traditional models of pathology and psychopathology to the prevention of sub-optimal functioning to incorporate not only sickness and disability management, but also incorporate enhancement of resilience and optimization of the individual's functioning with the recognition that it is not possible to abolish all pain.

In a recent series of reports, the Institute for Health and Productivity management has considered the issue of sub-optimal performance from an organizational perspective (Peterson and Travis, 2001). Although the report derives primarily from consideration of productivity and profit, there is much relevance to human performance. Indeed some of the solutions offered to optimize performance in the workplace offer potential solutions to the management of blue and black flags. Although their recommendations regarding the management of absenteeism are not a matter for this chapter, their recommendations in relationship to stress and performance optimization merit comment. In terms of management, they advocate screening for 'emotional intelligence' (Goleman, 1998).

Developing healthy organizational cultures in which people "experience greater personal control in how they do their work, are rewarded for de-veloping supportive rather than competitive relationships; are equipped with the skills to communicate effectively and manage differences among employees with high levels of trust and mutual respect" (Peterson and Travis, 2001, p. 31). They also advocate the development of 'work-life balance'. With regard to the rapid growth of employee assistance programs (EAPs), however, they offer the following caution: "Certainly the expansion of EAPs confirms the recognition by organizations of the need to take direct actions when they see employee emotional problems affecting work performance and organizational productivity and costs. Unfortunately, treating the problem (in this case rehabilitating the employee) is not the same as prevention", p. 31.

Pain is part of life. We need to incorporate optimal management of obstacles to recovery with facilitation of optimal functioning (in terms of personal well-being as well as productivity). Recent concepts of wellness and presenteeism have offered ways in which people can be helped. Seen from a health-care perspective, we need to enhance individual's positive or adaptive coping strategies. This focus has always been an important part of the pain management agenda. In several countries, new disability legislation requires opportunities for work to be accessible to LBP sufferers who previously might have been rejected.

12.3. Conclusions and recommendations

Health care and social systems are slow to change and the power of underling models of illness in directing the focus of attention needs to be recognized. The advent of evidence-based medicine has enabled a critical examination of the basis from which our therapeutic efforts are developed. In terms of prevention per se, there are many interesting new challenges, but they require reconsideration of our fundamental assumptions, not only regarding the objectives for intervention, but also the type of interventions.

The concept of prevention, within the field of musculoskeletal disorders, has developed mainly from a clinical perspective. We need to expand our role in terms of a 'systems' perspective. As clinicians, however, we need to re-examine our range of competencies in the light of such new challenges. There needs to be a focus on skills rather than just professional accreditation. We may need to expand our clinically derived concepts of prevention; broaden our skills and develop closer and more effective liaison with other agencies. This must, however, carried out within an evidence-based framework. We need to develop and validate new individualized and system measurement tools.

References

AHCPR (1994) Acute low back pain problems in adults. Clinical practice guidelines No. 14. Agency for Health Care Policy and Research. US Department of Health and Human Services, Rockville, MD.

Beck, A. (1976) Cognitive Therapy and Emotional Disorders. International University Press, New York.

Bigos, S.J., Battie, M.C., Nordin, M., Spengler, D.M. and Guy, D.P. (1990) Industrial low back pain. In: J. Weinstein and S. Wiesel (Eds.), The Lumbar Spine. W.B. Saunders, Philadelphia, PA, pp. 846–859.

Bongers, P.M., de Winter, C.R., Kompier, M.A.J. and Hildebrandt, V.H. (1993) Psychosocial factors at work and musculoskeletal disease. Scand. J. Work Environ. Health, 19: 297–312.

Burton, A.K. (1997) Back injury and work loss: biomechanical and psychosocial influences. Spine, 22: 2575–2580.

Burton, A.K., Battie, M.C. and Main, C.J. (1998) The relative importance of biomechanical and psychosocial factors in low back injuries. In: W. Karwowski and W.S. Marras (Eds.), The Occupational Ergonomics Handbook. CRC Press, Boca Raton, FL, pp. 1127–1138.

Burton, A.K., Symonds, T.L., Zinzen, E., Tillotson, K.M., Caboor, D., Van Roy, P. and Clarys, J.P. (1997) Is ergonomic intervention alone sufficient to limit musculoskeletal problems in nurses. Occup. Med., 47: 25–32.

Burton, A.K., Tillotson, K.M., Symonds, T.L., Burke, C.E. and Mathewson, T. (1996) Occupational risk factors for first onset of low back trouble: a study of serving police officers. Spine, 21: 2612–2620.

Burton, A.K. and Main, C.J. (2000a) Relevance of biomechanics in occupational musculoskeletal disorders. In: T.G. Mayer, R.J. Gatchel and P.B. Polatin (Eds.), Occupational Musculoskeletal Disorders. Lippincott, Williams and Wilkins, Philadelphia, PA, pp. 157–166.

Burton, A.K. and Main, C.J. (2000b) Obstacles to recovery from work-related musculoskeletal disorders. In: W. Karwowski (Ed.), International Encyclopaedia of Ergonomics and Human Factors. Taylor and Francis, London, pp. 1542–1544.

Carayon, P. and Lim, S.-Y. (1999) Psychosocial work factors. In: W. Karwowski and W. Marras (Eds.), The Occupational Ergonomics Handbook. CRC Press, Boca Raton, FL, pp. 275–283.

Carosella, A.M., Lackner, J.M. and Feuerstein, M. (1994) Factors associated with early discharge from a multidisciplinary work rehabilitation program for chronic low back pain. Pain, 57: 69–76.

Carter, J.T. and Birrell, L.N. (Eds.) 2000. Occupational health guidelines for the management of low back pain at work – principal recommendations. Faculty of Occupational Medicine, London.

Cats-Baril, W.L. and Frymoyer, J.W. (1991) Identifying patients at risk of becoming disabled because of low-back pain: The Vermont Rehabilitation Engineering Center predictive model. Spine, 16: 605–607.

Cox, T. (1993) Stress Research and Stress Management: Putting Theory to Work. H.S.E. Books, Sudbury.

Crombie, I. (1999) The potential of epidemiology. In: I. Crombie (Ed.), Epidemiology of Pain. IASP Press, Seattle, WA, pp. 1–5.

CSAG (1994). The Clinical Standards Advisory Group on Back Pain. HMSO, London.

Cyriax, J. (1969) Textbook of Orthopaedic Medicine. Williams and Wilkins, Baltimore, MD.

Davis, K.G. and Heaney, C.A. (2000) The relationship between psychosocial work characteristics and low back pain: underlying methodological issues. Clin. Biomechan., 15: 389–406.

Descartes, R. (1664) L'homme. E. Angot, Paris.

Feuerstein, M. and Huang, G.D. (1998) Preventing disability in patients with occupational musculoskeletal disorders. Am. Pain Soc. Bull., 8: 9–11.

Feuerstein, M., Menz, L., Zastowny, T.R. and Barron, B.A. (1994) Chronic back pain and work disability: vocational outcomes following multidisciplinary rehabilitation. J. Occup. Rehabil., 4: 229–251.

Feuerstein, M. and Zastowny, T.R. (1999) Occupational rehabilitation: multidisciplinary management of work-related musculoskeletal pain and disability. In: R. Gatchel and D.C. Turk (Eds.), Psychological Approaches to Pain Management: A Practitioner's Handbook. Guilford Press, New York, pp. 458–485.

Fordyce, W.E. (1976) Behavioral Methods for Chronic Pain and Illness. C.V. Mosby, St. Louis, MO.

Fordyce, W.E., Brockway, J., Bergman, J.A. and Spengler, D. (1986) Acute back pain: control group comparison of behavioral versus traditional management methods. J. Behav. Med., 9: 127–140.

Goleman, D.P. (1998) Working with Emotional Intelligence. Bantam Doubleday Dell.

Griffiths, A. (1998) The psychosocial work environment. In: R. McCaig and M. Harrington (Eds.), The Changing Nature of Occupational Health. H.S.E. Books, Sudbury, pp. 213–232.

Hadler, N.M. (1997) Back pain in the workplace. What you lift or how you lift matters far less than whether you lift or when. Spine, 22: 935–940.

Haazen, I.W.C.J., Vlaeyen, J.W.S., Kole-Snidjers, A.M.K., van

Eek, F.D. and van Es, F.D. (1994) Behavioral rehabilitation of chronic low back pain: searching for the predictors of treatment outcome. J. Rehabil. Sci., 7: 34–43.

Halpern, M. (1992) Prevention of low back pain: basic ergonomics in the workplace and clinic. In Nordin, M. and Vischer, T. (Eds). Common Low Back Pain: Prevention of Chronicity. Bailliere Tindall, London, pp. 705–730.

Herzberg, E. (1974) The wise old turk. Harvard Business Review, Sep/Oct.: 70–80.

Jones, J.R., Hodgson, J.T., Clegg, T. et al. (1998) Self-Report of Work-Related Illness in 1995. HSE, Sudbury, Suffolk.

Kendall, N.A.S., Linton, S.J. and Main, C.J. (1997) Guide to assessing psychosocial yellow flags in acute low back pain: risk factors for long term disability and work loss. Accident Rehabilitation and Compensation Insurance Corporation of New Zealand and the National Health Committee. Wellington, N.Z.

Lehmann, T.R., Spratt, K.F. and Lehmann, K.K. (1993) Predicting long term disability in low back injured workers presenting to a spine consultant. Spine, 18: 1103–1112.

Linton, S.J. and van Tulder, M.W. (2000) Preventative interventions for back pain and neck pain. In: A. Nachemson and E. Jonsson (Eds.), Neck Pain and Back Pain: The Scientific Evidence of Causes, Diagnoses and Treatment. Lippincott, Williams and Wilkins, Philadelphia, PA, pp. 127–147.

Magni, G., Moreschi, C., Rigatti-Luchini L, S. and Merskey, H. (1994) Prospective study on the relationship between depressive symptoms and chronic musculoskeletal pain. Pain, 56: 289–297.

Main, C.J. and Burton, A.K. (1998) Pain mechanisms. In: R. McCaig and M. Harrington (Eds.), The Changing Nature of Occupational Health. H.S.E. Books, Sudbury, pp. 233–254.

Main, C.J. and Spanswick, C.C. (2000) Pain Management: an Interdisciplinary Approach. Churchill Livingstone, Edinburgh.

Marras, W.S., Lavender, S.A., Leurgans, S., Rajulu, S., Allread, W.G., Fathallah, F. and Ferguson, S.A. (1993) The role of dynamic three-dimensional trunk motion in occupationally related low back disorders: the effects of workplace factors, trunk position and trunk motion characteristics on injury. Spine, 18: 617–628.

Mechanic (1968) Medical Sociology. Free Press, New York.

Melzack, R. and Wall, P.D. (1965) Pain mechanisms: a new theory. Science, 150: 971–979.

Melzack, R. and Casey, K.L. (1968) Sensory, motivational and central control determinants of pain. In: D.R. Kenshalo (Ed.), The Skin Senses. Charles C. Thomas, Springfield, IL, pp. 423–439.

Mixter, W.J. and Barr, J.S. (1934) Rupture of the intervertebral disc with involvement of the spinal canal. New Engl. J. Med., 211: 210–215.

Morley, S., Eccleston, C. and Williams, A. (1999) Systematic review and meta-analysis of randomized controlled trials of cognitive behaviour therapy and behaviour therapy for chronic pain in adults excluding headache. Pain, 80: 1–13.

Palmer, D.D. (1910) The Science, Art and Philosophy of Chiropractic. Portland Printing House, Oregon.

Payne, R. (1988) Individual differences in the study of occupational stress. In: C.L. Cooper and R. Payne (Eds.), Causes, Coping and Consequences of Stress at Work. Wiley and Sons, Chichester.

Peterson, K.W. and Travis, J.W. (2001) Health, Work and Productivity Management: Report Summaries from Centers of Inquiry. Institute for Health and Productivity Management. Scottsdale, AZ.

Pilowsky, I. and Katsikitis, M. (1994) A classification of illness behaviour in pain clinic patients. Pain, 57: 91–94.

RCGP (1996) Clinical Guidelines for the Management of Acute Low Back Pain. Royal College of General Practitioners, London.

Rudy, T.E., Kerns, R.D. and Turk, D.C. (1988) Chronic pain and depression: toward a cognitive–behavioral mediation model. Pain, 35: 129–140.

Smedley, J. and Coggan, D. (1994) Will the manual handling regulations reduce the incidence of back disorders. Occup. Med., 44: 63–65.

Still, A.T. (1899) Philosophy of Osteopathy, A.T. Still, Kirksville, MO.

Turk, D.C., Meichenbaum, D.H. and Genest, M. (1983), Pain and Behavioral Medicine: A Cognitive–Behavioral Perspective. The Guilford Press, New York.

Vingard, E. and Nachemson, A. (2000) Work related influences on neck and low back pain. In: A. Nachemson and E. Jonsson (Eds.), Neck Pain and Back Pain: The Scientific Evidence of Causes, Diagnosis and Treatment. Lippincott, Williams and Wilkins, Philadelphia, PA.

Virchow, R. (1858) Cellular pathologie in ihrer Begrundung auf physiologische and pathologische A. Hirschwald, Berlin.

Von Korff, M., Dworkin, S.F. and Le Resche, L. et al. (1988) An epidemiological comparison of pain complaints. Pain, 32: 173–183.

Waddell, G. (1996) Low back pain: a twentieth century health care enigma. Spine, 21: 2820–2825.

Waddell, G. (1998) The Back Pain Revolution. Churchill-Livingstone, Edinburgh.

Waddell, G., Bircher, M., Finlayson, D. and Main, C.J. (1984) Symptoms and signs: physical disease or illness behaviour. Br. Med. J., 289: 739–741.

Watson, P.J., Main, C.J., Gales, T., Waddell, G. and Purcell-Jones, G. (1997) Medically certified work loss, benefit claims and costs of back pain: a one year epidemiological study of the Bailiwick of Jersey. Br. J. Rheumatol., 37: 82–96.

Williams, R.A., Pruitt, S.D., Doctor, J.N., Epping-Jordan, J.E., Wahlgren, D.R., Grant, I., Patterson, T.L., Webster, J.S. and Slater, M.A. (1998) The contribution of job satisfaction to the transition from acute to chronic low back pain. Arch. Phys. Med. Rehabil., 79: 366–373.

Section II

Risk Factors and Mechanisms

An important prerequisite for prevention appears to be a good understanding of the process of chronification. This section provides an overview of why chronic pain may develop that attempts to integrate many of the findings in the scientific literature. Subsequent chapters provide in-depth reviews of a particularly relevant risk factor or mechanism.

Objectives are for the reader to:

- gain knowledge of what the known risk factors are
- understand how the risk factors may work to produce a persistent problem
- gain in-depth knowledge of particular factors so that the intricacies of the area are highlighted

New Avenues for the Prevention of Chronic Musculoskeletal Pain and Disability
Pain Research and Clinical Management, Vol. 12
Edited by S.J. Linton

CHAPTER 6

Why does chronic pain develop? A behavioral approach

Steven J. Linton [*]

Department of Occupational and Environmental Medicine, Örebro University Hospital, S-701 85 Örebro, Sweden

Abstract: Although chronic pain patients are well described and numerous 'risk' factors have been isolated, much less is known about why persistent pain and associated disability develop. This chapter analyzes the chronification of pain from a behavioral perspective. A brief review confirms that psychological variables, including behaviors, emotions, and cognitions are intricately related to the transition from acute to chronic pain. A psychological model of pain is also available that helps us to understand how nociceptive stimuli are processed psychologically. Recent data underscore the need for a dynamic model that takes into consideration the recurrent nature of the pain, learning factors, the gradual lifestyle changes propelled by critical events that characterize the problem, as well as the injury itself. When an injury occurs, psychological factors interact dynamically with other variables to shape the course of development. The analysis suggests that effective preventive methods must intervene with the right person, at the right point in development, and with a suitable intervention. Possible applications are presented.

1. Introduction

Recent research has shed new light on a central question: why does a seemingly normal acute musculoskeletal pain develop into a chronic problem? Despite the dire need for prevention, surprisingly few analyses of this process have been available. Yet, identifying the mechanisms involved should provide new insights that could culminate in more effective interventions. Innovative studies have now identified a number of risk factors and a picture of the development of chronic pain is steadily emerging. However, it is still a puzzle where each piece of evidence must be meticulously fitted together. Despite the difficulty in doing this, fitting the new evidence into a theoretical model might reap the benefit of seeing the 'whole picture' more clearly even if several pieces of the puzzle are not yet available. The purpose of this chapter is to examine the development of chronic pain where the available data are cast into a behavioral perspective that has implications for prevention.

A particular focus will be on the processes involved in the development of persistent pain. As background, the literature on psychological risk factors that have been scientifically established will first be reviewed. Next, various mechanisms that might explain how these risk factors operate will be investigated. This sets the stage for describing central processes that seem to be involved in the development of a chronic pain problem. Finally, the implications of this model will be explored with regard to interventions.

[*] Correspondence to: S.J. Linton, Department of Occupational and Environmental Medicine, Örebro University Hospital, S-701 85 Örebro, Sweden. Fax: +46 (19) 120404; E-mail: steven.linton@orebroll.se

The analysis highlights that successful secondary prevention must provide the correct intervention, at the right time point, for the right person. Although this may sound like common sense, it represents a critical change from current practice where patients are often provided with 'standard' medical procedures such as medications or 'physical therapy' and if this fails patients are provided with 'more of the same'. On the other hand, the current analysis keys on isolating the right person, at the right time point as well as providing the proper intervention to meet the patient's risk profile. Thus, this model sheds light on the classic problems of whom to offer an intervention to, when, as well as what the content of the intervention should be.

2. Psychological risk factors

Psychological factors play a significant role in chronic pain (Skevington, 1995), but they play a central role in the *transition* from acute to chronic problems. Because specific psychological variables are known to influence development, theoretical models need to incorporate these variables. Still, psychological factors in themselves only account for a portion of the variance, thereby highlighting a multidimensional view where biological and psychological factors interact. An overview of psychological factors that may influence pain and associated disability is provided in Table I (based on Linton and Skevington, 1999).

Even though back pain is a multidimensional process, psychological events are instrumental in the transition from an acute injury to a chronic disability. Indeed, the way we view our pain, the communication we have with loved ones and health-care professionals, the pain relief we receive, etc. may all affect the development of the problem. Although we clearly are a long way from fully understanding the process of chronification, psychological factors have nevertheless been reported to be more potent predictors than either biomedical or biomechanical factors (Turk, 1997; Burton et al., 1999; Linton, 2000b).

As a starting point, we may consider which psychological factors have been determined to be re-

lated to the development of pain problems. A model should explain or incorporate the main findings and may also serve as a mirror of the relevance of the model. A vast literature on the relationship between various psychological factors and back pain is available. In our recent review, over 900 articles were identified (Linton, 2000b). Unfortunately, there have been considerable methodological difficulties in studying psychological processes. These problems include sample composition and size, severity of the pain, inadequate measures of the predictors, time of outcome, outcome criteria, design of the study, possible treatment between assessments, and the use of self-ratings as both the independent and dependent variables (Turk, 1997; Linton, 2000b).

Given the methodological problems present, we reviewed the best available evidence, namely prospective studies, where the psychological variable was first measured and participants were then followed over time to determine whether a problem developed in the future. We located 37 such studies (Linton, 2000a,b). Of specific interest for this analysis are the 26 studies that actually examined the development of a back pain problem where outcome was either a new onset or the further development of a problem after acute onset. Psychological factors were consistently found to be related to the onset and development of back pain problems.

In our review, significant risk factors represented cognitive, emotional, and behavioral variables. For example, stress, distress or anxiety were found to be related to back pain in all of the studies investigating it. Moreover, mood and depression were consistently reported to be significant risk factors. Cognitive variables, such as beliefs about the pain, were related to outcome. In particular, fear–avoidance beliefs and catastrophizing were stable features having a particularly significant relationship with the development of dysfunction. Behavioral aspects included coping strategies where passive strategies were related to poor outcome. Finally, high levels of pain behavior and dysfunction were a risk factor for future back pain problems. Thus, psychological aspects were found to be related to back pain from its inception to the development of a persistent problem, and they

TABLE I

Overview of some psychological variables believed to be important in the development of chronic pain [a]

Psychological factor	Description
Pain behaviors	
Overt	Various ways in which one communicates to others that we are experiencing pain. Examples are grimacing, bracing, and rubbing.
Activity/function	Low levels of daily activities and high levels of "down time" signify a problem, but not necessarily related to pain level.
Avoidance	A learning paradigm where certain activities, places etc. are avoided. Behavior is maintained by reduction in fear, anxiety. Patients may avoid activity to reduce fear.
Cognitions	
Beliefs about pain	Strongly held views about pain and illness containing both cognitive and affective components. Socially and culturally generated and modifiable. May include beliefs about pain control (locus of control), pain modification (self-efficacy), health professionals and efficacy of treatments.
Catastrophizing	One of a number of maladaptive strategies for coping with pain, commonly related to the etiology of depression. Believed to be related to fear–avoidance vicious circle.
Cognitive distortion	Systematic errors in the thinking of people, particularly in the depressed. This may take the form of making arbitrary inferences or drawing mistaken conclusions in the absence of evidence. They may magnify the significance of an unpleasant event and minimize or discount a pleasant one. Commonly found in relation to pain and disability.
Locus of control	Beliefs concerning the place where the control of pain is based, e.g. personal responsibility for pain control, pain control by others (e.g. doctors), and pain control through chance happenings or misfortune. These beliefs may be the foundation for action to seek pain relief.
Coping strategies	A number of ways of managing or deflecting unwanted stress or pain. These may include cognitive, (distraction) and behavioral (take pill) aspects and they may be passive (hoping) or active strategies (relaxation).
Control	Belief that it is possible to respond to influence an aversive event. Desire to predict such an event. Control and predictability influence pain perception.
Attention	A type of vigilance or monitoring activity that can be harnessed in coping strategies either to divert or distract from the source of stress or to focus directly on the pain, stress, or anxiety. Choice of strategy depends on the circumstances.
Helplessness	A style of beliefs predominantly used by those who are prone to depression whereby negative events, such as the onset of pain, tend to be seen as likely to persist and generalize.
Emotions	
Mood	Depression, anxiety, but also fear, sadness, anger, frustration are associated with pain and disability. More likely to be a consequence of pain than a precursor to it.
Anxiety/somatic anxiety	Increased physiological arousal together with cognitive components like worry that enhance the detection of painful sensation and maintain perceived pain. Thus, a target for treatment. Somatic anxiety refers to the distress and concurrent symptoms.
Social	
Gender	Similarities and differences in the way women and men respond to pain sensations, interpret them and report them and styles of obtaining treatment. Formed in part by social and cultural frame.
Social comparison	Comparisons made with other people with different diseases or health states or with self (ideal self) at different times defined by health events, within the lifespan.
Social support	Any input directly provided by another person or group which moves recipients towards the goals they desire. For pain may be positive or negative.
Spouse relations	The interpersonal relationship between pain patient and spouse and the effect that this has on pain behaviors. A solicitous spouse may increase pain behaviors.
Work place	Relationships at work with management as well as coworkers may influence perceptions of injury as well as pain and disability.
Work management	The way in which a work place organizes and deals with pain problems and rehabilitation may influence pain perception and behavior.

[a] Based on Linton and Skevington, 1999.

seem to be pivotal in the transition from acute to chronic pain.

2.1. Psychological factors at work

As chronic pain problems often involve work disability, it is intriguing to examine the literature on the role of psychological work-place factors in disability due to pain. Fortunately, some reviews are available that summarize this literature.

In our clinic, we examined prospective studies where a psychological work-place factor was first measured and outcome was assessed at a later time point, usually 1 year later (Linton, 2001). Twenty-one such studies were located in a systematic literature search. Back pain was used as an outcome in some studies while function was used in others. Overall the evidence was compelling that psychological factors at work are related to future pain and disability. There was strong evidence indicating that job satisfaction, monotonous tasks, work relations, demand levels, stress, perceived health were related to future back pain problems. Moreover, there was moderate evidence that control, pace, emotional effort and the belief that work is dangerous are also associated with future back problems. We concluded that the psychological work environment plays a considerable role in the development of future back pain problems.

Other reviews in the literature draw similar conclusions. For example, Bongers et al. (1993) found that a lack of social support and low control were related to back pain, while Hoogendoorn et al. (2000) found strong evidence that social support at work and job satisfaction are risk factors, whereas there was insufficient evidence for work pace, perceived, demands, content, and job control. Indeed, the American National Research Council recognized in their report that several work-related psychosocial factors were associated with musculoskeletal disorders (National Research Council, 2001). Consequently, psychological and social factors at work appear to play a significant role in the development of persistent pain and disability.

In summary, there is considerable evidence linking psychological factors to the development of persistent pain problems including suffering, health-care consumption and work disability. One way this may operate is that such variables create *barriers* for a return to work. Several obstacles for return to work in fact appear to be related to the interaction between the individual patient and his/her psychological work environment (Marhold et al., 2002). However, while the reviews underscore the importance of these variables, they do not provide a theoretical model for how or why such problems develop.

3. Developmental mechanisms

In this section, we review some of the mechanisms that appear to be involved when spinal pain extends to a persistent problem. No such appraisal could possibly cover every conception of operative mechanisms as a seemingly infinite number has been proposed. However, many of these may overlap or simply be different labels and descriptions of a similar mechanism. In this section, an overview is provided focusing on some major categories of mechanisms. To provide an overview, I have put these into an historical perspective.

3.1. Learning

Despite the tremendous advances being made in the physiology of pain, most of what we do when we experience a painful stimulus is learned behavior. Whether we take an aspirin, go for a walk or attempt to think about something else, these activities are learned rather than innate. In essence, learning theory postulates that our behavior, including when we are in pain, is steered by its consequences and the situation in which it occurs. Early on, Fordyce and others (Fordyce, 1976; Keefe et al., 1978; Linton et al., 1984) described how learning factors influence behavior. He referred to 'pain' behavior as opposed to 'well' behavior. Since then, learning paradigms have been developed and tested. Clearly, pain behaviors are controlled in part by their consequences.

Interestingly, various sorts of pain-related behaviors are specific to the situation in which they occur (the setting or discriminative stimulus), but may generalize to other situations. By providing reinforcement according to certain schedules, the pain behavior may be maintained even though the nociceptive stimulus is no longer present. As a specific example, in one experiment, we provided positive feedback to normal subjects who received painful stimuli in the form of pressure. At the same time, as we systematically reduced the pressure, we provided reinforcement for high pain ratings and indeed, subjects continued to rate the stimulus as clearly 'painful' even though the pressure was reduced dramatically (Linton and Götestam, 1985).

Although this learning model neatly explains the increase in the frequency of behavior and has resulted in a revolution in the way we view pain, it does have certain limitations. First, the theory in its most adamant forms from the 1970s suggests that learning might be the same for all people. That is, that learning occurs in 'an empty box' and all people might react in the same way given the proper stimulus and consequences. However, learning appears to be more complex and there are numerous individual differences. Furthermore, the simple learning model did not seem to adequately explain why some people in fact increase their pain behavior while most people recover and their pain behavior decreases in frequency as the nociception dissipates. In other words, why do a few people increase their pain behavior while most do not, even though the Western World provides sympathy when we are in pain?

3.2. Cognitive and emotional factors

Psychologists in the 1980s attempted to expand the learning model by adding cognitive processes (Turk et al., 1983; Keefe et al., 1992; Turk, 1996a). In essence, they maintained that learning does not take place in an empty box, but instead is influenced by cognitive and emotional processes. These represent such things as beliefs, attitudes and emotional states. As an example, the interpretations that a patient makes concerning a perceived painful stimulus

influence coping behavior (i.e. how the pain is dealt with) as well as how environmental consequences are experienced. Interpretations of the cause of the pain are central. If a patient interprets the cause as being cancer, this is linked to a different emotional reaction than if the cause was interpreted as being benign (the garlic I ate last night). Indeed, our belief system seems to be associated with a host of factors that influence expectations about what constitute a proper assessment, treatment, response from friends and family as well as prognosis.

In the back pain literature, it has been found that the belief that an increase in activity increases pain is linked to several behaviors. As the review on fear–avoidance in Chapter 7 elucidates, back pain patients for example expect more pain when doing activities (even though the actual pain is less than expected) and higher levels of the belief are associated with lower activity levels. In other words, people who hold this belief tend to avoid movements and activities that they believe will increase the pain or result in injury.

People may have conceptions of how the spine works that enhance and reflect negative beliefs. As an illustration, a person may believe that the spine has a limited number of movements before it wears out, much like the miles on a car. Given this belief, a good strategy would be to conserve movements so as to not waste the precious few remaining. This results in avoidance. Consequently, examining beliefs about back pain seems to provide insights into how patients behave.

Furthermore, examining beliefs helps to explain how a given consequence may be experienced. That is, the same consequence, such as a stretching sensation in a muscle, may be experienced as positive or negative depending on the belief/cognitive system the person has. A person who believes there is a risk that the back may break would experience this sensation negatively and it might strengthen the idea that movement is indeed harmful. These beliefs in turn set the stage for avoidance behavior. On the other hand, a person who believes it is important with stretching may interpret the same sensation as positive. Thus, cognitive factors, like beliefs, provide a link between the environment and behavior.

Emotional factors are also tied to the development of persistent problems. Experiences, thoughts and cognitions trigger emotional responses. For example, the thought (expectation) that a movement will result in severe pain, triggers fear and worry. Worry in turn serves the purpose of being vigilant so that danger may be avoided. While this is ordinarily a helpful process, we know that for pain, vigilance seems to increase suffering. That is, when we focus our attention on a painful sensation it tends to magnify the pain. As a result, emotions that are linked to cognitions, might then be said to set the stage for a particular behavior and learning.

The fear–avoidance model is one concrete mechanism that illustrates the relationship between cognitions, emotions and behavior (see Chapter 7). The model features cognitions such as catastrophizing, emotions, such as fear, worry and associated vigilance, as well as behavior, such as avoidance. Thus, it is an important, specific model that may help us to understand how a persistent pain problem develops. Let us examine a model that summarizes the information thus far.

3.3. Psychology of pain model: cross-sectional view

Putting the evidence together, a model was developed that helps us understand the psychological processes involved in pain perception and behavior. This model, that might be described as a cross-sectional view since it deals with how a nociceptive stimulus is psychologically processed, is shown in Fig. 1 (Linton, 1994).

This model stresses the role of appraisal and beliefs that complement the roles of coping and learning. As the model illustrates, the first step is to attend to the noxious stimulus. This, in part, is controlled by psychological factors, e.g. whether a person's attention is focused inward or outward. Vigilance is a term used to denote to what extent a person focuses on internal stimuli with the specific aim of detecting signs of danger. In the second step, an appraisal of the stimulus is made. This attribution is influenced by a host of psychological factors and previous experiences. The noxious stimulus is given meaning

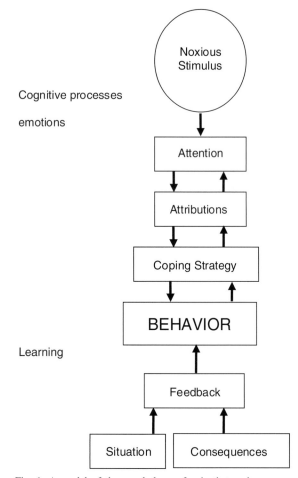

Fig. 1. A model of the psychology of pain that underscores a cross-sectional view of how pain is processed.

and is evaluated in the decision about whether it is harmful, unusual, or irrelevant and not worth further attention. This in turn influences coping strategies, i.e. the way we 'plan' to deal with the pain. These cognitive processes, according to the model, are important prerequisites to the next step, i.e. behavior. However, these cognitive processes are not always conscious 'thought' and may occur automatically.

Learning factors operate and influence 'pain' behaviors just as they do any other behavior. Consequently, behaviors designed to cope with a pain problem are influenced by the situation in which they occur as well as the consequences. Although the rules known to govern learning are very specific and intricate, simply put, behaviors that successfully reduce or eliminate pain will tend to increase in frequency in similar situations, that is they are reinforced. Likewise, behaviors that increase the pain will tend to decrease in frequency due to punishment. An example of how learning may affect pain behaviors is the avoidance paradigm. In the first stage, respondent conditioning occurs so that stimuli, such as a certain place, situation or activity (such as lifting), elicit a response, such as increased anxiety, fear, and muscle tension. In the second stage, this stimulus is experienced as a 'threat' ("Please help me lift this suitcase.") and this sets the stage for an avoidance response. The behavioral response of avoiding the situation ("I can't, I have back pain") is reinforced by the consequences, i.e. a reduction of the anxiety, tension and pain (Linton et al., 1984). Once learned, the person may never come in contact with the actual threatening situation (the lift). Moreover, this paradigm is related to certain cognitive thought patterns. The most conspicuous is so called catastrophizing, where the patient makes exaggerated and negative interpretations. This model then summarizes many of the known processes and provides a framework. However, this model is by nature static, while the chronification of pain appears to be a dynamic developmental process.

4. The process of chronification

Today we tend to view the development of chronic pain as a linear process that occurs relatively rapidly (e.g. 3 months), and that is directly related to a specific injury. However, musculoskeletal pain tends to be recurrent and the development of persistent disability gradual. In turn, this gradual change seems to be related to cognitive and learning factors. Let us examine a variety of aspects of the chronification process.

4.1. Individual process

Although we can describe some of the general process and mechanisms involved, it is important to accentuate that the process is unique to each individual. In fact, the differences between people may be quite large. This is not surprising since individual variation is true not only for psychological variables, but for physiological ones as well; diversity is a part of nature.

The actual factors that influence the development of persistent pain are peculiar to any given individual. While anxiety and fear–avoidance may be important for one person, monotonous work and a poor relationship with a supervisor may be critical for another. Likewise, the pertinent risk factors may change over time. For example, anxiety and fear may be crucial in the acute stage, while depression and catastrophizing may become more important as the problem becomes non-relenting.

4.2. Recurrent nature of back pain = repeated learning

A key to the model is an understanding of the natural history of back pain where recurrent problems are the rule. First, a bout of back pain normally takes about 8 weeks to reside (Van den Hoogen et al., 1998) even though patients may expect it to go away within a few days. Second, back pain is normally recurrent (Von Korff, 1994; Van den Hoogen et al., 1997, 1998). Thus, once a person has a problem there is great likelihood for a new bout, usually within a year; the average being 8 weeks (Van den Hoogen et al., 1998). In the development of a chronic problem, the interval between bouts may gradually become shorter and the length of the bouts longer. During the bouts people will attempt a variety of ways of coping with the pain and the resultant disability. The intensity of the pain itself may change thoughts and beliefs about the pain.

4.3. Gradual lifestyle changes

The recurrent nature of back pain allows ample opportunities for learning. Keeping in mind the large number of people who deal with their back pain effectively, this learning ordinarily seems to be helpful in coping with the problem. However, for some people, coping strategies that seem to work on the short term, may enhance the development of a persistent problem in the long term. The process is gradual. Rather than the 'straight line' often depicted in the literature, the road to chronic pain is crooked. It is not unusual for some periods with little or no pain. With small alterations taking place during bouts of pain, a change in lifestyle may occur. However, because of the gradual nature of the change, the person may not be aware of the process until a major development is already a fact.

Remember that gradual changes in lifestyle are particularly difficult to perceive. Therefore, on a cognitive–perceptual level, individuals may not become aware of the type and size of the change until it is quite advanced.

Contributing to this is the expectation that the pain will reside quickly and 'normality' will be restored. Patients may thereby incorporate coping strategies such as rest, taking medications and the reduction of social activities because they believe they will only be temporary. As an illustration, a father who normally plays with his small children each day upon returning home from work, may stop doing so when faced with back pain. He may believe that the pain will soon reside and then the play may be resumed exactly in its usual form. While this is but one small lifestyle change involving a few minutes, it is quite likely that other small changes will be made in other sectors of this man's life. When these small changes are pieced together, they involve a major change. The gradual character of the change may then short-cut feedback so that the problem continues to develop.

4.4. The role of injury and its resultant pain

Psychological models might be criticized because they always seem to assume that an injury has occurred, but often ignore this injury once the nociception has been initiated. Indeed, many psychological models seem void of the role of nociception. Nevertheless, a body of evidence indicates that the intensity, duration and quality of the pain seem to influence our psychological reaction. Thus, an intense 'jolt' of pain is experienced differently than a mild 'ache'.

These nuances have direct relevance for this model. First, pain sensations generate reactions including central emotional processes. Intense pain, or a hurt that is very different in character relative to earlier experiences are linked to fear and worry. This may in turn elicit beliefs (it must be dangerous or it wouldn't hurt so much). In addition, worry enhances vigilance that influences whether pain signals will be detected. Vigilance and worry, if sufficiently strong, are said to result in misinterpretations, i.e. where nonpainful signals such as pressure or movement are interpreted as painful.

Second, the pain signals from an injury are related to how the problem might best be dealt with. Coping is postulated to be directly related to the idiosyncrasies of the pain sensations. Distraction may work wonderfully to cope with low-intensity pain, but might be relatively useless for very intense pain. This may be the direct result of the fact that intense pain physiologically is programmed to elicit our attention or to the fact that it is difficult to maintain distraction techniques as intensity increases.

4.5. Critical events

The problem may reach a plateau where further development of the problem is subsequently triggered by a critical event. These events are decisive experiences that result in a new belief and/or behavior for the individual. In this section, we will concentrate on negative thoughts and behaviors, but 'positive' critical events also apply to the recovery process. An example of a negative critical event is when a patient attempts to return to work and the supervisor states, "Your back is too weak for this work". This event might be critical in changing the patient's beliefs about his/her back and ability to work ("If my supervisor doesn't believe I can do the job, I must be really bad.")

Another example might involve a visit to a healthcare practitioner. Let us assume that the person with back pain expects to get something to relieve the pain and that the pain will then go away within a few days. The provider, however, states that there is probably degeneration in the spine and that the person needs to rest to protect the back. This might trigger a dramatic change in beliefs and behavior where the patient now begins to entertain the thought that the pain may not reside, that permanent functional problems will develop and that it is necessary to restrict movement in order to 'save' on wear and tear.

Critical events emphasizes that development occurs in 'jumps' rather than in an even, linear fashion. The increments may be relatively small, but also large. Here again, we see the individual nature of the development, as the exact events that trigger the critical events appear to be peculiar to the individual.

4.6. Dynamic process

Models to date, by their nature, tend to be static, while a developmental process, by its nature, is dynamic. Consequently, if we are to understand how and why chronic pain develops, we need to consider the longitudinal aspects. Static models are quite good at isolating important variables and demonstrating links between them. This is vital for understanding which factors are involved and developing an understanding for the problem. However, static models are poor at elucidating the process involved. Indeed, if we consider the number of variables that may be important in the development of chronic pain and then multiply them by a time unit, such as hours or days, a tremendous number of events can occur. To understand development then, we need to know more about how these processes start and progress. A good model will incorporate dynamic aspects, although we certainly could not expect a detailed description of every possible road to a chronic problem.

Learning is an important concept as it incorporates a dynamic view. Thus, the person's interaction with pain as well as the interaction with the environment is included in a learning approach. Modern theories of learning include cognitive and emotional aspects. Their advantage is that they serve as an aid in understanding the dynamics of the process since different stimuli, thoughts, emotions, behaviors, and consequences may be placed into the scheme. In

this way, an individual's situation may be entered into the scheme and analyzed to determine a reasonable explanation for the development. At the present, however, it is difficult to generate scenarios of common paths for the development of persistent pain disability. Such information is vital in order to be able to identify people at risk of developing persistent pain as well as to develop effective preventive interventions. As a result, more work needs to be done so that we may understand better how a chronic problem develops.

4.7. Summary of development

The development of chronic pain is a complex, multidimensional process where psychological factors play an important role in enhancing or catalyzing the development of the problem. The evidence and theories available do not suggest that back pain is psychogenic. Rather, once an injury occurs, psychological factors may influence the course of development. Usually this is advantageous and quite often the person copes adequately and recovers. However, sometimes the process results in further development of the problem. Thus, psychological factors interplay with other types of variables. Rather than being static, the development involves a dynamic process where critical events trigger changes in beliefs and behavior. Small resultant changes in lifestyle may then gradually proceed without alarming the individual since they do not perceive the change. The recurrent nature of musculoskeletal pain is an important element as it presents numerous opportunities for learning.

Thus, psychological factors are therefore important in the development of a persistent pain problem. They are comparatively powerful in predicting disability and they may offer important insights as to how such problems might be prevented.

5. Implications

Although still not complete, our current understanding of how pain develops into a persistent problem highlights the *need to intervene with the right person, at the right time point, and with the proper intervention.* Common preventive strategies that are applied to 'everyone' in a given setting such as a work place have produced very disappointing results (Linton and Van Tulder, 2001). This may be due to the general nature of such programs where high and low 'risk' individuals regardless of the time point are provided with an 'average' intervention. Instead, the ideas put forward here suggest the need for targeting the population for people truly at risk of developing a persistent problem. A corollary is intervening at a correct point in time. The evidence to date suggests that once the process has reached a certain point, it is difficult to hinder. Likewise, even if certain risk factors are present, intervening too early may have limited success if the intervention in question is not an effective one. Furthermore, intervening too early may have the disadvantage of low engagement on the client's part. Selecting the proper intervention for the problem at hand is thus an extremely important aspect and our knowledge of the development of the problem shows that matching the intervention to the individuals needs may optimize intervention.

Psychological factors might be utilized for prevention in two fashions. First, since psychological factors are related to future disability, early identification is feasible. Psychological factors might serve to screen patients. Second, the content of early preventive interventions might be tailored after the psychological factors identified. To date most preventive interventions have been based on biomedical or biomechanical theories. A logical approach would be to provide an intervention that focuses on the psychological elements identified. This section explores what the implications of the analysis mean for secondary prevention in health-care settings.

5.1. Early identification

In order to utilize our limited resources, screening would help us converge our resources on the minority of people with back pain who risk developing persistent disability. Identifying the right person at the right point in time is a real challenge that appears to be attainable.

5.2. Right person

Screening refers to a first, gross evaluation. It is not a final product, but rather the start of a clinical process. Patients determined to be potentially at risk for developing problems, will need further attention to assess them properly. Consequently, screening allows clinicians to focus their time on further assessing only those individuals that indicate a risk for developing persistent problems. Additional evaluation may or may not show a need for early intervention. However, for those who are determined to have a need, the next step will be to address the specific problems isolated. Screening is therefore the first step in a health-care based preventive intervention.

Although psychological techniques are emphasized here, early identification also includes medical factors. To aid in applying this knowledge to clinical settings, the idea of red and yellow flags has been introduced (Kendall et al., 1997). 'Red flags' denote the rare, but serious, diseases that need to be addressed in a medical examination (Kendall et al., 1997). These include signs and symptoms related to fractures, tumors, neurological damage and infections. 'Yellow flags' on the other hand refer to the psychological factors described above that may enhance the development of a persistent problem.

Unfortunately, translating psychological risk factors into a perfect screening procedure is not an easy task. Health-care professionals, for example, do not believe that they can accurately predict which patients would develop chronic problems (Linton et al., 2002). This may well be because doctors and physical therapists are best acquainted with the biomedical variables that unfortunately are not particularly salient predictors. Moreover, evidence from an ongoing study at our clinic indicates that health-care providers are indeed not very accurate in predicting future disability. Lastly, some professionals may be concerned about how to bring up 'sensitive' psychological issues.

There are, however, instruments available to assist in assessing 'yellow flags' and more detailed examples are discussed elsewhere (see Chapters 12 and 13). For example, Main and colleagues (Main et al.,

1992; Main and Watson, 1995) developed an instrument based on measures of depression and distress (DRAM) and showed that it helped identify patients seeking orthopedic care who were at risk of a poor outcome. In an exciting development since it entails a method for use in primary care settings, Gatchel et al. (1995) employed the Minnesota Multiphasic Personality Inventory (MMPI), questionnaires, and a clinical diagnostic interview to assess patients seeking care for acute back pain. Scores on several psychological factors correctly classified 87% of the patients' work status 6 months later. Finally, the Örebro Screening Questionnaire for Pain is a 25-item instrument developed for use in primary care and it has shown a predictive validity of 0.83 (see Chapter 13). It appears then that by using a screening procedure, the 'right person' may be identified who is in need of a preventive intervention.

5.3. Right time point

In order to prevent long-term disability, the intervention needs to be initiated at an early time point, but when is the best time? One line of thought has been to 'wait out' the natural course of the problem as most people return to work relatively quickly. According to this idea, as most people recover from their back pain within a few weeks, early interventions might instead be oriented toward those with a problem persisting more than 6–8 weeks (Frank et al., 1996). Indeed, there is evidence that early, multidimensional rehabilitation produces significant improvements for this group (Frank et al., 1996; Turk, 1996b; Waddell, 1998; Morley et al., 1999; Van Tulder et al., 2000). Waiting too long is also devastating as results diminish and the opportunity to truly 'prevent' the problem dissipate.

An alternative view has been to intervene before the problem arises to attain true primary prevention. Sadly, the research to date shows that interventions aimed at non-patient populations, e.g. a workforce or the general population have had little success (Linton and Van Tulder, 2001). Indeed, our review found that people without a pain problem might not be motivated to participate as compliance is usually low. Worse, for some people, focusing on possible back problems may exacerbate the problem. Finally, providing help for all people, even those with no problem at all, would be resource intensive.

A health-care visit for spinal pain appears to represent an ideal time point for early identification and possible subsequent preventive intervention. First, although most people will 'recover' from their current bout of pain, there is no innate reason for waiting until the problem persists several weeks before beginning. This is particularly true since back pain tends to be recurrent in nature. Second, limiting the process to those who seek medical help will, in itself, greatly reduce the number of people in need of the service. Third, as medical care has been sought, the patient has indicated an interest and might therefore be better engaged to participate. Thus, rather than simply 'referring' patients to an early intervention, screening should also encompass the patient's goals and interest in participating in a preventive intervention.

5.4. Proper content

Once the right person has been identified at the right time point, the next step is to provide an effective intervention. In this vein, I suggest that the reason early, preventive interventions often fail is because they do not directly deal with the factors associated with the development of a persistent disability. A traditional approach de facto has been simply providing 'more of the same'. That is, as the problem progresses and the patient gets worse, there is a tendency to prescribe more of the same therapies tried early on. Thus, if physical therapy was given for three sessions, the 'dose' might be increased to 10 sessions. Similarly, if prescribed pain killers were not solving the problem the dose or type of drug would be altered. Although this may sometimes be helpful, it may not address the actual factors that are catalyzing the development of the problem. The evidence presented thus far in this chapter shows that psychological factors are key ingredients in the transition from an acute to a chronic pain problem. Consequently, a significant part of the treatment might be psychological in nature.

Early, health-care based preventive interventions usually involve two basic approaches. These are certainly not exclusive. The first focuses on the initial meetings with the patient. It involves addressing the patient's concerns and providing a working relationship with the patient and may be applied to all patients seeking care for musculoskeletal pain. The second converges on those patients with a clear risk for developing a persistent problem. Here, special interventions are initiated that are designed to specifically deal with the problem including the psychological aspects.

5.5. Initial visit

Developing a 'preventive' approach to the first health-care visit provides a unique opportunity to provide effective treatment as well as to hinder the development of a persistent problem. The model above suggests that patients may begin to have thoughts and behaviors very early on that, if reinforced, may lead to the development of dysfunctional behaviors. In this light we may also consider what patients desire from a first consultation with a health-care provider; most often a doctor or physical therapist. An excellent study has shown that patients in primary care are interested in receiving a diagnosis (why it hurts), reassurance that it is not serious, a cure, and information (Von Korff, 1999) (see Chapter 15). The information desired features pain management with and without analgesics, as well as advice on how to resume normal activities. Yet, this same research demonstrates that only a relatively small minority actually receives this when visiting their physician. Moreover, patients may not have modern information about back pain. For example, a study in Belgium found that 42% of the general population believed that the *cause* of back pain could always be identified with an X-ray and 35% reported that bedrest was the mainstay of treatment (Geert Crombie, personal communication). What may we learn from this and how might the first meeting be organized to be preventive in nature?

Rather than simply alleviate the pain, the goal of a prevention-oriented consultation is also to educate

and shape behavior. In fact, the first consultation seems to offer a short, but decisive opportunity for providing patients with valuable advice on how to cope with the problem. This is particularly central since musculoskeletal pain is normally recurrent. Since patients are interested in why they have pain and whether it involves a 'serious' problem, the first consultation should include an examination focusing on red flags. Given that no red flags exist, the consultation should provide information on 'why it hurts', and reassurance that it is not a serious disorder. Information and recommendations that relieve the fear that the problem is dangerous are appropriate. Next, 'yellow flags' may be ascertained in an interview format that focuses on the main issues. Often examining the consequences of the problem for the individual may start the section on yellow flags. Finally, advice on self-management may be offered where the message is to remain active. We recommend that patients maintain their everyday routines as well as possible. Although pain may set some limitations, normal activities are not harmful, but rather enhance recovery. Advice about pain relief should include the role of pharmacological and non-pharmacological options. Many patients do not understand that a possible objective for taking analgesics is that it will allow them to partake in physical activities so this should be accentuated.

One objective in discussing these issues with the patient is to provide a framework for cooperative effort. Without having a 'shared understanding' of the problem, it is difficult to engage the patient in treatments that require his/her participation.

Another objective is to prevent fear–avoidance behaviors from developing. Thus, the discussion focuses on relieving fears as well as enhancing self-management and activity. Although this sounds elaborate, experience suggests that it can often be achieved in a few minutes. Indeed, modern, behaviorally oriented information has been developed to assist in this process and to provide patients with concrete advice they can refer to at home (see Chapters 15 and 16). Consequently, the first visit is an opportunity to educate patient about back pain, relieve fears and provide specific plans for recovery.

Some studies have attempted to apply this approach. Interestingly, the first published evaluation of this approach came out already in 1986 in a study with patients seeking medical help for acute back pain (Fordyce et al., 1986). Low activity levels and the misuse of medications characterize persistent pain. Therefore, Fordyce keyed on preventing these. Doctors learned to provide patients with specific advise about activities focusing on what patients should do and being specific about any limitations. In addition, doctors were taught to limit sick leave and restrict prescription medications to a limited number (if needed at all) taken on a time rather than pain contingency. The results of this randomized controlled study indicated that disability levels 1 year later were lower in the experimental group. Thus, the study shows that the way clinicians deal with patients with acute pain can have a significant effect on outcome. In addition, it supports the idea that prevention is possible by addressing some behavioral aspects, such as medications and activities.

In our own work, we attempted to improve the care provided during the first visit according to the principles described above. For those seeking care for the first time for their back pain, a doctor carried out a medical examination focusing on possible 'red' flags. The doctor also provided information and the message that activity was a good preventive treatment. Patients also saw a physical therapist who conducted an examination but mainly provided information about the cause of the problem and self-management methods. The message was that patients should maintain their everyday routines and remain active. This preventive approach was compared to treatment as usual in a randomized study that demonstrated a significantly lower rate of sick absenteeism over the course of the following year (Linton et al., 1989).

Another indication of the impact of the initial meetings with the patient is reflected in what advice patients are provided with. The results of the Belgian study described earlier indicated that a third of the population believed that bed rest is a treatment of choice. Furthermore, patients reported that they were very keen to have information on returning to normal activities (Von Korff, 1999). This highlights the need for providing clear and practical advice about activity. Consider the review conducted by Waddell et al. (1997), for example, on the effects of providing advice for back pain patients. They found that advice for bed rest was counterproductive while advice to remain active despite the pain produced a significantly better long-term result with regard to pain and disability. Information about activity may also have an impact as described in Chapter 16. Consequently, the content and manner in which patients are cared for may offer an opportunity for prevention.

5.6. Specific interventions: CBT as prevention

However good the skills at the first consultation, a few patients will nevertheless proceed down the avenue towards chronicity. Screening procedures may help identify those at risk. In addition, the screening procedure may help to identify important psychological factors that may be contributing to the problem. This information is crucial in determining which preventive interventions might be useful. Should the patient indicate problems such as fear–avoidance or a lack of coping skills, a behaviorally oriented intervention may be of help. Matching the intervention to the problem appears to be essential for best results. In fact, the level of risk as indicated by yellow flags seems to be associated with the success level of a behaviorally oriented preventive intervention (Linton, 2002).

As cognitive behavioral treatments have been successful for persistent pain problems (Compas et al., 1998; Morley et al., 1999; Van Tulder et al., 2000), several attempts have been made to emulate these in a preventive intervention. For example, Von Korff and associates employed a technique based on lay-led groups for arthritic pain as a preventive intervention for patients seeking care for acute back pain (Von Korff et al., 1998). A four-session program including problem-solving skills, activity management and educational videos was offered to patients with acute back pain. An evaluation conducted on 255 primary care back pain patients in a randomized design showed that the cognitive-behavioral group had significantly reduced worry and disability relative to the treatment as usual control. Participants in the lay-led group also had a significantly more positive view toward self-care, but there was no significant difference with regard to pain intensity or medication use. Similar results have been reported in two other reports using similar methods (Saunders et al., 1999; Moore et al., 2000).

We have developed a six-session program for participants that enable them to derive their own coping program designed to prevent future back pain related problems. This program is described in detail in Chapter 18. Briefly, participants met in groups of 6–10 people for 2 h once a week for 6 weeks. Each session contains a review of homework, a short presentation of educational material, problem solving, the presentation of new skills, and individualized homework assignments. The end product for participants was a personalized coping program.

To test the utility of this approach, we compared this approach to treatment as usual in three randomized controlled trials (Linton and Andersson, 2000; Linton and Ryberg, 2001; Marhold et al., 2001). These studies have all demonstrated that this intervention has a clear preventive effect on sick absenteeism and function. For example, in the Linton and Andersson (2000) study, the risk for having a long-term sick absenteeism at the 1-year follow-up was more than 8-fold lower in the cognitive behavioral group. More details of the results are provided in Chapter 18.

Thus, there appears to be implications for the model developed for both the identification of 'at risk' patients as well as for the implementation of effective early, preventive interventions.

6. Conclusions

This chapter has highlighted cognitive–behavioral factors in the development of a chronic pain problem that are also pertinent for prevention. It is now clear that psychological variables including behaviors, emotions, and cognitions are intricately related to the transition from acute to chronic pain. Psychological factors enhance or catalyze the problem. A psychological model of pain helps us to understand how nociceptive stimuli are processed psychologically. However, while models are static, this developmental process is quite dynamic. Because musculoskeletal pain is recurrent in nature, this provides ample opportunities for learning to deal with occurrences. Recent data suggest that the process of chronification is highly individual, but normally involves a gradual change in lifestyle. These changes are propelled by certain critical events. The role of the injury and pain is vital. The experience of the pain interacts with other psychological variables influencing our emotions, cognitions and behaviors. Thus, when an injury occurs, psychological factors interact with other variables to shape the course of development.

This analysis of the development of chronic pain has several implications for prevention. It suggests that effective preventive methods must intervene with the right person, at the right point in development, and with a suitable intervention. Our knowledge about psychological processes may be utilized in the early identification of patients who are likely to develop problems as well as in the design of preventive interventions. Improving the content of the first visit with the patient, for example, may have considerable preventive consequences. Moreover, providing psychologically oriented early interventions for those patients with a psychological risk profile might also produce preventive results. Future efforts should be directed at developing a sound theory concerning the development of chronic pain. As this develops, additional investigations will be needed to test the new preventive methods isolated in the theories.

References

Bongers, P.M., de Winter, C.R., Kompier, M.A. and Hildebrandt, V.H. (1993) Psychosocial factors at work and musculoskeletal disease. *Scand. J. Work Environ. Health*, 19: 297–312.
Burton, A.K., Battié, M.C. and Main, C.J. (1999) The relative importance of biomechanical and psychosocial factors in low back injuries. In: W. Karwowski and W. Marras (Eds.), The Occupational Ergonomics Handbook. CRC Press, Boca Raton, FL, pp. 1127–1138.
Compas, B.E., Haaga, D.A.F., Keefe, F.J., Leitenberg, H. and

Williams, D.A. (1998) A sampling of empirically supported psychological treatments from health psychology: smoking, chronic pain, cancer, and bulimia nervosa. J. Consult. Clin. Psychol., 66: 89–112.

Fordyce, W.E. (1976) Behavioral Methods for Chronic Pain and Illness. Mosby, St. Louis, MO.

Fordyce, W.E., Brockway, J.A., Bergman, J.A. and Spengler, D. (1986) Acute back pain: a control-group comparison of behavioral vs traditional management methods. J. Behav. Med., 9: 127–140.

Frank, J.W., Brooker, A.S., DeMaio, S.E., Kerr, M.S., Maetzel, A., Shannon, H.S., Sullivan, T.J., Norman, R.W. and Wells, R.P. (1996) Disability resulting from occupational low back pain: Part II: What do we know about secondary prevention? A review of the scientific evidence on prevention after disability begins. Spine, 21: 2918–2929.

Gatchel, R.J., Polatin, P.B. and Kinney, R.K. (1995) Predicting outcome of chronic back pain using clinical predictors of psychopathology: a prospective analysis. Health Psychol., 14: 415–420.

Hoogendoorn, W.E., Van Poppel, M.N.M., Bongers, P.M., Koes, B.W. and Bouter, L.M. (2000) Systematic review of psychosocial factors at work and in the personal situation as risk factors for back pain. Spine, 25: 2114–2125.

Keefe, F.J., Kopel, S. and Gordon, S.B. (1978) A Practical Guide to Behavioral Assessment. Springer, New York.

Keefe, F.J., Dunsmore, J. and Burnett, R. (1992) Behavioral and cognitive–behavioral approaches to chronic pain: recent advances and future directions. J. Consult. Clin. Psychol., 54: 776–783.

Kendall, N.A.S., Linton, S.J. and Main, C.J. (1997) Guide to assessing psychosocial yellow flags in acute low back pain: risk factors for long-term disability and work loss. Accident Rehabilitation and Compensation Insurance Corporation of New Zealand and the National Health Committee. Wellington, New Zealand.

Linton, S.J. (1994) The role of psychological factors in back pain and its remediation. Pain Rev., 1: 231–243.

Linton, S.J. (2000a) Psychologic risk factors for neck and back pain. In: A. Nachemson and E. Jonsson (Eds.), Neck and Back Pain: The Scientific Evidence of Causes, Diagnosis, and Treatment. Lippincott, Williams and Wilkins, Philadelphia, PA, pp. 57–78.

Linton, S.J. (2000b) A review of psychological risk factors in back and neck pain. Spine, 25: 1148–1156.

Linton, S.J. (2001) Occupational psychological factors increase the risk for back pain: a systematic review. J. Occup. Rehabil., 11: 53–66.

Linton, S.J. (2002) Early identification and intervention in the prevention of musculoskeletal pain. Am. J. Indust. Med., 41(5): 433–442.

Linton, S.J. and Andersson, T. (2000) Can chronic disability be prevented? A randomized trial of a cognitive–behavior intervention and two forms of information for patients with spinal pain. Spine, 25: 2825–2831.

Linton, S.J., Bradley, L.A., Jensen, I., Spangfort, E. and Sundell,

L. (1989) The secondary prevention of low back pain: a controlled study with follow-up. Pain, 36: 197–207.

Linton, S.J. and Götestam, K.G. (1985) Controlling pain reports through operant conditioning: a laboratory demonstration. Percept. Motor Skills, 60: 427–437.

Linton, S.J., Melin, L. and Götestam, K.G. (1984) Behavioral analysis of chronic pain and its management. Prog. Behav. Modif., 18: 1–42.

Linton, S.J. and Ryberg, M. (2001) A cognitive–behavioral group intervention as prevention for persistent neck and back pain in a non-patient population: a randomized controlled trial. Pain, 90: 83–90.

Linton, S.J. and Skevington, S.M. (1999) Psychological factors and the epidemiology of pain. In: I. Crombie, P.R. Croft, S.J. Linton, L. LeResche and M. Von Korff (Eds.), The Epidemiology of Pain. IASP Press, Seattle, WA, pp. 25–42.

Linton, S.J. and Van Tulder, M.W. (2001) Preventive interventions for back and neck pain: what is the evidence. Spine, 26: 778–787.

Linton, S.J., Vlaeyen, J.W.S. and Ostelo, R. (2002) The back pain beliefs of general practitioners and physical therapists. Are professionals fear-avoidant? manuscript submitted for publication.

Main, C.J. and Watson, P.J. (1995) Screening for patients at risk of developing chronic incapacity. J. Occup. Rehabil., 5: 207–217.

Main, C.J., Wood, P.L.R., Hollis, S., Spanswick, C.C. and Waddell, G. (1992) The distress and risk assessment method: a simple patient classification to identify distress and evaluate the risk of poor outcome. Spine, 17: 42–52.

Marhold, C., Linton, S.J. and Melin, L. (2001) Cognitive behavioral return-to-work program: effects on pain patients with a history of long-term versus short-term sick leave. Pain, 91: 155–163.

Marhold, C., Linton, S.J. and Melin, L. (2002) Identification of obstacles for chronic pain patients to return to work: evaluation of a questionnaire. J. Occup. Rehabil., 12(2): 65–75.

Moore, J.E., Von Korff, M., Cherkin, D., Saunders, K. and Lorig, K. (2000) A randomized trial of a cognitive–behavioral program for enhancing back pain self care in a primary care setting. Pain, 88: 145–153.

Morley, S., Eccleston, C. and Williams, A. (1999) Systematic review and meta-analysis of randomised controlled trials of cognitive behaviour therapy and behaviour therapy for chronic pain in adults, excluding headache. Pain, 80: 1–13.

National Research Council (2001) Musculoskeletal Disorders and the Workplace. National Academy Press, Washington, DC.

Saunders, K.W., Von Korff, M., Pruitt, S.D. and Moore, J.E. (1999) Prediction of physician visits and prescription medicine use for back pain. Pain, 83: 369–377.

Skevington, S.M. (1995) Psychology of Pain. Wiley, London.

Turk, D.C. (1996a) Biopsychosocial perspective on chronic pain. In: R.J. Gatchel and D.C. Turk (Eds.), Psychological Approaches to Pain Management: A Practitioner's Handbook, Vol. 1. Guilford Press, New York, pp. 3–32.

Turk, D.C. (1996b) Efficacy of multidisciplinary pain centers in the treatment of chronic pain. In: M.J.M. Cohen and J.N. Campbell (Eds.), Pain Treatment Centers at a Crossroads: A Practical and Conceptual Reappraisal, Vol. 7. IASP Press, Seattle, WA, pp. 257–273.

Turk, D.C. (1997) The role of demographic and psychosocial factors in transition from acute to chronic pain. In: T.S. Jensen, J.A. Turner and Z. Wiesenfeld-Hallin (Eds.), Proceedings of the 8th World Congress on Pain, Progress in Pain Research and Management, Vol. 8. IASP Press, Seattle, WA, pp. 185–213.

Turk, D.C., Meichenbaum, D. and Genest, M. (1983) Pain and Behavioral Medicine: A Cognitive–Behavioral Perspective. Guilford, New York, 452 pp.

Waddell, G. (1998) The Back Pain Revolution. Churchill Livingstone, Edinburgh.

Waddell, G., Feder, G. and Lewis, M. (1997) Systematic reviews of bed rest and advice to stay active for acute low back pain. Br. J. Gen. Pract., 47: 647–652.

Van den Hoogen, H.J.M., Koes, B.W., Devillé, W., Van Eijk, J.T.M. and Bouter, L.M. (1997) The prognosis of low back pain in general practice. Spine, 22: 1515–1521.

Van den Hoogen, H.J.M., Koes, B.W., Van Eijk, T.M., Bouter, L.M. and Devillé, W. (1998) On the course of low back pain in general practice: a one year follow up study. Ann. Rheum. Dis., 57: 13–19.

Van Tulder, M.W., Ostelo, R., Vlaeyen, J.W.S., Linton, S.J., Morely, S.J. and Assendelft, W.J.J. (2000) Behavioral treatment for chronic low back pain: a systematic review within the framework of the Cochrane Back Review Group. Spine, 25: 2688–2699.

Von Korff, M. (1999) Pain management in primary care: an individualized stepped/care approach. In: R.J. Gatchel and D.C. Turk (Eds.), Psychosocial Factors in Pain. Guilford Press, New York, pp. 360–373.

Von Korff, M., Moore, J.E., Lorig, K., Cherkin, D.C., Saunders, K., González, V.M., Laurent, D., Rutter, C. and Comite, F. (1998) A randomized trial of a lay-led self-management group intervention for back pain patients in primary care. Spine, 23: 2608–2615.

Von Korff, M. (1994) Perspectives on management of back pain in primary care. In: G.F. Gebhart, D.L. Hammond and T.S. Jensen (Eds.), Proceedings of the 7th World Congress on Pain: Progress in Pain Research and Management, Vol. 2. IASP Press, Seattle, WA, pp. 97–110.

New Avenues for the Prevention of Chronic Musculoskeletal Pain and Disability
Pain Research and Clinical Management, Vol. 12
Edited by S.J. Linton

CHAPTER 7

Pain-related fear and its consequences in chronic musculoskeletal pain

Johan W.S. Vlaeyen [1,2,*] and Steven J. Linton [3]

[1] *Pain Management and Research Center, University Hospital Maastricht, P.O. Box 5800, 6201 AZ Maastricht,*
The Netherlands
[2] *Department of Medical, Clinical and Experimental Psychology, Maastricht University, P.O. Box 616,*
6200 MD Maastricht, The Netherlands
[3] *Department of Occupational and Environmental Medicine, Örebro University Hospital, S-701 85 Örebro, Sweden*

Abstract: In an attempt to explain how and why some individuals with musculoskeletal pain develop a chronic pain syndrome, Lethem et al. (1983) introduced a so-called 'fear–avoidance' model. The central concept of their model is fear of pain. 'Confrontation' and 'avoidance' are postulated as the two extreme responses to this fear, of which the former leads to the reduction of fear over time. The latter, however, leads to the maintenance or exacerbation of fear, possibly leading to a phobic state. In the last decade, an increasing number of investigations have corroborated and refined the fear–avoidance model. The aim of this paper is to review the existing evidence for the mediating role of pain-related fear, and its immediate and long-term consequences in the initiation and maintenance of chronic pain disability. We will first highlight possible precursors of pain-related fear including the role negative appraisals of internal and external stimuli, negative affectivity and anxiety sensitivity. Subsequently, a number of fear-related processes will be discussed including escape and avoidance behaviors resulting in poor behavioral performance, hypervigilance to internal and external illness information, muscular reactivity, and physical disuse in terms of deconditioning and guarded movement. We will also review the available assessment methods for the quantification of pain-related fear and avoidance. Finally, we will discuss the implications of the recent findings for the prevention and treatment of chronic musculoskeletal pain. Although there still are a number of unresolved issues which merit future research attention, pain-related fear and avoidance appear to be an essential feature of the development of a chronic problem for a substantial number of patients with musculoskeletal pain.

1. Introduction

Pain is a common and universal experience and leads to the urge to escape the situation in which pain has emerged. As such, pain can best be concep-tualized as an emotional experience, as emotions are believed to be drives for action. Not surprisingly, the etymologic meaning of the word 'emotion' also comes from the latin 'movere' which means 'to act'. In acute injury, the escape from the harm-

---

* Correspondence to: J.W.S. Vlaeyen, Pain Management and Research Center, University Hospital Maastricht, P.O. Box 5800, 6201 AZ Maastricht, The Netherlands. E-mail: j.vlaeyen@dep.unimaas.nl

ful situation and the associated withdrawal behavior promotes the healing process. In the majority of the cases, healing occurs within a couple weeks and the pain resides quickly. However, in some individuals with pain, the immediate withdrawal behaviors do not lead to the anticipated reduction of pain, which then is interpreted as a signal of a continuous threat to the integrity of the body. In fact, a mismatch occurs between what the patient expects (quick decrease of pain) and what actually happens (increasing or lasting pain). Such a negative interpretation may not always reflect the real threat, and in such cases catastrophic misinterpretations of benign physical sensations may occur. Sometimes, these misinterpretations may be fueled by external information, such as unfavorable pain histories of relatives or acquaintances, verbal and/or visual information provided by health-care providers suggesting the probability of a serious illness causing the pain complaints. Catastrophic interpretations always lead to an increase of the individual distress level, and fear reactions in particular. In pain patients, the interpretational errors, such as catastrophizing, inevitably result in pain-related fear: fear of pain, fear of injury, fear of physical activity etc. depending on the anticipated source of threat. There now is accumulating evidence that these misinterpretations and the associated pain-related are likely to cause a cascade of psychological and physical events including hypervigilance, muscular reactivity, avoidance and guarding behaviors, physical disuse, which in turn are responsible for the maintenance of the pain problem.

The purpose of this paper therefore is to present the current state-of-the-art regarding the role of pain-related fear in musculoskeletal pain, and its relevant consequences. We will review the concept and theoretical underpinnings of the fear–avoidance model and the existing evidence for the main predictions that originate from this model. In addition, we shall critically appraise the currently available data relevant to assessment methods and interventions based on the fear–avoidance model. Finally we will provide some direction for future research.

2. Theoretical models

Although the idea of a relationship between fear and pain is not new, it was not until modern times that a model was developed which relates fear and pain. One of the first contributions conceptualized that fear would be linked through chronic pain behaviors through 'avoidance'. Avoidance is a psychological term with a relatively long history, but the term 'fear–avoidance' applied to the field of pain first appeared in an article by Lethem et al. in 1983. These authors described a model explaining how fear of pain and avoidance result in the perpetuation of pain behaviors and experiences, even in the absence of demonstrable organic pathology (Lethem et al., 1983). Avoidance behavior, presumably fueled by fear, has been intensively studied since the 1960s (e.g. Rachlin, 1980). It refers to a type of learned behavior, which postpones or averts the presentation of an aversive event. Avoidance learning occurs when the undesirable event has been successfully avoided by the performance of a certain (avoidance) behavior. Already in 1976, Fordyce devoted nearly 10 pages to avoidance learning to explain various pain behaviors in chronic pain patients. Fordyce et al. (1982) also described how individuals learn that the avoidance of pain-provoking or pain-increasing situations reduces the likelihood of new pain episodes of increased suffering. The authors also proposed behavioral treatment approaches how to modify these learned behaviors. In synchrony with the so-called 'cognitive revolution' in behavioral science, Turk et al. (1983) emphasized the role of attributions, efficacy expectations, and personal control within a cognitive–behavioral perspective on chronic pain. The basic new assumption of this approach is that individuals actively process information regarding internal stimuli and external events. In this context, Philips (1987) argued in favor of a cognitive approach of avoidance behavior, rather than an instrumental one. She took the view that avoidance is associated with the expectancy that further exposure to certain stimuli will promote pain and suffering.

Both the 'instrumental' and 'cognitive' approach

have led to influential fear–avoidance models explaining how pain behaviors can be maintained in chronic musculoskeletal pain. We will subsequently describe these models.

2.1. Model 1: the 'activity'–avoidance model

Fig. 1 shows the basic fear–avoidance conditioning model specific for activities or movement and pain (Linton et al., 1984). Generally, two components are distinguished: a classical and an operant one. The classical component refers to the process in which a neutral stimulus receives a negative meaning or valence. The person learns to predict events in his/her environment. An injury elicits an automatic response such as muscle tension and sympathetic activation including fear and anxiety. An external stimulus may, through classical conditioning, elicit a similar response. Conditioning may take place through direct experience, or by information (vicarious learning) or even observation (modeling). For example, a person involved in a traffic accident may develop a fear of driving as a result of the traumatic experience. Likewise, a back pain patient may develop a fear of lifting after experiencing pain while lifting or after receiving information from a doctor that lifting can damage nerves in the spinal cord. The same type of fear can also develop if a person witnesses another

person having an acute pain attack as the result of lifting.

When the stimulus, which precedes the noxious or painful experience, begins to predict the pain, avoidance learning begins. The discriminative stimulus takes on negative valence that activates muscle reactivity, fear, anxiety etc. in itself. Avoiding the threatening situation, as illustrated in Fig. 1, is reinforced by reductions e.g. in pain, fear, tension and anxiety. Once established, avoidance behavior is extremely resistant to extinction (Rachlin, 1980). This is because successful avoidance prevents the person from coming into contact with the actual consequences of the threatening situation. Moreover, fear will return whenever the avoidance behavior cannot be carried out.

2.2. Model 2: the 'fear'–avoidance model

A more cognitively oriented model of pain-related fear, which builds upon the previous model, is presented in Fig. 2 (Vlaeyen et al., 1995a,b). This model serves as a heuristic aid and ties several findings in the more recent literature together concerning the role of fear–avoidance in the development of musculoskeletal pain problems. It postulates two opposing behavioral responses: confrontation and avoidance, and presents possible pathways by which injured pa-

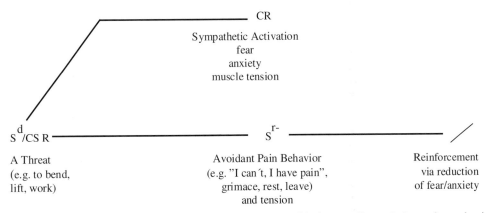

Fig. 1. The 'activity' avoidance model, combining classical and operant conditioning paradigms. A threatening and pain producing situation (S^d/CS) elicits a conditioned response (CR) of sympathetic activation including fear, which in turn leads to avoidance of the situation (R). The avoidance behavior is reinforced by a reduction of the unpleasant stimuli. CS refers to 'conditioned stimulus' and CR to 'conditioned response' in the classical paradigm. S^d refers to 'discriminative stimulus', R to 'response' and S^{r-} to reinforcement consequences. Reproduced with permission from Elsevier Science.

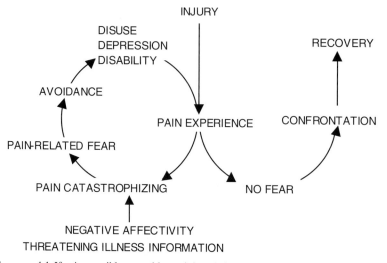

Fig. 2. The 'fear'–avoidance model. If pain, possibly caused by an injury, is interpreted as threatening (pain catastrophizing), pain-related fear evolves. This leads to avoidance behaviors, followed by disability, disuse and depression. The latter will maintain the pain experiences thereby fueling the vicious circle of increasing fear and avoidance. In non-catastrophizing patients, no pain-related fear and rapid confrontation with daily activities is likely to occur, leading to fast recovery. Pain catastrophizing is assumed to be also influenced by negative affectivity and threatening illness information. Reproduced with permission from Elsevier Science.

tients get caught in a downward spiral of increasing avoidance, disability and pain. The model, which was based on the work of Lethem et al. (1983), Philips (1987) and Waddell et al. (1993), predicts that there are several ways by which pain-related fear can lead to disability. (1) Negative appraisals about pain and its consequences, such as catastrophic thinking, is considered a potential precursor of pain-related fear. (2) Fear is characterized by escape and avoidance behaviors, of which the immediate consequences are that daily activities (expected to produce pain) are not accomplished anymore. Avoidance of daily activities results in functional disability. (3) Because avoidance behaviors occur in anticipation of pain rather than as a response to pain, these behaviors may persist because there are fewer opportunities to correct the (wrongful) expectancies and beliefs about pain as a signal of threat of physical integrity. In this case, fearful beliefs may become dissociated from actual pain experiences. (4) Long-standing avoidance and physical inactivity has a detrimental impact on the musculoskeletal and cardiovascular systems, leading to the so-called 'disuse syndrome' (Bortz, 1984), which may further worsen

the pain problem. In addition, avoidance also means the withdrawal from essential reinforcers leading to mood disturbances, such as irritability, frustration and depression. Both depression and disuse are known to be associated with decreased pain tolerance level (Romano and Turner, 1985; McQuade et al., 1988), and hence they might promote the painful experience.

From a cognitive–behavioral perspective, there are a number of additional predictions that can be derived from this model. (5) Just like other forms of fear and anxiety, pain-related fear interferes with cognitive functioning. Fearful patients will attend more to possible signals of threat (hypervigilance) and will be less able to shift attention away from pain-related information. This will be at the expense of other tasks including actively coping with problems of daily life. (6) Pain-related fear will be associated with increased psychophysiological reactivity, when the individual is confronted with situations that are appraised as 'dangerous'.

In the next section, we will review the existing evidence in support of the above-mentioned predictions, point to lacunas and discuss future directions.

3. Negative appraisals as precursors of pain-related fear

"An ache beneath the sternum, in connoting the possibility of sudden death from heart failure, can be a wholly unsettling experience, whereas the same intensity and duration of ache in a finger is a trivial annoyance easily disregarded." With this statement, Henry Beecher, 1959 (p. 159) emphasized the importance of cognitive processes in the pain experience since pain lacks an external standard of reference thus allowing considerable room for interpretation; more so than, for example, normal vision or touch. A recent cognitive–behavioral theory of anxiety, the so-called 'four-factor theory' assumes that the emotional experience of anxiety is influenced by four different sources of information of which the cognitive appraisal of the situation is considered the most important. The other three, which are indirectly dependent on the first, are the level of physiological arousal, cognitions based on information stored in long-term memory, and action tendencies and behavior (Eysenck, 1997). In chronic pain, there is ample evidence that certain pain-specific beliefs have an impact on chronic pain adjustment (for a review, see Jensen et al., 1991, 1994; Jensen and Karoly, 1992a,b), but there are almost no studies on the specific beliefs that influence pain-related fear. In fact, with the statement cited above, Beecher gives an early example of what is now called a catastrophic (mis)interpretation of a bodily sensation.

There is some evidence that catastrophizing thoughts may be considered a precursor of pain-related fear. Pain catastrophizing is considered an exaggerated negative orientation toward noxious stimuli, and has been shown to mediate distress reactions to painful stimulation (Sullivan et al., 1995). McCracken and Gross (1993) found a significant correlation between the catastrophizing scale of the Coping Strategies Questionnaire and the scores on the Pain Anxiety Symptoms Scale, a recently developed measure of fear of pain. Vlaeyen et al. (1995a,b) found that pain catastrophizing, measured with the Pain Cognition List was superior in predicting pain-related fear than biomedical status and pain

severity. In further support of this idea, Crombez et al. (1998) found that pain-free volunteers with a high frequency of catastrophic thinking about pain became more fearful when threatened with the possibility of occurrence of intense pain than students with a low frequency of catastrophic thinking.

A prospective study by Burton et al. (1995) concerning predictors of back pain chronicity at 1 year after the acute onset is also worth mentioning in this context. These researchers found that catastrophizing, as measured by the Coping Strategies Questionnaire (Rosenstiel and Keefe, 1983) was the most powerful predictor: almost 7 times more important than the best of the clinical and historical variables for the acute back pain patients. Additional evidence of the importance of catastrophizing is provided in a study comparing chronic pain patients seeking help (consumers) with people with chronic pain who were not having treatment, and who were recruited via advertisements in local newspapers (non-consumers). The results revealed that the consumers reported much higher levels of pain catastrophizing than the non-consumers did (Reitsma and Meijler, 1997).

Constructs that appear to overlap considerably with catastrophizing, are negative affectivity and anxiety sensitivity. *Negative affectivity* can be seen as a moderating variable in the emergence of pain-related fear. According to Watson and Pennebaker (1989), persons with high negative affectivity are hypervigilant for all forms of (external and internal) threat, and therefore are considered more vulnerable to develop specific fears (Eysenck, 1992). For individuals with high negative affectivity who also experience pain, pain may be the most salient threat, and as a consequence, pain-related fear may emerge. Reiss and McNally (1985) introduced a fear–expectancy model of avoidance behavior which is based on the idea that anxiety disorders occur more frequently in patients with a specific personality characteristic which they called '*anxiety sensitivity*'. This should be seen as a specific tendency to react anxiously to one's own anxiety and anxiety-related sensations (fear of fear). Asmundson and Norton (1995) found that chronic back pain patients with high anxiety sensitivity reported more fear of pain and tended to have greater avoidance of activities than those with lower anxiety sensitivity, despite equal levels of pain. In a subsequent study using structural equation modeling, Asmundson and Taylor (1996) corroborated the finding that anxiety sensitivity directly exacerbates fear of pain, even after controlling for the effects of pain severity on fear of pain. However, anxiety sensitivity affected escape and avoidance behaviors indirectly, via fear of pain. These findings would support the view of Reiss (1991) that more basic fears underlie many fears, and that these should be considered a more general vulnerability factor for the development of more specific fears (see Asmundson et al., 1999).

Fears can also originate from traumatic experience. Within 1–4 months of their motor vehicle accident, 39% of these victims develop a post-traumatic stress disorder (Blanchard et al., 1996). Turk and Holzman (1986) suggested that fear–avoidance beliefs in chronic pain patients may especially be the case when the original acute pain problem resulted from sudden traumatic injury. Further evidence for this assumption was found by Vlaeyen et al. (1995b) and Crombez et al. (1999). Chronic low back pain patients who retrospectively reported a sudden traumatic pain onset, scored higher on the Tampa Scale for Kinesiophobia than patients who reported that the pain complaints started gradually. Additionally, there is evidence that a large percentage of people with chronic musculoskeletal pain meet DSM-IV criteria for post-traumatic stress disorder (Asmundson et al., 1998).

4. Pain-related fear and the overprediction of pain

Almost half a century ago, Hill et al. (1952) observed in their study on the effects of anxiety and morphine on discrimination of intensities of painful stimuli that under conditions promoting anxiety or fear of pain, subjects tended to overestimate the intensities of painful stimuli. More recently, in a series of studies with laboratory-induced pain, Arntz et al. (1990) concluded that anxious subjects pro-

duced more overpredictions of pain and that these overpredictions were less easily disconfirmed than those of the nonanxious subjects were. In a clinical setting, McCracken et al. (1993) investigated associations among predictions about pain, pain-related fear using the Pain Anxiety Symptoms Scale and range of motion in 43 chronic back pain patients who were exposed to pain during a physical examination. During the examination, patients were requested to repeatedly raise the extended leg to the point of pain tolerance. They found that anxious patients showed a tendency to overpredict pain early in the sequence of pain, while the low anxious patients underpredicted pain. Moreover, a significant relation between prediction of pain and range of motion during the straight leg raise was found, suggesting that those who expect more pain avoid pain increase by terminating the leg raise earlier. Of interest, however, is that patients tend to correct their pain expectancies when they are given the opportunity to repeat the same pain-eliciting activity. When chronic back pain patients were requested to perform four exercise bouts consisting of flexing and extending the knee three times at maximal force (with a Cybex 350 system), Crombez et al. (1996) found that after overpredicting the pain experienced during the first exercise bout, the reported pain expectancy was corrected during the next exercise bout. In other words, after some exposures, overpredictions of pain intensity tended to match with the actual experience. The important clinical implication is that fearful patients may benefit from graded exposure to movements and activities that they previously avoided.

5. Attention to bodily sensations

The cognitive theory of anxiety put forward by Eysenck (1997) makes the assumption that the most important function of anxiety is to facilitate the early detection of potentially threatening situations. In other words, highly anxious individuals demonstrate hypervigilance, both generally and specifically. General hypervigilance (or distractibility) refers to the propensity to attend to any irrelevant stimuli being presented. Specific hypervigilance involves the inclination to attend selectively to threat-related rather than to neutral stimuli. In laboratory studies with healthy subjects and experimentally induced pain stimuli, there is evidence that the role of anxiety on pain perception is mediated by attentional processes (Arntz et al., 1994). There is very little research that directly examined hypervigilance in pain patients who report pain-related fear. Based on their study investigating the construct validity of the McGill Pain Questionnaire, Pearce and Morley (1989) suggested that patients with chronic pain are characterized by a selective attention towards cues that are thematically related to pain and its consequences. A more recent replication with the dot–probe paradigm, Asmundson et al. (1997b) found that individuals with chronic pain with low anxiety sensitivity were able to shift their attention away from stimuli related to pain, in contrast to the subjects with high pain sensitivity. In other words, they found evidence for a specific form of hypervigilance. These findings are in line with the observation by Crombez et al. (1998) that chronic back pain patients who avoid back straining activities not only report high fear of pain and fear of (re)injury, but also high attention to back sensations. In line with this finding, McCracken (1997) reported that attention to pain as reported with the Pain Vigilance and Awareness Questionnaire (PVAQ) was most strongly associated with pain-related fear, and to a somewhat lesser degree, but still significantly, with depression, physical and psychosocial disability and health-care utilization. Using the PVAQ and a measure of more general body vigilance (BVS: Body Vigilance Scale), Peters et al. (2000, 2002) have shown that within a group of patients with fibromyalgia and low back pain, respectively, significant differences were found between patients with high and low pain-related fear (see Fig. 3).

Eccleston et al. (1997) used a primary task paradigm, in which subjects are requested to direct their attentional focus towards a mental task while receiving painful stimuli. Degradation in task performance on the mental task is also taken as an

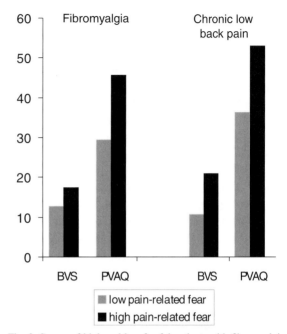

Fig. 3. Scores of high and low fearful patients with fibromyalgia and chronic low back pain on the Body Vigilance Scale (BVS) and the Pain Vigilance and Awareness Questioniare (PVAQ). Data based on Peters et al. (2000, 2002).

index of attentional interference due to body hypervigilance. These researchers found that disruption of attentional performance was most pronounced in chronic pain patients who reported high negative affect, somatic awareness and high pain intensity (Eccleston and Crombez, 1999). These attentional processes not only apply to clinical pain or painful stimulation but also appear to hold for more ambiguous bodily sensations. One way of examining body scanning is the application of a reaction time paradigm. At four body locations (both arms and both legs), electrodes were attached by means of which innocuous electrical stimulation was provided with gradually increasing amplitude, but always below the pain threshold. Patients are requested to respond as fast as possible to stimulus detection by pressing a button corresponding to the correct body location. In a group of fibromyalgia patients, detection latency for innoxious electrical stimuli in the arm was predicted by scores on the Pain Anxiety Symptoms Scale, and most consistently by the cognitive anxiety subscale (Peters et al., 2000). Other methods have also been utilized to study selective attentional processes in pain-related fear, such as the dot–probe paradigm, have shown similar results (e.g. Keogh et al., 2001).

A conclusion that may be drawn is that although the majority of studies have used experimental pain with healthy volunteers, there is good evidence that pain-related fear leads to increased attention toward the source of threat, in casu bodily sensations (hypervigilance). This is at the cost of other tasks, such as usual everyday activities or the voluntary use of pain-coping strategies. An interesting question to be answered is whether, through attentional demands, pain-related fear hampers adjustment to chronic pain, at worst resulting in persisting disability.

6. Symptom-specific muscular reactivity

In addition to the attentional processes, pain-related fear can also lead to increasing pain through its concomitant muscular reactivity. When individuals are confronted with anxiety-eliciting stimuli, a number of changes occur in autonomic nervous system including skin conductance levels, muscular reactivity and heart rate. Extensive research by Flor and Turk (1989) and Flor et al. (1992) suggests that psychophysiological responses in chronic pain are symptom specific and stress-related. For example, compared to healthy controls, chronic low back pain patients showed elevated reactivity in the paralumbar musculature when confronted with a personally relevant stressor, and not with stressors in general. Similar elevations were found at symptom-specific body musculature for tension headache patients (musculus frontalis) and patients with temporomandibular pain dysfunction (musculus masseter). This response stereotypy appears to be limited to the muscular system and was not observed in measures of the autonomic system. Similarly, for the subgroup of chronic low back pain patients with substantial pain-related fear, one can predict elevated paraspinal EMG-levels to occur in fearful chronic low back pain patients when confronted with movements which they be-

lieve are harmful. This muscular reactivity to stress may further maintain the pain problem.

Psychophysiologic reactivity in fearful chronic low back pain patients was studied in an experiment where the subjects were presented a video recording including a neutral situation (a nature documentary) followed by a physical activity being performed rigorously by a dummy patient (Vlaeyen et al., 1999). The patients remained seated during the 6-min video exposure, and the instruction was given to watch carefully as they would be asked to perform the same activity at the end of the video presentation. EMG activity of four muscles were recorded continuously: lower paraspinal muscles and tibialis anterior muscles (both bilaterally). The results were partly as predicted, partly surprising. Although self-reported subjective tension increased from nature documentary to the activity exposure in the fearful chronic low back pain patients, there was a decrease in muscular reactivity across both stimuli. This decrement, however, was significantly less in fearful patients who remained at about the same reactivity level. As predicted, the reactivity was symptom-specific: only the reactivity of the left erector spinae was predicted by fear of movement/(re)injury. Extending the diathesis-stress model described by Flor et al., reactivity of other than paraspinal muscles (in casu the tibialis anterior muscles) were also influenced by pain-related fear, but only in the subgroup of patients reporting high negative affectivity. In addition, change in lower paraspinal EMG predicted subsequent pain report during a lifting task in the expected direction: fewer decreases in EMG readings predicted higher pain ratings. Although these results are in line with the series of carefully designed studies by Flor and Turk (1989); Flor et al. (1992), further studies are needed to fully understand what the consequences for this muscular reactivity could be.

7. Pain-related fear and physical performance

Does pain-related fear also affect physical performance? One of the main features of fear and anxiety is the tendency to avoid and escape from the perceived threat. Although chronic pain in itself cannot always be avoided, the activities assumed to increase pain or (re)injury may be. One of the consequences, however, is that daily activity levels decrease, possibly resulting in functional incapacity. A number of studies have investigated the association between pain-related fear and physical performance. McCracken et al. (1992) found a significant correlation between fear of pain and range of motion during physical examination as measured with a flexometer. Vlaeyen et al. (1995a) used a simple lifting task during which patients were asked to lift a 5.5-kg weight with the dominant arm and hold it until pain or physical discomfort made it impossible for the patient to continue. A significant correlation was found between lifting time and the Tampa Scale for Kinesiophobia (TSK). In addition, the TSK correlated significantly with a single visual analog scale measuring the fear of (re)injury just after completion of the lifting task. However, in this study, pain intensity was not measured. As a consequence, it might be possible that the poor performance was due to increased pain rather than escape or avoidance. To rule out this possibility, Crombez et al. (1998) conducted a similar study using the knee extension–flexion unit (KEF; Cybex 350 system) as the behavioral task. They purposely chose a performance test of which patients believed that it was minimally back straining. The researchers again found a significant association between performance level and pain-related fear, and not pain intensity. In a replication study using linear regression, Crombez et al. (1999) showed the performance during a trunk extension–flexion and weight lifting task that pain-related fear was the best predictor of behavioral performance, even after partialling out the effects of pain intensity. Similarly, In a spinal isometric strength test measured by the Medx lumbar extension machine, Al-Obaidi et al. (2000) found that the anticipation of pain and the fear–avoidance beliefs about physical activities were the strongest predictors of the variation in physical performance. In summary, there is now ample evidence that pain-related fear is associated with escape/avoidance of physical activities resulting in poor behavioral performance.

Do the results of these studies also generalize to everyday situations in the home environment? A quite robust measure of activity levels in daily life consists of the quantification of energy expenditure, for example with the use of the doubly-labeled water technique (Westerterp and Wouters, 1995). Energy expenditure may be calculated by analyzing the excretion of isotopes in urine samples during a number of consecutive days. The method has not been utilized in pain patients, and has the disadvantage of being expensive. In patients who underwent coronary bypass surgery, energy expenditure on postoperative leisure activities has been reported to be associated to fear of injury (O'Connor, 1983). Alternatively, quantification of physical activity can be done with activity diaries (Fordyce, 1976) or with the more advanced automated activity monitors (Bussman et al., 1998).

8. Pain-related fear and self-reported disability

A key issue is how pain-related fear actually affects daily activities and the development of disability. Studies investigating the effects of pain-related fear on measures of escape/avoidance appear to generalize to disability levels in daily life are quite convincing. Philips and Jahanshahi (1986) found that in a group of headache sufferers, avoidance of activities, and withdrawal from social situations was the most prominent behavior reported by these individuals. One salient stimulus may be work or the workplace as patients often associate their pain with work (Linton and Buer, 1995). Waddell et al. (1993) reported that fear–avoidance beliefs about physical activities and work are strongly related to disability and work loss in the previous year, more so than biomedical variables and characteristics of pain and concluded that "fear of pain and what we do about it is more disabling than the pain itself" (p. 164, Waddell et al., 1993). In a study that compared people matched for pain intensity and duration, fear–avoidance beliefs (Pain and Impairment Relationship Scale) were found to be an important factor discriminating between people with no sick leave and those with considerable sick leave (Linton and Buer, 1995). However, when 252 patients presenting with low back pain at a primary health-care facility were studied in an effort to isolate risk factors, the results did not support the pain-related fear concept (Burton et al., 1995). Although the Fear Avoidance Beliefs Questionnaire (FABQ) was employed, the final discriminate analysis on disability showed that psychosocial factors e.g. coping and distress were related, but not pain-related fear. This may indicate differences between studies in outcome variables e.g. disability versus work, but it may also indicate that the fear–avoidance concept is closely related to other psychosocial terms. Pain-related fear has been included in a screening questionnaire designed to detect patients at risk of developing persistent problems. Not only were 'fear–avoidance beliefs' related to future pain and function, but also it was the most salient variable related to future sick absenteeism (Linton and Halldén, 1997, 1998).

With their Survey of Pain Attitudes (SOPA), Jensen et al. (1994) examined the relationship of pain-specific beliefs to chronic pain adjustment. They found that the SOPA Harm scale (the specific belief that pain is a signal for damage) made a unique contribution to the prediction of physical dysfunction, as measured by the Sickness Impact Profile (SIP; Bergner et al., 1981). However, this relationship was substantial only for patients reporting pain duration of less than about 2.4 years. Using linear regression, Vlaeyen et al. (1995b) found that fear of movement/(re)injury is a better predictor of self-reported disability levels as measured with the Roland Disability Questionnaire (RDQ; Roland and Morris, 1983; Beurskens et al., 1996) than biomedical findings and pain intensity levels. These findings were successfully replicated by Crombez et al. (1999). Asmundson et al. (1997a) described a cohort of chronic pain patients with the Multidimensional Pain Inventory (MPI; Kerns et al., 1985) and found that patients who were classified as 'dysfunctional', and hence considered most disabled, scored the highest on the Pain Anxiety Symptoms Scale. In their study comparing pain-specific fear measures with more general anxiety questionnaires,

McCracken et al. (1996) showed that disability was most strongly correlated with the more specific pain-related fear measures, as compared to a more general measure of anxiety. These researchers also showed that pain-related fear not only predicts disability levels, but also non-specific physical complaints other than the primary pain complaints in patients with chronic pain, thereby complicating the pain problem (McCracken et al., 1998). A recent study in chronic back pain patients who recently went on sick leave because of their pain complaints shows that besides experienced pain, intensity and pain catastrophizing, pain-related fear additionally predicted disability levels (Van de Hout et al., 2001). Similar results have now been reported in a sample of acute pain patients, suggesting that pain-related fear affects behavior early on (Ciccone and Just, 2001). All of these studies are cross-sectional in nature and positive correlations or regression weights should not be confused with causal effects. Pain-related fear is likely to cause increased avoidance of activity and disability, but theoretically, the opposite might be true as well, or both may be related to a third variable (e.g. traumatic experience).

The prospective study by Klenerman et al. (1995), however, supports the idea that pain-related fear is a precursor of disability, rather than a consequence of it. In this study, which employed acute back pain patients in a primary care setting, a set of psychological variables (including fear–avoidance indicators) turned out to be one of the most powerful predictors of chronic disability 1 year later. One problem with this study, however, is that the authors did not actually use a standardized measure of pain-related fear and avoidance. A similar study, but employing the TSK as measure of pain-related fear found that pain-related fear at first consultation with the GP was the best predictor of levels of disability 3 and 12 months later (Sieben et al., 2002). Linton et al. (1999) included a large sample from the general population in their prospective cohort study with the aim to examine whether pain catastrophizing and fear–avoidance in pain-free individuals predict subsequent episodes of musculoskeletal pain. They found that individuals who scored above the median score of a modified version of the FABQ (Waddell et al., 1993) had twice as much chance of having a pain episode in the following year.

In summary, there is considerable evidence that pain-related fear not only leads to poor physical performance as measured in the laboratory, but that these effects also generalize to activities of daily life including activities at the workplace. In addition, fear–avoidance beliefs may be an important predictor of pain episodes, early on in pain-free people.

9. The 'disuse' syndrome

Although escape and avoidance may be an effective and appropriate coping response in the short term (Wall, 1979), exclusive reliance on it may result in a variety of negative repercussions. There is surprisingly little research focused on the negative effects of avoidance behavior in humans. As pointed out above, a strong correlation has been found between fear–avoidance beliefs, behavioral performance and self-reported disability. However, no study directly assessing the physiological consequences of fear–avoidance in the pain situation could be located. Prolonged avoidance of movements and activities is assumed to cause detrimental changes in the musculoskeletal system, often referred to as 'disuse syndrome' (Kottke, 1966; Bortz, 1984). Although we have not been able to find a more specific definition than 'the detrimental consequences of long-term inactivity', the term disuse is being used in the pain literature in at least two different ways: (a) physical deconditioning as a consequence of reduced use of the musculoskeletal system (e.g. Wagenmakers et al., 1988) and (b) impairments in muscle coordination, leading to guarded movements (e.g. Main and Watson, 1996).

9.1. Deconditioning

There is a plentitude of studies demonstrating that exercise and fitness are beneficial in a biomedical sense to maturation, strength, and healing of bones, tendons and muscles. Exercise is found to be associated with psychological benefits, possibly mediated by neuroendocrine responses (Bouchard et al., 1994; Morgan, 1997). Likewise, bedrest and other forms of immobilization are pernicious for disks, muscles, joints, bones, ligaments, and tendons. Deconditioning refers to a progressive process of worsening physical fitness as a result of reduced muscular activity.

A classic method for the assessment of muscle strength is based on dynamometry. Patients are requested to perform maximally on a bicycle ergometer or Cybex machine. For example, Wagenmakers et al. (1988) found that during incremental cycle ergometry and as compared to healthy but untrained controls, patients with non-specific muscle pains had were unable to exercise at high intensities, showed decreased endurance and an increased dependence on glycolysis at low intensities. Biopsies revealed that these patients also had a lower content of mitochondria in their muscles, and the authors suggested that these biochemical changes were a consequence of their reduced habitual activities. However, the assumption that lumbar dynamometry provides objective and unbiased measures that can quantify functional capacity is now being challenged. Against the common belief that patients with chronic low back pain have low fitness levels as a result of inactivity because of pain, a comparison of predicted maximum oxygen consumption (VO_{2max}) between patients and healthy controls yielded no significant differences (Wittink et al., 2000). One possible explanation might be that the variation within the patients group is larger than the variation between groups of patients and normals. For example, Menard et al. (1994) found a difference in the pattern of dynamometry in two groups of LBP patients who differed only in the propensity of abnormal illness behavior (as indicated by the Waddell score). Lee et al. (1995) found a generalized strength reduction (of both trunk and knee muscles) in chronic low back patients as compared to healthy controls, with significant correlations between trunk and knee strength in both groups. Both Menard et al. (1994) and Lee et al. (1995) proposed that fear of pain or (re)injury might be one of the possible explanations. Unfortunately, neither of the above-mentioned studies included a measure of pain-related fear.

A major problem with dynamometry is that pain-related fear or pain intensity may inhibit muscle activation (Verbunt et al., submitted). A relatively easy technique to detect the discrepancy between muscle force during voluntary contraction and the maximum available muscle force is the percutaneous twitch superimposition technique (Rutherford et al., 1986; Mannion et al., 1997). During voluntary contraction, the motor nerves are stimulated percutaneously (twitch). During a truly maximum contraction, no extra force is generated by the twitch. This method provides a way to predict maximum force from submaximal efforts, and can be considered a promising tool in assessing muscle weakness in cases where muscle activation is inhibited for example by pain-related fear. However, it still needs to be demonstrated that pain-related fear is a significant predictor of the extra force generated by the twitch.

9.2. Guarded movement

The second meaning of disuse involves disordered coordination and electromyography (EMG) patterns during movement such as walking. For example, Arendt-Nielsen et al. (1995) have shown in their gait study on disordered trunk movements that in chronic low back pain patients and individuals with experimentally induced muscle pain, the EMG patterns of the musculus erector trunci show less modulation and more continuous activity during gait as compared to healthy subjects. Koelman et al. (1996) reported that a number of chronic low back pain patients do not allow a counter-rotation between transversal pelvic and thoracic rotation when increasing walking speed. Patients who experienced less pain showed more counter-rotation at higher walking speeds. The inability to make a counter-rotation was often accompanied by a hyperstability of the pelvic and thoracic rotation, leading to 'guarded movements'. Keefe and Hill (1985) have provided early evidence that asymmetries in gait are correlated with pain behavior, and Fordyce (1976) advocated the use of 'speed walking' in reducing pain behaviors of chronic low back pain patients. Main and Watson (1996) suggested that guarded movements are likely

to be moderated by pain-related fear, and elaborated on the Flexion Relaxation Phenomenon (FRP). The FRP refers to the sudden cessation of muscle activity during the activity of forward flexion from the standing position. In subjects with back pain, the FRP is frequently absent. The FRP has been observed to return to normal as symptoms resolve after an acute injury (Haig et al., 1993) and as a result of treatment (Triano and Schultz, 1987). Watson et al. (1997) demonstrated that the loss of the FRP can be reliably measured over time by the use of the Flexion Relaxation Ratio (FRR) which compares the amount of EMG activity in the paraspinal muscles at maximal activity during forward flexion and the activity at the fully flexed position. In a subsequent study, Watson et al. (1997) examined the role of pain-related fear and self-efficacy beliefs on guarded movement, as measured by the FRR. They found the FRR to be significantly correlated with fear–avoidance beliefs, and not with current pain intensity or disability level. Moreover, following a pain management program, significant correlations were discovered for between reductions in fear–avoidance beliefs, increases in pain self-efficacy beliefs and increased FRRs on movement. No such associations were identified between EMG measures and changes in range of movement, pain report or disability. This study suggests that pain-related fear plays an important role in the development of guarded movement, and more so than pain severity or disability levels.

In summary, pain-related fear may also be responsible for the worsened physical condition and the occurrence of guarded movement patterns displayed by a number of chronic musculoskeletal pain patients. These effects are likely be mediated by avoidance behaviors and poor physical performance, which are considered as the more immediate consequences of pain-related fear.

10. Pain-related fear and the role of the health-care provider

In individuals with pain-related fear, the threat value of pain may also be influenced by external illness information, such as feedback about diagnostic tests. In the field of health anxiety (e.g. Warwick and Salkovskis, 1990), a number of studies have examined cognitive responses to different kinds of information about diagnostic tests. In general, individuals who are anxious about their health tend to use avoidant strategies when receiving negative test results, but are hypervigilant when perceiving positive and ambiguous test results. In non-anxious individuals, almost the opposite seems to occur: positive test results elicit minimization of the seriousness of the condition, and doubts about the validity of the information (Ditto et al., 1988). In a well-designed study in individuals with subclinical health anxiety, Hadjistavropoulos et al. (1998) examined responses to a cold pressor task after the subjects received feedback on an ostensible diagnostic measure, indicating positive, negative or ambiguous risk for health complications. Overall, health anxious individuals interpreted the diagnostic information more negatively, reported more catastrophizing, sought more reassurance, and were less able to engage in protective strategies during the cold pressor task. Surprisingly, the moderating effect of the positive or ambiguous diagnostic information was not found. It still needs to be seen whether the findings can be replicated in a clinical sample health anxious individuals, and more particularly chronic pain patients who report substantial pain-related fear. Based on the available literature, it is likely that pain-related fear has implications for how individuals respond to diagnostic information and attend to pain. Therefore, fearful patients may benefit from clear and unambiguous information, not only about the diagnostic tests but also about possible strategies that can be used to cope with daily life situations. This is an area on which more research effort needs to be devoted (e.g. Turner et al., 1998).

The review thus far as demonstrated the possible importance of fear–avoidance in chronic pain. This evidence is so compelling that it has become relevant to work routinely with it in research as well as in the clinic. This section surveys techniques for measuring fear–avoidance while treatment is dealt with in the final section.

11. Assessment of pain-related fear

Measuring fear–avoidance is an important, but sometimes a difficult task in clinical and research settings. Fortunately, there is considerable relevant experience in measuring avoidance available in the psychological literature. It is generally agreed that assessment should strive to cover objective and subjective aspects falling within the cognitive, behavioral, and physiological realm. Thus, while self-report is an important part of assessment, behavioral observation and psychophysiological recordings may also be valuable in determining the qualities of pain-related fear.

11.1. Self-report

A basic question that may be asked is what the patient is afraid of, or in other words what is the nature of the perceived threat? The most common answer would be pain. Nevertheless, the relationship between avoidance behavior and specific fears appears to be more complex than the model may insinuate. Patients, for example, may not view their problem as involving fear at all and may simply see difficulty in performing certain movements or activities. Other patients may fear not so much current pain, but pain that will be experienced at a later time, for example the day after a physical exercise. Finally, patients may not fear pain itself, but the impending (re)injury that it is supposed to indicate. The literature reflects this lack of clarity by discussing measures for the assessment of fear of pain, fear of work and physical activity, and fear of (re)injury as a result of movement. Overall, these pain-specific measures of pain-related fear are better predictors of pain, disability and pain behavior compared with more general anxiety measures or measures of negative affect (McCracken et al., 1996; Crombez et al., 1999).

11.2. Fear of pain

An early attempt is the *Pain and Impairment Relationship Scale (PAIRS)* developed to study chronic pain patient's attitudes concerning activity and pain (Riley et al., 1988). The scale has 15 items which are rated on 7-point Likert scales and it has been found to have good psychometric characteristics (DeGood and Shutty, 1992). The original study demonstrated that beliefs that activity would increase pain were related to physical impairment.

In 1992, the *Pain Anxiety Symptoms Scale* (PASS, McCracken et al., 1992) was developed to measure cognitive anxiety symptoms, escape and avoidance responses, fearful appraisals of pain and physiologic anxiety symptoms related to pain. It is a 40-item questionnaire with internally consistent subscales (McCracken et al., 1993). The validity of the PASS has been supported by positive correlations with measures of anxiety, cognitive errors, depression, and disability (McCracken et al., 1996). A more recent exploratory factor analysis (Larsen et al., 1997) revealed five factors which could be labeled as catastrophic thoughts, physiological anxiety symptoms, escape/avoidance behaviors, cognitive interference and coping strategies.

11.3. Fear of work-related activities

The *Fear-Avoidance Beliefs Questionnaire* (FABQ), developed by Waddell et al. (1993), focuses on the patient's beliefs about how work and physical activity affect his/her low back pain. The FABQ consists of two scales, fear–avoidance beliefs of physical activity and fear–avoidance beliefs of work, of which the latter was consistently the stronger. The authors found that fear–avoidance beliefs about work are strongly related with disability of daily living and work lost in the past year, and more so than biomedical variables such as anatomical pattern of pain, time pattern, and severity of pain. On the other hand, the FABQ-physical subscale is much stronger in predicting behavioral performance tests (Crombez et al., 1999).

11.4. Fear of movement/(re)injury

The *Survey of Pain Attitudes* (SOPA: Jensen et al., 1987) was developed to assess patients attitudes

towards five dimensions of the chronic pain experience: pain control; pain-related disability; medical cures for pain; solicitude of others; and medication for pain. Because of the authors' clinical observation of an association between chronic patients' hesitancy to exercise and the expressed fear of possible injury, a new scale (Harm) was added to the original instrument (Jensen et al., 1994). As well as the Disability and Control scales, the Harm scale appeared to independently predict levels of dysfunction.

The *Tampa Scale for Kinesiophobia* (TSK; Kori et al., 1990) is a 17-item questionnaire that is aimed at the assessment of fear of (re)injury due to movement. Each item is provided with a Likert scale with scoring alternatives ranging from 'strongly agree' to 'strongly disagree'. Most psychometric research has been carried out with the Dutch version of the TSK (Vlaeyen et al., 1995a). The TSK appears to be sufficiently reliable ($\alpha = 0.77$) and valid. Modest, but significant, correlations were found with measures of pain intensity, catastrophizing, impact of pain on daily life activities and generalized fear. Regression analyses revealed that levels of disability were best predicted by pain-related fear, and that the latter was best predicted by catastrophizing. Pain intensity levels and biomedical findings were significantly less predictive of both pain-related fear and disability levels (Vlaeyen et al., 1995b). Moreover, the TSK discriminated well between avoiders and confronters during a behavioral performance task (Vlaeyen et al., 1995a). A factor analysis revealed four nonorthogonal factors, to which following labels were assigned: harm; fear of (re)injury; importance of exercise; and avoidance of activity (Vlaeyen et al., 1995b). Because of the relatively high intercorrelations among the subscales, the more favorable internal consistency of the TSK total score, and the good construct validity of the total score, the total score is preferable to the subscales. The TSK-total score has been shown to be associated with behavioral performance tests and self-reported disability (Crombez et al., 1999).

In summary, questionnaires for the assessment of pain-related fear are now available, although the validity of some of them need to be further explored.

For clinical purposes, these questionnaires seem to be appropriate as a first screening to identify patients who suffer excessive pain-related fear. However, the questionnaires do not tell us what the individual is exactly fearful of. To identify the idiosyncratic aspects of the fear, and the essential fear-provoking stimuli in a particular patient, new assessment methods will need to be developed.

11.5. Observational methods

The observational measure most frequently used in fear is the Behavioral Approach (or Avoidance) Test (BAT). A BAT is a behavioral measure in which a fear-eliciting stimulus is placed in a standardized environment. The patient is instructed to approach the stimulus and engage in progressively more bold interactions with it (Bellack and Hersen, 1988). The test is particularly useful in that it elicits specific thoughts, bodily sensations and other experiences that may complete the assessment procedure. Although BATs have been extensively used in fear and anxiety assessment, their application in the area of chronic pain has been scarce. A variant of the test has been described by Fordyce (1976), who called it an activity (in)tolerance test. To assess activity or exercise intolerance, patients are asked to perform the target exercise "Until pain, weakness, or fatigue causes him or her to stop" (p. 170). Consequently, a BAT assessment might include movements for which the patient is fearful could be chosen as the target exercises. Since we could find no report of an observational method for evaluating fear–avoidance, there appears to be a dire need for further work in this area.

11.6. Psychophysiological methods

Besides symptom-specific muscular reactivity, fear conditioning can also be demonstrated using the so-called startle probe. The startle response is a primitive defensive reflex that serves a protective function, avoiding organ injury and acting as a behavioral interruption that prepares the individual in dealing with possible threat. According to a number of animal and

human experiments, the magnitude of the startle reflex is found to be related to the emotional valence of the foreground stimulus (Vrana et al., 1988; Lang, 1995). There is also evidence that the startle is potentiated when anxious subjects are anticipating a threatening stimulus (Grillon et al., 1991). In a recent experiment, Crombez et al. (1997) exposed healthy volunteers to different heat stimuli. The researchers observed an intensification of the startle reflex to a noise burst during the more threatening high intensity stimuli as compared to the low intensity stimuli. Likewise, it is hypothesized that startle responses may provide an psychophysiological index of the threat value of pain, movements or activities that are reported to be threatening in pain patients. Some evidence was found in a study in which high and low fearful chronic low back pain patients were given video-exposure with vigorous movements performed by a dummy patient. After the video-exposure, patients were also requested to actually perform the movements. While they were anticipating the performance, a number of noise bursts were delivered. The results showed a trend in which the high-fearful patients had larger amplitudes than the low fearful patients (Beisiegel, 1997).

12. Clinical management of pain-related fear

What can be the implications of the current findings for the treatment of musculoskeletal pain? Keeping in mind that the relatively small percentage of chronic back pain patients are responsible for 75–90% of the societal costs (Van Tulder et al., 1995), the early identification of patients at risk of becoming disabled might lead to more specific and preventive interventions, the reduction of disability, and associated costs (Linton, 1998). Pain-related fear, and fear of movement/(re)injury in particular, must be considered such a risk factor. Pain-related fear may be an essential aspect of a broader early assessment of psychosocial 'yellow flags' (Kendall et al., 1997). Both the FABQ and the TSK have the potential to identify a subgroup of back pain patients whose level of disability may be mainly determined by pain-related fear, and not by pain intensity or biomedical status. For this subgroup, an early cognitive–behavioral intervention might be warranted. According to the suggestions made by Turner (1996) and Von Korff (1996) for behavioral interventions in primary care, such an intervention could be designed in three steps: screening, education, and exposure.

In terms of screening, both the TSK and FABQ are relatively short questionnaires that are appropriate for use in a primary care setting. In case of elevated scores, it is worth inquiring about the essential stimuli: what is the patient actually afraid of? So far, there is a lack of standardized tools for identifying these stimuli. In addition to checklists of daily activities, the presentation of visual materials such as pictures of back-stressing activities and movements might be worthwhile. They can be quite helpful in the development of graded hierarchies, reflecting the full range of situations avoided by the patient, beginning with those that provoke only mild discomfort, and ending with activities or situations that are well beyond the patient's present abilities. Each item is then rated by the patient on a 0–100 scale according to the amount of fear it would cause. In our experiences, abrupt changes in movements (e.g. suddenly being hit) or activities consisting of repetitive spinal compressions (riding a bicycle on a bumpy road) are frequently mentioned stimuli in chronic back pain patients who score high on the pain-related fear measures. These situations are feared because of beliefs about the causes of pain, such as ruptured or severely damaged nerves. ("If I lift heavy weights, the nerves in my back might be damaged"). Such a screening may also be supplemented by information about the precipitants (situational or internal) of the pain-related fear, and about the direct and indirect consequences. This screening might also include other areas of life stresses, as they might increase arousal levels and indirectly also fuel pain-related fear.

The second step consists of unambiguously educating the patient in a way that the patient views his pain as a common condition that can be self-managed, rather than as a serious disease or a condition that needs careful protection. Although cognitive–perceptual factors, such as catastrophizing in particular, are associated with pain-related fear, didactic lectures and rational argument may facilitate behavior change, but are not as effective as first-hand evidence. For a fearful patient, it is far more convincing to actually experience him/herself behaving differently than it is to be told that he/she is capable of behaving differently (Bandura, 1977). Graded exposure to the feared stimulus has proven to be the most effective treatment ingredient for individuals suffering from excessive fears and phobias (Davey, 1997). The reason is that it provides a unique way of challenging the credibility of the patients (maladaptive) fear–avoidance beliefs system.

Therefore, the third, and probably most essential step, consists of graded exposure to the situations the patients has identified as 'dangerous' or 'threatening'. Such a cognitive–behavioral approach always is introduced with a careful explanation of the fear–avoidance model (Fig. 2), using the patient's individual symptoms, beliefs and behaviors to illustrate how vicious circles maintain the pain problem. Subsequently, the most common approach would be to devise individually tailored practice tasks based on a graded hierarchy of fear-eliciting situations. Such a graded exposure is quite similar to the graded activity programs in that it gradually increases activity levels despite pain (Fordyce et al., 1982, 1986; Lindström et al., 1992), but is quite dissimilar in that it pays special attention to the idiosyncratic aspects of the pain-related fear stimuli. For example, if the patient fears the repetitive spinal compression produced by riding a bicycle on a bumpy road, then the graded exposure should include an activity that mimics that specific activity, and not just a stationary bicycle. Such an approach gives the individual an opportunity to correct the inaccurate predictions about the relationship between activities and harm. A preliminary study using a replicated single case cross-over experimental design in four patients with chronic low back pain who were offered a treatment outlined above showed promising results (Vlaeyen et al., 2001). After a no-treatment baseline measurement period, the fearful patients were randomly assigned to one of two interventions.

In intervention A, patients received the grade exposure in vivo first, followed by graded activity. In intervention B, the sequence of treatment modules was reversed. As predicted, improvements only occurred during the graded exposure in vivo, and not during the graded activity, irrespective of the treatment order. Analysis of the pre–post treatment differences also revealed that decreases in pain-related fear also concurred with decreases in pain catastrophizing and pain disability. Similar findings were reported in a replication study in which activity levels at the home situation were assessed by means of an activity monitor. (Vlaeyen et al., 2002) also suggest that treatment gains produced during the exposure to activities typical of the treatment setting do generalize to the home setting and in the absence of therapists. This is of particular interest in the light of experimental data showing that in chronic back pain patients, effects of exposure to one movement not easily generalizes towards another, dissimilar movement (Goubert et al., 2002). It is plausible that in our study, generalization has been facilitated by the repeated exposure to essential and individually identified stimuli as measured with PHODA.

Although such a cognitive–behavioral approach would appear highly applicable in most treatment settings, it has not been implemented and studied systematically. Randomized prospective studies including extended follow-up assessments and cost-effectiveness analyses demonstrating the impact of such a customized approach are likely to promising, and badly needed.

13. Conclusions

The idea that fear of pain and (re)injury may be more disabling than pain (Waddell, 1996, 1998; Crombez et al., 1999) refutes the early notion that the lowered ability to accomplish tasks of daily living in chronic pain patients is merely the consequence of pain severity. The accumulating research evidence seems to corroborate this. A large number of mainly cross-sectional studies have shown that pain-related fear is indeed one of the most potent predictors of observable physical performance and self-reported disability levels. There is also preliminary evidence that pain-related fear predicts new back pain episodes in pain-free people and that in chronic pain patients, it is associated with collateral non-specific physical complaints than the primary pain compliant. Possible mechanisms reviewed here are misinterpretations of bodily sensations, inaccurate predictions about pain, hypervigilance, physical deconditioning processes, and psychophysiologic reactivity. The evidence gathered in the last decennium also favors a cognitive–behavioral model first forwarded by Lethem et al. (1983) and later, in a refined version, put forward by Vlaeyen et al. (1995a).

There still are a number of unresolved issues, which merit future research attention. They concern the origins of pain-related fear, the role of illness information and feedback about diagnostic tests provided by medical specialists and therapists, the early identification of individuals with pain-related fear, the identification of the essential fear-stimuli, the relationship between pain-related fear and aspects of muscular disuse and reactivity, and finally, the development and evaluation of systematic treatment of patients with chronic pain who suffer from pain-related fear.

Pain-related fear and avoidance appears to be an essential feature of the development of a chronic problem for at least some patients. Indeed, this line of research may unlock the mysterious transition from acute to chronic pain. This in turn promises to provide a new foundation for the early identification of risk patients, prevention, assessment and treatment. The cognitive–behavioral conceptualization also not only contributes to the differential diagnosis of the heterogeneous group of patients with chronic musculoskeletal pain, but also constitutes possible explanations for the patients' symptoms, and hence successful treatment suggestions. Yet, we just scratched the surface of this area so that the implications and conclusions we may draw are limited. Given the compelling evidence reached to date, however, fear–avoidance needs to be considered in clinical practice and given priority in research.

Acknowledgements

Work related to this paper was, in part, supported by grant 904-65-090 of the Council for Medical and Health Research of the Netherlands (MW-NWO) to J.W.S.V. and by a grant of the Swedish Fund for Working Life Research to S.J.L.

References

Al-Obaidi, S.M., Nelson, R.M., Al-Awadhi, S. and Al-Shuwaie, N. (2000) The role of anticipation and fear of pain in the persistence of avoidance behavior in patients with chronic low back pain. Spine, 25: 1126–1131.

Arendt-Nielsen, L., Graven-Nielsen, T., Svarrer, H. and Svensson, P. (1995) The influence of low back pain on muscle activity and coordination during gait. Pain, 64: 231–240.

Arntz, A., Van Eck, M. and Heijmans, M. (1990) Predictions of dental pain: the fear of any expected evil, is worse than the evil itself. Behav. Res. Ther., 28: 29–34.

Arntz, A., Dreesen, L. and De Jong, P. (1994) The influence of anxiety on pain: attentional and attributional mediators. Pain, 56: 307–314.

Asmundson, G.J.G. and Norton, G.R. (1995) Anxiety sensitivity in patients with physically unexplained chronic back pain: a preliminary report. Behav. Res. Ther., 33: 771–777.

Asmundson, G.J.G. and Taylor, S. (1996) Role of anxiety sensitivity in pain-related fear and avoidance. J. Behav. Med., 19: 577–586.

Asmundson, G.J.G., Norton, G.R. and Allerdings, M.D. (1997a) Fear and avoidance in dysfunctional chronic back pain patients. Pain, 69: 231–236.

Asmundson, G.J.G., Kuperos, J.L. and Norton, G.R. (1997b) Do patients with chronic pain selectively attend to pain-related information? Preliminary evidence of the mediating role of fear. Pain, 72: 27–32.

Asmundson, G.J.G., Norton, G.R., Allerdings, M.D., Norton, P.J. and Larsen, D.K. (1998) Post-traumatic stress disorder and work-related injury. J. Anxiety Disord., 12: 57–69.

Asmundson, G.J.G., Norton, P.J. and Norton, G.R. (1999) Beyond pain: the role of fear and avoidance in chronicity. Clin. Psychol. Rev., 19: 97–119.

Bandura, A. (1977) Self-efficacy: toward a unifying theory of behavioral change. Psychol. Rev., 84: 191–215.

Beecher, H.K. (1959) Measurement of Subjective Responses. Oxford University Press, Oxford.

Beisiegel, E. (1997) De startle respons als maat voor kinesiofobie [The startle response as a measure of kinesiophobia]. Unpublished thesis, University of Maastricht.

Bellack, A.S. and Hersen, M. (1988) Behavioral Assessment, A Practical Handbook. Pergamon Press, New York.

Bergner, M., Bobbit, R.A., Carter, W.B. and Gibson, B.S. (1981) The sickness impact profile: development and final revision of a health status measure. Med. Care, 19: 787–805.

Beurskens, A., de Vet, H. and Köke, A. (1996) Responsiveness of functional status in low back pain: a comparison of different instruments. Pain, 65: 71–76.

Blanchard, E.B., Hickling, E.J., Taylor, A.E., Loos, W.R., Forneris, C.A. and Jaccard, J. (1996) Who develops PTSD from motor vehicle accidents. Behav. Res. Ther., 34: 1–10.

Bortz, W.M. (1984) The disuse syndrome. West. J. Med., 141: 691–694.

Bouchard, C., Shephard, R.J. and Stephens, T. (Eds.) (1994) Physical Activity, Fitness and Health. Human Kinetics Publishers, Champaign, IL.

Burton, A.K., Tillotson, K.M., Main, C.J. and Hollis, S. (1995) Psychosocial predictors of outcome in acute and subchronic low back trouble. Spine, 20: 722–728.

Bussman, J.B.J., Van de Laar, Y.M., Neleman, M.P. and Stam, H.J. (1998) Ambulatory accelerometry to quantify motor behaviour in patients after failed back surgery: a validation study. Pain, 74: 153–161.

Ciccone, D.S. and Just N. (2001) Pain expectancy and work disability in patients with acute and chronic pain: A test of the fear avoidance hypothesis. J. Pain, 2: 181–194.

Crombez, G., Vervaet, L., Lysens, R., Eelen, P. and Baeyens, F. (1996) Do pain expectancies cause pain in chronic low back patients? A clinical investigation. Behav. Res. Ther., 34: 919–925.

Crombez, G., Baeyens, F., Vansteenwegen, D. and Eelen, P. (1997) Startle intensification by painful heat stimuli. Eur. J. Pain, 1: 87–94.

Crombez, G., Vervaet, L., Lysens, R., Baeyens, F. and Eelen, P. (1998) Avoidance and confrontation of painful, back straining movements in chronic back pain patients. Behav. Modif., 22: 62–77.

Crombez, G., Vlaeyen, J.W.S., Heuts, P.H.T.G. and Lysens, R. (1999) Fear of pain is more disabling than pain itself. Evidence on the role of pain-related fear in chronic back pain disability. Pain, 80: 329–340.

Davey, G.C.L. (1997) Phobias. A Handbook of Theory, Research and Treatment. Wiley, Chichester.

DeGood, D.E. and Shutty, M.S. (1992) Assessment of pain beliefs, coping and self-efficacy. In: D.C. Turk and R. Melzack (Eds.), Handbook of Pain Assessment. Guilford Press, New York.

Ditto, P.H., Jemmott, J.B. and Darley, J.M. (1988) Appraising the threat of illness: a mental representation approach. Health Psychol., 7: 183–200.

Eccleston, C. and Crombez, G. (1999) Pain demands attention: a cognitive–affective model of the interruptive function of pain. Psychol. Bull., 125: 356–366.

Eccleston, C., Crombez, G., Aldrich, S. and Stannard, C. (1997) Attention and somatic awareness in chronic pain. Pain, 72: 209–215.

Eysenck, M.W. (1992) Anxiety: The Cognitive Perspective. Lawrence Erlbaum Associates, Hillsdale, NJ.

Eysenck, M.W. (1997) Anxiety and Cognition. A Unified Theory. Psychology Press, Hove.

Flor, H. and Turk, D.C. (1989) Psychophysiology of chronic

pain: do chronic pain patients exhibit symptom-specific psychophysiological responses. Psychol. Bull., 105: 215–259.

Flor, H., Birbaumer, N., Schugens, M.M. and Lutzenberger, W. (1992) Symptom-specific psychophysiological responses in chronic pain patients. Psychophysiology, 29: 452–460.

Fordyce, W.E. (1976) Behavioral Methods for Chronic Pain and Illness. Mosby, St. Louis.

Fordyce, W.E., Shelton, J.L. and Dundore, D.E. (1982) The modification of avoidance learning in pain behaviors. J. Behav. Med., 5: 405–414.

Fordyce, W.E., Brockway, J., Bergman, J. and Spengler, D. (1986) A control group comparison of behavioral versus traditional management methods in acute low back pain. J. Behav. Med., 2: 127–140.

Goubert, L,. Francken, G., Crombez, G., Vansteenwegen, D. and Lysens, R. (2002) Exposure to physical movement in chronic back pain patients: no evidence for generalization across different movements. Behav. Res. Ther., 40(4): 415–429.

Grillon, C., Ameli, R., Woods, S.W., Merikangas, K. and Davis, M. (1991) Fear-potentiated startle in humans: effects of anticipatory anxiety on the acoustic blink reflex. Psychophysiology, 28: 588–595.

Hadjistavropoulos, H.D., Craig, K.D. and Hadjistavropoulos, T. (1998) Cognitive and behavioral responses to illness information: the role of health anxiety. Behav. Res. Ther., 36: 149–164.

Haig, A.J., Weisman, G., Haugh, L.D., Pope, M. and grobler, L.J. (1993) Prospective evidence for change in paraspinal muscle activity after herniated nucleus pulposus. Spine, 18: 926–930.

Hill, H.E., Flanary, H.G., Kornetsky, C.H. and Wikler, A. (1952) Effects of anxiety and morphine on discrimination of intensities of painful stimuli. J. Clin. Invest., 31: 473–480.

Jensen, M.P. and Karoly, P. (1992a) Pain-specific beliefs, perceived symptom severity, and adjustment to chronic pain. Clin. J. Pain, 8: 123–130.

Jensen, M.P. and Karoly, P. (1992b) Self-report scales and procedures for assessing pain in adults. In: D.C. Turk and R. Melzack (Eds.), Handbook of Pain Assessment. Guilford Press, New York, pp. 135–151.

Jensen, M.P., Karoly, P. and Huger, R. (1987) The development and preliminary validation of an instrument to assess patients' attitudes toward pain. J. Psychosom. Res., 31: 393–400.

Jensen, M.P., Turner, J.A. and Romano, J.M. (1991) Self-efficacy and outcome-expectancies: relationship to chronic pain coping strategies and adjustment. Pain, 44: 263–269.

Jensen, M.P., Turner, J.A., Romano, J.M. and Lawler, B.K. (1994) Relationship of pain-specific beliefs to chronic pain adjustment. Pain, 57: 301–309.

Keefe, F.J. and Hill, R.W. (1985) An objective approach to quantifying pain behavior and gait patterns in LBP patients. Pain, 21: 153–161.

Kendall, N.A.S., Linton, S.J. and Main, C.J. (1997) Guide to assessing psychosocial Yellow Flags in acute low back pain: risk factors for long-term disability and work loss. Accident rehabilitation and Compensation Insurance Corporation of New Zealand and the National Health Committee, NZ.

Kerns, R.D., Turk, D.C. and Rudy, T.E. (1985) The West Haven-Yale Multidimensional Pain Inventory (WHYMPI). Pain, 23: 345–356.

Keogh, E., Ellery, D., Hunt, C. and Hannent, I. (2001) Selective attentional bias for pain-related stimuli amongst pain fearful individuals. Pain, 91: 91–100.

Klenerman, L., Slade, P.D., Stanley, I.M., Pennie, B., Reilly, J.P., Atkinson, L.E., Troup, J.D.G. and Rose, M.J. (1995) The prediction of chronicity in patients with an acute attack of low back pain in a general practice setting. Spine, 4: 478–484.

Koelman, T.W., Kwakkel, G. and Wagenaar, R.C. (1996) Het fysiotherapeutisch pijnmanagement: lage rugklachten als voorbeeld. [Physiotherapeutic management: low back pain as an example]. In: Mattie et al. (Eds.), Pijninformatorium. Bohn Stafleu Van Loghum, Houten.

Kori, S.H., Miller, R.P. and Todd, D.D. (1990) Kinisophobia: a new view of chronic pain behavior. Pain Management, Jan/Feb: 35–43.

Kottke, F.J. (1966) The effects of limitation of activity upon the human body. J. Am. Med. Assoc., 196: 117–122.

Lang, P.J. (1995) The emotion probe. Studies of motivation and attention. Am. Psychol., 50: 372–385.

Larsen, D.K., Taylor, S. and Asmundson, G.J.G. (1997) Exploratory factor analysis of the Pain Anxiety Symptoms Scale in patients with chronic pain complaints. Pain, 69: 27–34.

Lee, J.H., Ooi, Y. and Nakamura, K. (1995) Measurement of muscle strength of the trunk and the lower extremities in subjects with history of low back pain. Spine, 20: 1994–1996.

Lethem, J., Slade, P.D., Troup, J.D.G. and Bentley, G. (1983) Outline of a fear–avoidance model of exaggerated pain perceptions. Behav. Res. Ther., 21: 401–408.

Lindström, I., Öhlund, C., Eek, C., Wallin, L., Peterson, L., Fordyce, W.E. and Nachemson, A.L. (1992) The effect of graded activity on patients with sub-acute low back pain: a randomized prospective clinical study with an operant conditioning behavioral approach. Phys. Ther., 72: 279–290.

Linton, S.J. (1998) The socioeconomic impact of chronic back pain: is anyone benefiting. Pain, 75: 163–168.

Linton, S.J. and Buer, N. (1995) Working despite pain: factors associated with work attendance versus dysfunction. Int. J. Behav. Med., 2(3): 252–262.

Linton, S.J. and Halldén, K. (1997) Risk factors and the natural course of acute and recurrent musculoskeletal pain: developing a screening instrument. In: T.S. Jensen, J.A. Turner and Z. Wiesenfeld-Hallin (Eds.), Proceedings of the 8th World Congress on Pain: Progress in Pain Research and Management, Vol. 8. IASP Press, Seattle, WA, pp. 527–536.

Linton, S.J. and Halldén, K. (1998) Can we screen for problematic back pain? A screening questionnaire for predicting outcome in acute and subacute back pain. Clin. J. Pain, 14(3): 209–215.

Linton, S.J., Melin, L. and Gotestam, K.G. (1984) Behavioral Analysis of Chronic Pain and its Management. Progress in Behavior Modification, Vol. 18. Academic Press, New York, p. 1.

Linton, S.J., Buer, N., Vlaeyen, J.W.S. and Hellsing, A.-L. (2000) Are fear–avoidance beliefs related to a the inception of an episode of back pain? A prospective study. Psychol. Health, 14: 1051–1059.

Main, C.J. and Watson, P.J. (1996) Guarded movements: development of chronicity. J. Musculoskelet. Pain, 4: 163–170.

Mannion, A.F., Dolan, P., Adam, G.G., Adams, M.A. and Cooper, R.G. (1997) Can maximal back muscle strength be predicted from submaximal efforts. J. Back Musculoskelet. Rehabil., 9: 49–51.

McCracken, L.M. (1997) Attention to pain in persons with chronic pain: a behavioral approach. Behav. Ther., 28: 271–284.

McCracken, L.M. and Gross, R.T. (1993) Does anxiety affect coping with pain. Clin. J. Pain, 9: 253–259.

McCracken, L.M., Zayfert, C. and Gross, R.T. (1992) The Pain Anxiety Symptoms Scale: development and validation of a scale to measure fear of pain. Pain, 50: 63–67.

McCracken, L.M., Gross, R.T., Sorg, P.J. and Edmands, T.A. (1993) Prediction of pain in patients with chronic low back pain: effects of inaccurate prediction and pain-related anxiety. Behav. Res. Ther., 31: 647–652.

McCracken, L.M., Gross, R.T., Aikens, J. and Carnkike Jr., C.L.M. (1996) The assessment of anxiety and fear in persons with chronic pain: a comparison of instruments. Behav. Res. Ther., 34: 927–933.

McCracken, L.M., Faber, S.D. and Janeck, A.S. (1998) Pain-related anxiety predicts non-specific physical complaints in persons with chronic pain. Behav. Res. Ther., 36: 621–630.

McQuade, K.J., Turner, J.A. and Buchner, D.M. (1988) Physical fitness and chronic low back pain. Clin. Orthop. Rel. Res., 233: 198–204.

Menard, M.R., Cooke, C., Locke, S.R., Beach, G.N. and Butler, T.B. (1994) Pattern of performance in workers with low back pain during a comprehensive motor performance evaluation. Spine, 2: 1359–1366.

Morgan, W. (1997) Physical Activity and Mental Health. Taylor and Francis, London.

O'Connor, A.M. (1983) Factors related to the early phase of rehabilitation following aortocoronary bypass surgery. Res. Nurs. Health, 6: 107–116.

Pearce, J. and Morley, S. (1989) An experimental investigation of the construct validity of the McGill Pain Questionnaire. Pain, 39: 115–121.

Peters, M.L., Vlaeyen, J.W.S. and Van Drunen, C. (2000) Do fibromyalgia patients display hypervigilance for innoxious somatosensory stimuli? Application of a body scanning reaction time paradigm. Pain, 86: 283–292.

Peters, M.L., Vlaeyen, J.W.S. and Kunnen, A.M. (2002) Is pain-related fear a predictor of somatosensory hypervigilance in chronic low back pain patients. Behav. Res. Ther., 40: 85–103.

Philips, H.C. (1987) Avoidance behaviour and its role in sustaining chronic pain. Behav. Res. Ther., 25: 273–279.

Philips, H.C. and Jahanshahi, M. (1986) The components of pain behaviour report. Behav. Res. Ther., 24: 117–125.

Rachlin, H. (1980) Behaviorism in Everyday Life. Prentice-Hall, Englewood Cliffs, NJ.

Riley, J.F., Ahern, D.K. and Follick, M.J. (1988) Chronic pain and functional impairment: assessing beliefs about their relationship. Arch. Phys. Med. Rehabil., 69: 579–582.

Reiss, S. (1991) Expectancy theory of fear, anxiety, and panic. Clin. Psychol. Rev., 11: 141–153.

Reiss, S. and McNally, R.J. (1985) The expectancy model of fear. In: S. Reiss and R.R. Bootzin (Eds.), Theoretical Issues in Behavior Therapy. Academic Press, New York, pp. 107–121.

Reitsma, B. and Meijler, W.J. (1997) Pain and patienthood. Clin. J. Pain, 13: 9–21.

Roland, M. and Morris, R. (1983) A study of the natural history of back pain. Part I: Development of a reliable and sensitive measure of disability in low back pain. Spine, 8: 141–144.

Romano, J.M. and Turner, J.A. (1985) Chronic pain and depression. Does the evidence support a relationship. Psychol. Bull., 97: 311–318.

Rosenstiel, A.K. and Keefe, F.J. (1983) The use of coping strategies in chronic low back pain patients: relationship to patient characteristics and current adjustment. Pain, 17: 33–44.

Rutherford, O.M., Jones, D.A. and Newham, D.J. (1986) Clinical and experimental application of the percutaneous twitch superimposition technique for the study of human muscle activation. J. Neurol. Neurosurg. Psychiatry, 49: 1288–1291.

Sieben, J.M., Vlaeyen, J.W.S., Tuerlinckx, S. and Portegijs, P. (2002) Pain-related fear in acute low back pain: the first two weeks of a new episode. Eur. J. Pain, in press.

Skevington, S.M. (1995) Psychology of Pain. Wiley, Chichester.

Sullivan, M.J.L., Bishop, S.R. and Pivik, J. (1995) The pain catastrophizing scale: development and validation. Psychol. Assess., 7: 524–532.

Triano, J.J. and Schultz, A.B. (1987) Correlation of objective measures of trunk motion and muscle function with low back disability ratings. Spine, 12: 561–565.

Turk, D.C. and Holzman, A.D. (1986) Chronic pain: interfaces among physical, psychological and social parameters. In: A.D. Holzman and D.C. Turk (Eds.), Pain Management. A Handbook of Psychological Treatment Approaches. Pergamon, New York.

Turk, D.C., Meichenbaum, D. and Genest, M. (1983) Pain and Behavioral Medicine. A Cognitive–Behavioral Perspective. Guilford Press, New York.

Turner, J.A. (1996) Educational and behavioral interventions for back pain in primary care. Spine, 21: 2851–2857.

Turner, J.A., LeResche, L., Von Korff, M. and Ehrlich, K. (1998) Back pain in primary care. Patient characteristics, content of initial visit, and short-term outcomes. Spine, 23: 463–469.

Van den Hout, J.H., Vlaeyen, J.W., Houben, R.M., Soeters, A.P. and Peters, M.L. (2001) The effects of failure feedback and pain-related fear on pain report, pain tolerance, and pain avoidance in chronic low back pain patients. Pain, 92: 247–257.

Van Tulder, M.W., Koes, B.W. and Bouter, L.M. (1995) A cost-of-illness study of back pain in the Netherlands. Pain, 62: 233–240.

Verbunt, J., Van der Heijden, G., Vlaeyen, J.W.S., Seelen, H.A.M., Heuts, P.H.G.T., Pons, C. and Knottnerus, A. (2002)

Disuse and deconditioning in chronic low back pain. Submitted for publication.

Vlaeyen, J.W.S., Kole-Snijders, A.M.J., Boeren, R.G.B. and Van Eek, H. (1995a) Fear of movement/(re)injury in chronic low back pain and its relation to behavioral performance. Pain, 62: 363–372.

Vlaeyen, J.W.S., Kole-Snijders, A.M.J., Rotteveel, A., Ruesink, R. and Heuts, P.H.T.G. (1995b) The role of fear of movement/(re)injury in pain disability. J. Occup. Rehab., 5: 235–252.

Vlaeyen, J.W.S., Seelen, H.A.M., Peters, M., De Jong, P., Aretz, E., Beisiegel, E. and Weber, W. (1999) Fear of movement/(re)injury and muscular reactivity in chronic low back pain patients: an experimental investigation. Pain, in press.

Vlaeyen, J.W.S., de Jong, J., Geilen, M., Heuts, P.H.T.G. and Van Breukelen, G. (2002) The treatment of fear of movement/(re)injury in chronic low back pain: Further evidence on the effectiveness of exposure in vivo. Clin J. Pain, in press.

Von Korff, M. (1996) A research program for primary care pain management: back pain. In: J. Campbell (Ed.), Pain 1996 — An Updated Review. IASP Press, Seattle, WA, pp. 457–465.

Vrana, S.R., Spence, E.L. and Lang, P.J. (1988) The startle probe response: a new measure of emotion. J. Abnorm. Psychol., 97: 487–491.

Waddell, G. (1996) Keynote address for primary care forum. Low back pain: a twentieth century health care enigma. Spine, 21: 2820–2825.

Waddell, G. (1998) The Back Pain Revolution. Churchill Livingstone, Edinburgh.

Waddell, G., Newton, M., Henderson, I., Somerville, D. and Main, C. (1993) A Fear–Avoidance Beliefs Questionnaire (FABQ) and the role of fear–avoidance beliefs in chronic low back pain and disability. Pain, 52: 157–168.

Wagenmakers, A.J.M., Coakley, J.H. and Edwards, R.H.T. (1988) The metabolic consequences of reduced habitual activities in patients with muscle pain and disease. Ergonomics, 31: 1519–1527.

Wall, P.D. (1979) On the relation of injury to pain. Pain, 6: 253–264.

Warwick, H.M. and Salkovskis, P.M. (1990) Hypochondriasis. Behav. Res. Ther., 28: 105–117.

Watson, D. and Pennebaker, J.W. (1989) Health complaints, stress, and distress: exploring the central role of negative affect. Psychol. Rev., 96: 234–254.

Watson, P., Booker, C.K., Main, C.J. and Chen, A.C.N. (1997) Surface electromyography in the identification of chronic low back pain patients: the development of the flexion relaxation ratio. Clin. Biomech., 12: 165–171.

Westerterp, K.R. and Wouters, L. (1995) The Maastricht protocol for the measurement of body composition and energy expenditure with labeled water. Obesity Res., 3: 49.

Wittink, H., Hoskins Michel, T., Wagner, A., Sukiennik, A. and Rogers, W. (2000) Deconditioning in patients with chronic low back pain: fact or fiction? Spine, 25: 2221–2228.

New Avenues for the Prevention of Chronic Musculoskeletal Pain and Disability
Pain Research and Clinical Management, Vol. 12
Edited by S.J. Linton

CHAPTER 8

Depression and mood

Zoë Clyde [1,*] and Amanda C.deC. Williams [2]

[1] *INPUT Pain Management Unit, Guys and St. Thomas' NHS Hospital Trust, London SE1 7EH, UK*
[2] *Division of Psychological Medicine, GKT School of Medicine, Dentistry and Biomedical Sciences, INPUT Pain Management Unit, Guys and St. Thomas' NHS Hospital Trust, London SE1 7EH, UK*

Abstract: There is long-standing confusion regarding the relationship between pain and depression, and indeed about what constitutes depression of clinical concern in the context of the widespread impact of chronic pain. We address models of depression in pain and related problems around measurement, which continue to obscure the relationship. The dominant psychological model of diathesis and stress is discussed, with particular considerations concerning pain as a stressor, and adaptive processes such as acceptance. Information processing paradigms are described as a means to discover what distinguishes different profiles of depressive thinking in chronic pain and what uniquely characterises depression in chronic pain. Reformulated models in the light of these differences are used to examine current and potential treatment practices within pain management.

1. Introduction

By definition, chronic pain is prolonged and aversive, generally causing considerable disruption to the sufferer's life. Pain can present insurmountable obstacles to normal activities: work, leisure, and relationships with family and friends. Certain treatment attempts, and many adaptations generated by the sufferer, may unwittingly create further problems. In such a situation, feelings of hopelessness, lack of control, loss, frustration and anger are common. The subjectivity of the experience can impose real isolation, and the personal meaning of pain and its impacts may threaten the individual's sense of who he or she is. It would be surprising in such a predicament if sufferers were not to express feelings of unhappiness and depression. However, these feelings are not universal, nor are they directly proportional to pain severity or the extent of disability associated with the pain. The relationship between chronic pain and depression is complex, with much debate about its nature and extent (Banks and Kerns, 1996) and research findings which are inconsistent and whose interpretation may be controversial (Sullivan et al., 1992).

Biological and evolutionary models pose questions about the function of depression, and while most current biological models (based on shared neurotransmitters) lack specificity and are selective in the symptoms they claim to explain (Van Praag, 1993), evolutionary models (Gilbert, 1992; Nesse and Lloyd, 1992; Klinger, 1993) propose that in the face of serious loss or forced disengagement from previously high priority goals, survival may de-

* Correspondence to: Z. Clyde, INPUT Pain Management Unit, Guys and St. Thomas' NHS Hospital Trust, London SE1 7EH, UK. Tel.: +44 (207) 922 8107; Fax: +44 (207) 922 8229; E-mail: zoe.clyde@gstt.sthames.nhs.uk

pend on conserving physical resources and minimising risk of conflict, social rejection, or further loss. Much of this model is strikingly similar to descriptions of people and animals in severe pain (Wall, 1979), emphasising the phenomenological overlap described below. Mineka and Sutton (1992) contrasted the evolutionary functions of anxiety and depression: the cognitive biases of depression focus on themes of self-evaluation and loss as an aid to reflective learning about failures and losses, while those of anxiety promote rapid processing of potential threat.

Pain and depression as traditionally defined by diagnostic criteria such as DSM-IV (1994) (see Box 1) overlap somewhat, involving disruption of normal biological, psychological and social functioning. The overlap complicates the definition of depression in pain, and the construction and use of measurement tools which originate from those definitions and models (Sullivan et al., 1992; Williams, 1998). Further, assumptions of homogeneity of both depression

and pain, necessary for initial exploration of the association, have been overextended to the point where they confound the field (Sullivan et al., 1992; Pincus and Williams, 1999).

Research findings depend critically on design issues: definitions, classification criteria, measures and the population investigated. Although for certain purposes these concerns can be suspended and considerations of heterogeneity disregarded, the resulting picture still shows little consensus on prevalence and association. Reviews of the relationship between chronic pain and depression (Romano and Turner, 1985; Sullivan et al., 1992; Banks and Kerns, 1996; Fishbain et al., 1997) show a statistical association of a size which varies with definitions, instruments and populations (Atkinson et al., 1991; Polatin et al., 1993; Magni et al., 1994; Dohrenwend et al., 1999), but is consistently higher than in the general population, and often higher than in other medically ill populations (Romano and Turner, 1985; Banks and Kerns, 1996), posing the question as to what it is

---

Box 1   DSM-IV criteria for major depressive episode

A. Five or more of the following symptoms have been present over two weeks and represent a change from previous functioning.
  (1) depressed mood, most of the day, nearly every day
      and/or
  (2) markedly diminished interest or pleasure in all, or almost all, activities most of the day, nearly every day
  (3) significant weight loss when not dieting or weight gain or decrease or increase in appetite nearly every day
  (4) insomnia or hypersomnia nearly every day
  (5) psychomotor agitation or retardation nearly every day (observable)
  (6) fatigue or loss of energy nearly every day
  (7) feelings of worthlessness or excessive or inappropriate guilt nearly every day (not merely self-reproach or guilt about being sick)
  (8) diminished ability to think or concentrate, or indecisiveness, nearly every day
  (9) recurrent thoughts of death, recurrent suicidal ideation without a plan or a suicide attempt or specific plan for committing suicide.

B. The symptoms cause clinically significant distress or impairment in social, occupational, or other important areas of functioning.

C. The symptoms are not due to the direct physiological effects of a substance or a general medical condition (e.g. hypothyroidism).

D. The symptoms are not better accounted for by bereavement.

about chronic pain that causes such distress. This is addressed below.

Patient samples in prevalence studies vary enormously, as in all chronic pain research, and while narrowing the sample is an obvious solution, imposing constraints would require a conceptual or empirical basis. However, insofar as these questions have been addressed, the most common subsample is selected by diagnosis. There is neither a coherent hypothesis about why depression should vary with diagnosis (rather than, say, pain severity or resulting disability), nor any clear evidence for it (Pincus and Morley, 2001). Fewer studies have focussed on the incidence of chronic pain in depressed populations than on depression in chronic pain (Romano and Turner, 1985). Among the latter, samples are recruited from chronic pain clinics, from primary care, and from general population surveys, with highest rates of depression in clinic populations.

If symptomatology in depression and depressed mood is no longer considered to be homogeneous in the absence of pain (Costello, 1993), in its presence (Magni et al., 1994), or in chronic illness (Brewin, 1988), it makes sense either to investigate symptoms singly (Costello, 1993), or more helpfully for treatment purposes, to search for sub-populations which differ significantly in aetiology, mechanisms, contributory and precipitating factors, and in the relationship with depression.

2. Methodological problems and measurement

Central to the issue about the prevalence of depression in pain is the definition and hence measurement of depression. Reliable calculations of the prevalence of 'depression' in chronic pain are problematic because of measurement and sample selection. There are difficulties in the assessment of both pain and depression. There are variations in the requirements of what counts as a 'case', and problems with measurement, both in the way information is obtained, usually self-report, and in the content of what is presented. This is especially true for depression as classically defined and the overlap with

the somatic symptoms (e.g. sleep disturbance, low energy) present in chronic pain (Williams, 1998). In turn, pain is a psychological experience as well as a physical one (Melzack and Wall, 1988) and cannot be fully described without reference to the sufferer's emotional state.

However, attempts to measure and define depression in people with chronic pain draw on models of depression developed in mental health settings from which those with physical disease/disability have been excluded. Most studies use brief self-report measures of psychopathology (for instance, in the systematic review by Morley et al. (1999), 14 trials used the Beck Depression Inventory, two the Centre for Epidemiological Study Depression scale, one the Depressive Adjective Checklist, and four the depression scales from multicomponent pain impact scales; others in widespread use in pain include the Symptoms Check List 90/90R, the Minnesota Multiphasic Personality Inventory Depression Scale, and the Hospital Anxiety and Depression Scale). Standard diagnostic criteria (such as DSM-IV) are rarely used. The somatic symptoms of depression on the self-report and diagnostic criteria may also occur as part of various physical disorders. Only the HAD was developed for medical patients by excluding somatic symptoms (and consistent with its authors' anhedonia model, it also excludes cognitive items); other questionnaires were validated on populations without significant medical problems. Alternatively, standardised diagnostic criteria and the Hamilton Rating Scale for Depression require the interviewer to attribute symptoms to physical or psychological origins. The choice of measure often depends on the relative importance of false negatives versus false positives.

Investigations of chronic pain patients' responses to common depression measures such as the BDI frequently, but not always, show a different structure (Novy et al., 1995; Geisser et al., 1997; Williams, 1998; Williams et al., 2000), with high scores on somatic factors and low scores on self-denigratory cognitive items, unlike the unidimensional structure characteristic of depressed populations in which affective and cognitive items dominate. A recent study

(Wilson et al., 2001) demonstrates a significant difference in the prevalence of major depressive disorder depending on how symptoms are classified: by including all symptoms regardless of presumed etiology; or by counting only those symptoms which were not attributed to pain by the patient at interview, which produced a prevalence of nearly half the inclusive estimate. Use of cognitive and affective self-report items appeared adequately to differentiate those who met depression criteria by either method from those who were not depressed by either method, and avoided a large proportion of possible false positives. Thus the interpretation of commonly used depression measures in pain remains problematic. An alternative approach acknowledges that while some patients meet diagnostic criteria for depression, there is a level of depressed mood which is far more common (Skevington, 1995) but does not qualify as major depressive disorder (Calfas et al., 1997); it is important that measurement of depression does not disregard this group, and measurement problems are more complex than for major depressive disorder, if not so clinically urgent.

Measures arise from the theory of the state under investigation. If, as is suggested (Skevington, 1995; Williams, 1998; Clyde, 2000; Pincus and Morley, 2001), depression in chronic pain is qualitatively different in terms of cognitive content to classical depression, then appropriate measures should be used. As discussed above, until recently classification has involved trying to make existing definitions of depression fit, rather than asking the questions of who gets depressed, in what circumstances, and what is their experience. Patients' accounts can provide a wealth of information, yet there is little qualitative work in this area as applicability of existing models has largely been uncritically questioned. Those who have had previous episodes of depression may describe a qualitative difference between previous episodes of clinical depression and their current depressed mood, which they attribute to their pain and its impact; it is not uncommon when completing self-report measures for patients to comment that few of the items capture their mood adequately. A cognitive model promises not only a more heteroge-

neous representation of depression in chronic pain, but the possibility of developing more adequate measures. We argue that listening to the content of what patients say, and the ways in which they construe everyday experience, is more helpful than listening for diagnostic criteria and has implications for treatment. To reflect this, we have included quotes from patients' accounts of pain and depression.

3. Models

Use of the concept of depression without sufficient regard for its origins and development has unfortunately provided support for unscientific and unhelpful models of chronic pain and treatment practices. The question arises how one might reconsider the commonly formulated non-exclusive hypotheses concerning the relationship in the light of a focus on content and process. Accumulating evidence (Rudy et al., 1988; Brown, 1990; Gamsa, 1990; Atkinson et al., 1991; Magni et al., 1994; Fishbain et al., 1997; Dohrenwend et al., 1999) suggests that pain onset more commonly precedes than follows depression, although it is acknowledged that it is unlikely to be a straightforward causal relationship (Rudy et al., 1988). The age of onset of chronic pain varies widely but is on average about a decade later than that of depression (Atkinson et al., 1991) for which the median age is generally considered to be in the early to mid-twenties (Ingram et al., 1998). In addition, some previously and currently depressed people will develop chronic pain, a situation which might make both more liable to recurrent or prolonged depression.

The onset of depression prior to pain is more likely to be associated with a family history of depression, while onset of depression after pain is less likely to be so (Dohrenwend et al., 1999), and may be more to do with the nature of pain as a stressor. The suggestion that chronic pain and depression are somehow different aspects of the same pathology finds scant empirical or theoretical support (Turk and Salovey, 1984); nevertheless, it has attracted surprisingly little criticism and is widely used, risking exacerbating patients' distress and disability, and undermining its appropriate treatment. Despite consistent findings that psychosocial factors predict the development and maintenance of disability in chronic pain, the specific hypothesis that previous or current depression predisposes those with an acute pain episode to develop chronic pain remains unsubstantiated.

A majority of the prevalence studies are cross-sectional in design, requiring retrospective accounts of symptoms which fall short of answering the question of causality. Prospective studies have not produced compelling evidence to suggest that there is a simple causal relationship between depression and pain or vice versa. Von Korff et al. (1993) found in a community sample that moderate to severe depressive symptoms at baseline were a risk factor for developing headache or chest pain, but not other pain conditions. By contrast, the presence of a pain condition at baseline was a better predictor of the development of a new pain condition than was depression. In a general population sampled with an interval of eight years, Magni et al. (1994) found that while chronic pain predicted later depression and depressive symptoms at baseline predicted subsequent pain, each accounted only for a small amount of shared variance. A further question concerns the use of appropriate comparison groups. Healthy controls differ in multiple ways from chronic pain patients, while other chronic illness populations in which pain is absent or well controlled differ in specific ways: for example, having a well-recognised diagnosis (e.g. diabetes), or a clear if pessimistic prognosis (e.g. certain cancers).

Models of vulnerability and risk of depression have been applied to elucidate the relationship (Banks and Kerns, 1996), although they conclude that insufficient attention has been paid to pain as stressor. The fact that chronic pain does not universally cause depression can be attributed to differences in vulnerability, but it also makes sense to examine the stresses associated with pain in terms of its meaning for the individual (i.e. not pain per se). Social models, which particularly emphasised loss, are now refined and focus on loss which is associated with humiliation and entrapment, with chronic illness a key exemplar of the latter (Brown et al., 1995).

Whatever the content and extent of vulnerability and stress, the model is incomplete without some notion of process. Rudy et al. (1988) used a modelling approach to emphasise that neither pain nor associated loss is a sufficient condition for the subsequent development of depression, but that the relationship is mediated by perceived interference by pain with everyday life and loss of control. Therefore, we question whether the proposed psychological factors which mediate the relationship between pain and depression constitute more than the mechanism by which diathesis and stress affect people differently. The characteristics of vulnerability, pain as stress, and their cognitive representation and processing which increase the risk of depression remain unidentified.

3.1. Vulnerability to depression

"I have suffered from depression on and off, not always attributable to the pain"

(53 year old woman).

Vulnerability to depression is partly predicted by distal factors (Ingram et al., 1998), such as childhood experiences, previous episodes of depression, or a family history of depression. Diathesis can be expressed in terms of long-standing cognitive content and process, established as a result of such distal experiences, such as the belief that "I'm not strong enough to cope", or "I'm not worth other people trying to help me". Previous depression is an established risk factor for the development of clinical depression in psychiatric populations, but it is not known whether those who have experienced depression prior to the onset of pain are more likely to become depressed subsequently than those who have not. Nor is it clear to what extent such a post-pain-onset depression is comparable with the depression previously experienced. The study by Dohrenwend et al. (1999) found that the incidence of depression prior to pain was associated with a family history of depression; the incidence of depression after pain onset was less likely to be so. It may well be that different subtypes of depression are associated with different vulnerabilities but share a final common cognitive pathway (Ingram et al., 1998). There is a dearth of research on protective factors against the development of depression in people who might be considered vulnerable, both within and outside the pain field.

3.2. The nature of the stressor

". . . it's the pain that really gets you down"
(60 year old lady)

"you feel in limbo, at a total loss, restricted"
(48 year old man)

In Banks and Kerns' (1996) account, the unrelenting nature of the physical symptoms, combined with the impairment and disability, secondary losses and experience with the medical system, all interact to impact on the self. The negative interpersonal aspects of chronic pain, particularly not being believed or feeling understood, are also part of the pain experience. The constant cognitive burden and increasing behavioural disruption, often beginning during the most active adult years, cause a major disruption of life expectations; patients often describe feeling much older than they are, as if prematurely aged.

Questions remain, however, about relevant variables to investigate in relation to risk of depression in the presence of chronic pain. Duration since onset may be an important variable in relation to factors such as loss, adaptation and acceptance. However, it is rather the processes which occur, the search for a diagnosis and/or for relief or palliation of multiple problems, and the associated striving for credibility and an understandable status in the patient's own eyes and in those of others, which matter rather than simply the time they take. The impact of treatment variables on the development of depression may well be underestimated: uncertainties around pain and its implications for the patient are exacerbated if s/he does not feel believed or heard, or receives conflicting information on diagnosis and prognosis, multiple

referrals, and ineffective treatments, leading to feelings of powerlessness, helplessness and decreased control (Reid et al., 1991; Walker et al., 1999). In a comparison of patients according to whether their elicited description of their pain problem matched the case note diagnosis, Geisser and Roth (1998) found that those who effectively disagreed with their diagnosis were most distressed, but that those who were unsure (nearly one half the sample) had least sense of control over pain, were more convinced that pain implied harm, and reported themselves more disabled than those who were certain of their diagnosis, whether they agreed or disagreed with their notes.

"It's the psychological side that is worse then the pain. I can accept the pain for the pain itself, but it stops you from living your life. You go to hospital, and they tell you to come back in 6 months to a year. There is no consideration about what you are going to do in the meantime"
(43 year old man).

Uncertainty about diagnosis and prognosis leaves pain sufferers doubtful about how best to proceed. Pain creates physical and practical obstacles, but in addition the chronic pain sufferer who is unsure of what is wrong, and who may have had too little information or too much which is inaccurate or conflicting, is subject to fears about activity resulting in damage and/or increased pain. Trial and error is unlikely to disconfirm those fears, and patients frequently describe the dilemma of trying to remain active, only to suffer increased pain, but finding that rest brings little benefit and compounds their isolation.

The cognitive set which reflects these experiences and generates pessimistic expectations of the consequences of the individual's efforts to manage has been captured by a measure called catastrophising (Rosenstiel and Keefe, 1983; Sullivan et al., 2001). Despite its power to predict longer-term distress and disability, and its apparent similarity to cognitive distortion (within a Beckian model of depression) or a depressive schema, its relationship with depression is unclear and it remains somewhat unintegrated with existing theories of information processing and mood (Sullivan et al., 2001).

The model of loss, as a precipitant of depression, is used in chronic pain in relation to abandoned roles, hopes, ambitions and satisfactions. What distinguishes this loss from bereavement is that patients often retain some hope that they may obtain pain relief and thereby recover their previous lifestyle: adjusting to the loss can feel like voluntarily relinquishing that possibility, while a focus on pain relief leads to multiple unsuccessful medical interventions. A third possibility, offered by pain management, of partial or substantial recovery of previous lifestyle without pain relief, can be hard to contemplate.

3.3. The process of acceptance and adaptation

The limitations imposed by chronic pain may strongly affect the chance of a person attaining their goals (or ideal self), and the discrepancy between this and their actual self may lead to depression (Higgins, 1987). A similar model is proposed by Chapman and Gavrin (1999), who describe discrepancies between self-expectations and current performance as a threat to the integrity of the self, and constituting suffering. The process of reevaluating self-expectations and goals in life often involves is a change in the sense of self to incorporate pain, which is an important part of acceptance of chronic pain. Skevington (1995) suggests that cognitive complexity is protective, since with many aspects to the self, adverse life events will have fewer cognitive ramifications.

Research in this area in relation to pain has focussed on the concepts of acceptance of pain, and on the associated adaptation of roles and goals. McCracken (1998) defines acceptance of pain as: "acknowledging that one has pain, giving up on unproductive attempts to control pain, acting as if pain does not necessarily imply disability, and being able to commit one's efforts to living a satisfying life despite the pain". Acceptance of pain does not mean resignation. There are few studies which directly address this concept; McCracken (1998) found that acceptance of pain was a significant predictor of

several physical and psychosocial variables including depression. Acceptance of chronic pain would be expected to occur more easily for the patient who is believed, who receives adequate information and explanation, and is actively engaged in treatment. The process of acceptance may require abandonment of previous expectations, roles or goals, or their reassessment. Implicit in much pain management is that patients should aspire to achieving their existing goals despite continuing pain. However, Schmitz et al. (1996) found less distress among those pain patients who modified existing goals or substituted new ones (accommodation) than among those who pursued unmodified goals, relying on the eventual relief of pain to enable them to realise them.

"I was really [depressed] especially when I finished my job, what do I do next? I explored new roles. . . ."
(49 year old man, not currently depressed).

Models of adjustment exist for other chronic illnesses such as cancer (Moorey, 1996), but apply to patients who have a recognisable diagnosis, even if an uncertain prognosis. However, adjustment cannot proceed without some certainty about the starting point, which in chronic pain may be much more uncertain. Even where there is some understanding, the unpredictable course presents patients with new challenges to acceptance and thus to any process of adjustment.

"27 years ago I had a melanoma and had radical treatment. This [chronic pain] is harder to deal with as I can't do anything about it"
(45 year old lady).

3.4. Social context

The emphasis on the personal meaning, content and process of thoughts and their relationship to emotions, risks losing the interpersonal and social dimension of depression. However, this dimension plays an important part in the maintenance, exacerbation, or reduction of depressed mood. Gotlib and Hammen (1996) argue that it is important to integrate the inner experiences of depressed people with their interactions with the environment and emphasise the importance of cognitions which mediate the emotional impact of external circumstances.

Feeling believed emerges as a central issue, somewhat in contrast to the focus in pain research on instrumental help (solicitousness). As a subjective complaint with no external referents, it is not only hard to communicate quality and quantity of pain to others, but it is more easily discounted or dismissed by others, particularly given lay and medical theories that it can be psychologically generated or serve as a proxy complaint for psychopathology ('all in the mind'). It can be doubly stigmatised: as a psychological or psychiatric problem, and as dishonesty or suspected malingering. The dilemma of whether to tell others about the chronic pain, risking listeners' negative judgements about veracity of pain and its disabling effects, or to say nothing, worsening isolation and sacrificing the chance of help or comfort, was eloquently expressed by interviewees in a paper by Hilbert (1984). A study by James and Large (1992) found that closest others located physical illness as more central to the chronic pain patient's sense of self than did the patient. Closest others also believed that they, and the patient's doctor, understood pain well, in contradiction to the patient's account. Not feeling understood or believed about their pain was a major reason given by chronic pain sufferers for not communicating (Morley et al., 2000), and reference was made to the impact on self-worth of such experience. Family interactions characterised by high conflict and lack of mutual support were found to be related to higher levels of depression in a chronic pain sample (Tota-Faucette et al., 1993).

The main theories concerning social support and physical and psychological health are of a main effect, which promotes wellbeing, and a stress-buffering effect which mitigates the negative impact of stresses when they occur. Although they pay increasing attention to important psychological differences such as perceived versus actual support, and social versus instrumental transactions, concepts such as obligations and indebtedness, which the pain sufferer with a poor self-concept feels s/he can never discharge, are largely lacking, as is the potential for unasked help

to be experienced as intrusive and undermining of confidence (Revenson et al., 1991; Paulsen and Altmaier, 1995). In addition, there is evidence from a meta-analysis of social support literature that those with physical health problems gain from experts' advice and help at least as much as from emotional support (Schwarzer and Leppin, 1992). Fitzpatrick et al. (1991) found in a sample of rheumatoid arthritis patients that depression was partly predicted over 6 months by the adequacy of relationships with friends and neighbours; close attachments appeared to be little affected by disability, and the effects on depression of pain and disease variables were negligible. They encourage the recognition of the importance of social support given by health professionals and other carers, alongside treatment.

Chronic pain has been shown to have an impact on the mood and health of spouses and family members of pain patients (Flor et al., 1987). Marital satisfaction, and the physical and emotional health of spouses suffer. Appropriate help is not, however, straightforward, with differences between intentions and effects both of help giving and receiving. Cognitive behavioural intervention tends to be prescriptive about spouses reducing practical help to patients, which may promote disability, but pays little attention to emotional support and problem sharing, or to the beliefs of spouses which underpin their behaviours. In relation to social behaviour, a depressed patient, preoccupied with pain and/or unable to take part in group activities, may find him or herself avoided by others, compounding isolation (Feldman and Gotlib, 1993).

4. Cognitive models

When chronic pain develops in a previously healthy individual, the huge impact of chronic pain on many aspects of his or her life may evoke feelings of being frustrated, restricted, and disappointed in existing and anticipated roles and expectations. However, one individual will retain a sense of self-worth while another will feel diminished, his or her sense of who s/he is completely undermined by the changes brought about by pain. By contrast, in individuals who have had previous episodes of depression, the experience of chronic pain may reactivate negative schemata, that is, beliefs concerning their worthlessness and certainty of failure in all endeavours. While roles and expectations were satisfactorily met such beliefs were relatively dormant, but when reactivated they trigger another episode of depression. These hypotheses predict differences in cognitive style and so may be tested by looking in more detail at cognitive content and processing.

4.1. Cognitive content and processing

The application of paradigms from cognitive science to clinical studies has been very productive in contributing to the understanding of the information processing and cognitive content involved in clinical fears and depression (Alloy et al., 1997; Pincus et al., 1998). Individuals actively process incoming stimuli using pre-existing mental structures (schemata) constructed through experience. These schemata play an important role in organising and integrating information, including in memory, but with bias built in. Many different terms are used when referring to cognitive structures, input and output. A 'meta-construct' framework (Ingram et al., 1998) suggests three categories for particular groups of constructs: cognitive structures (e.g. memory) and propositions or content (e.g. knowledge) which includes schema-based models; cognitive products (e.g. attributions, thoughts and beliefs), some of which are thought to be accessible to conscious awareness; and cognitive processes (e.g. encoding, retrieval) which occur at a subconscious level.

4.2. Content and processing in depression

Beck's cognitive theory of depression (Beck, 1976) proposed that the core problems in depression stemmed from thinking distortions due to the dominance of certain negative schemata. The problems arise as a result of the negative way in which the depressed person views him/herself, his/her current experiences and future. All incoming information is subject to these biases and subject to selective attention. Experimental studies that have been conducted to provide evidence for these will be discussed below.

Key models such as Beck's cognitive theory were developed for specific clinical problems including depression. Evidence for the validity of such models relies largely on self-report measures, thus on conscious cognitive products such as beliefs and coping attempts (Alloy et al., 1997; Calfas et al., 1997). Certain experimental methods offer a way of investigating information processing biases that arise as a consequence of the self-schemata, and are not ordinarily accessible to conscious awareness. Particular biases in processing information tend to be associated with specific psychological problems (Williams et al., 1988): empirical work suggests characteristic attentional and perceptual processes in anxiety (e.g. Matthews and MacLeod, 1985), including in pain (Eccleston and Crombez, 1999; Vlaeyen and Linton, 2000), and memory biases in depression (e.g. Williams, 1992).

Empirical studies, mainly using recall of presented material, support Beck's notion of preferential processing of self-referential material consistent with the negative self-schemata of depressed people (Derry and Kuiper, 1981). To some extent such processing even occurs in those with previous but not current depression (Bradley and Matthews, 1988) and in those who may be at high cognitive risk to depression as measured by the content of self-statements (Alloy et al., 1997). Greater recall in self-referential encoding tasks provides evidence for the self-schema model of information processing. The increased recall of specific, relevant adjectives suggest that content is important to information processing biases. Further evidence for content specificity has been demonstrated by Barton and Morley (1999) using a sentence completion task. In sentences containing self as the agent, depression was significantly correlated with negative self, world and future completions but not with past or other people. When other people were in the agent role the significant correlation with depression was for self completions.

Barton (2000) expresses concern over the relative neglect of content (thus of meaning) in depression, in comparison with fears and phobias (including in pain: Vlaeyen and Linton, 2000) where the personal meaning of self-statements is central (Clark and Steer, 1996). A focus on the negativity of statements without reference to their accuracy or personal significance, or to their potential association with depressed mood, does not constitute effective therapy: material needs to be relevant and emotionally significant.

4.3. Content and processing in pain

These cognitive experimental approaches have been applied to patients with chronic pain both with and without current depression (for a review see Pincus and Morley, 2001). People with chronic pain show preferential recall for pain-related words compared to neutral words when rating the degree to which these words refer to themselves, whereas normal controls show no differential recall (Pincus et al., 1993). A common criticism of such studies is that the bias is due to the effect of mood (Edwards et al., 1992), so the methodology was further refined to try to tease out the bias attributable to pain or depression. Pincus et al. (1995) found that whereas depressed chronic pain patients selectively endorse and recall self-referent pain information, non-depressed patients do not. There was no difference between the groups on the depression related words. However, findings in this area are not entirely consistent, and it is suggested that the differences may be due to the nature of the words used, which lends further support to the importance of cognitive specificity. To explain these findings, conclusions have been drawn (Clemmy and Nicassio, 1997) about the existence of an illness self-schema in people with chronic pain.

Cognitive measures may be useful when investigating qualitative differences in depressive thinking as they are free from the confound of the somatic symptoms that characterise chronic pain and depression. As discussed earlier, sentence completion tasks have performed well in generating individual cognitive content related to specific patterns of neg-

ative thinking in depression: completed sentences in depressed people reveal negative reference to self, future and world in depressive thinking (Barton and Morley, 1999), and to interpersonal difficulties. Research is underway to explore the use of sentence completion tasks in chronic pain patients. A study looking at cognitive bias in chronic pain patients, using personal and general vignettes, found that compared with depressed patients, depressed chronic pain patients displayed high levels of cognitive distortion in pain-related situations and less in non-pain-related situations (Smith et al., 1994): that is, the depressed pain group showed situational (pain) specificity whereas the depressed group generalised their distortions to hypothetical situations (e.g. being in pain).

Therefore it seems that it is possible to distinguish between depressed and non-depressed pain patients on differences in information processing and content. However, there has been little thought given to the possibility of differences *within* groups of people with chronic pain and depression. A focus on meaning would suggest differences in the representation of pain and depression in self-schemata depending on past experience. In people with a past history of depression, the experience of pain may reactivate their depressive representations producing a more clinical depression; in people without previous depression, the pain and its immediate practical effects may constitute the grounds for their distress, without their drawing conclusions about their self-worth.

Work examining the cognitive content of currently depressed, previously depressed (recovered) and never depressed chronic pain patients found situationally specific rather than global negative adjectives applied to the self by depressed patients, and fewer positive somatic adjectives (Clyde, 2000). The depressed group showed a distinct lack of self-denigratory endorsements characteristic of major depression in psychiatric samples. However, the patients were classified into groups on the basis of semi-structured diagnostic interviews which, as discussed earlier, are problematic. In addition in Clyde's study, current pain rating (similar across groups) was inversely related to the endorsement of positive bodily and situational adjectives, although pain ratings were not significantly correlated with depression score and controlling for depression score abolished the relationship, suggesting that reporting of pain intensity and adjective endorsement were mediated by current mood. It was also interesting that it was the recovered group who were the least negative about adjectives with bodily content. It may be that recovery from depression is associated with some adaptation to the negative aspects of pain, although moderate levels of distress suggest one should be aware of the risk of future episodes. The suggestion of a qualitatively different type of depression from that in physically healthy subjects is supported by a study by Smith et al. (1994) described above, and by findings in patients with Parkinson's Disease (Gotham et al., 1986).

5. Reformulations of models

How can the dynamic interplay between pain, mood and circumstances be represented in cognitive terms (Pincus and Williams, 1999). There is the need for a new model to aid understanding and treatment of pain and depression. This needs to incorporate several factors.

- The relationship between pain and depression is not a straightforward causal one.
- The development of depression is not inevitable in the context of chronic pain.
- There is a need to take into account both vulnerability to depression, and the nature of the individual experience of pain (the stressor).
- There may be several pathways by which pain and depression co-occur, resulting in qualitatively different subtypes of depression.

It is suggested that differences in cognitive content and processing may reflect both vulnerabilities to depression and the personal meaning of chronic pain and its wider impact. Vulnerability to depression, as discussed, may take the form of a 'cognitive scar' representing long-standing cognitive content and processing bias, established as a result of prior experiences. Beliefs such as "I'm not strong enough

to cope", or "I'm not worth other people trying to help me" may be activated by the situation of being in pain. Alternatively, as also discussed, the nature of chronic pain as a stressor, interference with everyday life and the process of acceptance may produce negative patterns of thinking.

The task of acceptance may come about by the process of accommodation and the development of new or revised schemata for chronic pain, incorporating new ideas about illness: for example, the transition from acute to chronic pain in terms of meaning and management and revised self-expectations (for instance, no longer an active, healthy person). Chronic pain thus presents a challenge to the individual's view of him/herself, the world, the future, and how others perceive him/her, and demands that individuals adjust their internal working models to fit the new information.

Pincus and Morley (2001) have postulated a schema enmeshment model of chronic pain. Three self-schemata interact: those pertaining to pain (sensory features), illness consequences (behavioural and emotional), and self (a dynamic, multifaceted structure including evaluation of self-worth). In construction of any experience, but particularly in situations of uncertainty, existing associative networks (Melzack, 1996) — effectively schemata — are used to assign meaning to external information. In the Pincus and Morley model of depressed mood in chronic pain, elements of schemata which are regularly associated are incorporated into one another, described as enmeshment (see Chapter 9). Only when the pain and illness schemata become enmeshed with the self-schema does distress result.

Pincus and Morley compare their model with that of Banks and Kerns by making processing of the stresses of pain crucial in the development of depression: the difficulties, limitations and disappointments have to be construed in a way which confirms a self-denigratory self-schema, rather than a self-schema of doing as well as possible under difficult circumstances, and there is selective attention to information content which is relevant to that self-schema, such as others' apparent criticism or disbelief, or stigmatising of disabled people. To account for the lack of self-denigration in distressed chronic pain patients, it is suggested that beliefs about the responsibility of pain for current difficulties and disappointments might 'protect' from the sense of worthlessness of clinical depression. For example, if limitations and restrictions are attributed to the effect of the pain, rather than to limitations of the self per se, then feelings of worthlessness and guilt may not occur: "I'm a failure because of the pain" rather than "I'm a failure and nothing can change that".

An advantage of this kind of formulation is that a focus on cognitive content and process, not least in measurement, bypasses the problems caused by the confound of somatic symptoms in both pain and depression. In addition, there are implications for treatment and possible interventions at different levels, which may help prevent subsequent distress.

6. Clinical implications

6.1. Medical assessment and treatment

Given what has been said about the importance for patients of feeling believed, and that their doctors are exerting themselves on their behalf, the possibilities for primary and secondary prevention probably lie mainly in the area of medical assessment and treatment of pain problems. Accounts of the difficulties faced by pain patients in relation to their doctors (e.g. Reid et al., 1991; Walker et al., 1999) contain descriptions of feeling understood and cared for, whether or not the doctor has initiated any effective pain treatment, as well as descriptions of feeling disbelieved, suspected, and neglected. The patient who experiences his or her doctor as a partner in the attempt to find the best solution to the problem of pain, even if it falls far short of pain relief, is far less subject to uncertainty, unwarranted fears and associated behaviour, may be able to work steadily on goals which are satisfying despite continued pain. Thus the recommendations for secondary prevention of chronic pain [refer to chapters in section 3] likely apply to some extent to the prevention of depression,

or its recurrence. It would be encouraging to see attempts to inform the patient about pain and agree the aims and methods of treatment used as often as are antidepressant drugs, widely prescribed although often in anomalous doses whether as analgesics (low dose) or antidepressants.

6.2. Suicide risk

There is relatively little guidance in the literature on the assessment of suicide risk in chronic pain, an appropriate concern for the treating physician, particularly if s/he is prescribing drugs which might be used in an attempt. Unfortunately, without an accurate assessment of depression, and a suitable comparison or normative group, estimates of risk in chronic pain are subject to the same problems as prevalence estimates, as described above. Normal good communication and questioning, as recommended in many professional guidelines, is adequate to elicit active suicidal intentions and plans, and these should be distinguished from statements such as "I sometimes wish I wouldn't wake up next morning", or "My family would be better off without me, I'm just a burden", both of which require exploring but tend to express hopelessness about the pain and its restrictions.

6.3. Pain programmes

In view of the strong association between pain and depression, it would be expected that treatment of depression would be an integral part of the management of chronic pain. A review by Sullivan et al. (1992) concluded that this was not the case: that little attempt was made to address depressive symptomatology and patients were treated as a homogenous group whether or not they were depressed. In studies examined for a recent systematic review (Morley et al., 1999), the cognitive content of the large majority consisted of attention management techniques taught and practiced during the programme; the educational component, if present at all, varied from specific information about pain and disease to comprehensive information about pain and treatments which introduced the rationale of pain management. Nearly half fell substantially short of a thorough examination along Beckian lines of automatic thoughts, with attempted identification and modification of unhelpful schemata. It is likely that the cognitive component of many multi-component group programmes for chronic pain is too brief, unchallenging and/or dilute for severely distressed and depressed patients. This practice is probably driven both by the tenet that if depression is secondary to pain then addressing pain is a proper aim (Maruta et al., 1989), but also by a relative neglect of cognitive content in the 'coping' and practical/behavioural elements of treatment: both may undermine adherence to treatment and its effectiveness.

6.4. Evidence-based treatments for depression

In reviews in the mid-1990s (Scott, 1995; Roth and Fonagy, 1996) of the large and evidence-rich field of depression treatment (in the absence of pain), equal benefits resulted from cognitive therapy (CT), behavioural therapy (BT), and interpersonal therapy: all are superior to pharmacotherapy in recovery from an acute episode of depression. At 2-year follow-up, CT-treated patients show less relapse than those who had received pharmacotherapy. Overall, efficacy supports the use of psychological therapies, but cost and time favour the use of pharmacotherapy; however, when relapse is taken into account, the saving in time and cost of pharmacotherapy is smaller.

All three psychological therapies share an understandable model of depression which underpins the structure of treatment and methods for change, all encourage the independent use of skills (in homework assignments) to make changes and those changes are attributed by the patient to him/herself, improving self-efficacy. In individual therapy, CT and BT aim to achieve collaborative hypothesis testing; this is not necessarily so easy in a group setting as is common in the pain field, and while BT is equally effective delivered in a group as to individuals, CT is less so (Scott, 1995). Other variables affecting efficacy should be taken into account when applying these findings to the design of pain

programmes. Therapist skill and adherence to the therapeutic model (independently assessed in trials) consistently account for up to 30% of variance in outcome (Scott, 1995). The drive to lower costs by recruiting undertrained and inexperienced therapists may thereby undermine the overall aims of treatment. Similarly, reducing therapeutic input has effects on efficacy. A dose–response effect emerged in one depression study (Barkham et al., 1996), with more rapid change in symptoms of acute distress (crying, pessimism, sadness) and slower change in characterological symptoms (self-accusation, work problems) and most somatic symptoms, so that although briefer therapy was effective, longer treatment brought about clinically significant change in a larger proportion of patients. Replication of such studies in chronic pain patients with current, previous and no history of depression would help to assign patients to appropriate treatment more accurately than use of current total depression score.

While Beck's cognitive model of depression remains central in the treatment of depression, further 'fine-tuning' is appropriate. Barton (2000) distinguished between negative thinking and depressive thinking, that is, the specific content of the negative thoughts. While experienced therapists can anticipate many of the commoner concerns, effective cognitive therapy must elicit from patients the emotionally laden content which is associated with distress. An undue focus on practical coping, particularly on attention diversion (for which the evidence supports use for mild to moderate pain, acute and predictable, rather than for unremitting or severe pain), characterised early pain management programmes. Latterly, cognitive therapeutic methods used for depression in the absence of pain have been more widely adopted, but there is still surprisingly little discussion of appropriate methods, either for those patients who meet criteria for depression or for those who do not but show some depressive thinking about pain. In a somewhat similar area, that of cognitive therapy with cancer patients, Moorey (1996) discusses the role of 'depressive realism', when it is acknowledged that the patient is contending with major difficulties. Similarly, addressing realistic rather than 'positive' thinking, which for many patients approximates an idealised view, and bias in thinking rather than distortion or error, demonstrates the therapist's commitment to comprehending the patient's perspective, an important ingredient of therapeutic alliance. In addition, depression and depressed mood can, despite the comments above, seem an overly narrow focus in the context of patients' reported emotions, and it is unfortunate that there is virtually no psychology of frustration, the most commonly named emotion associated with chronic pain (Price, 1999).

> *"there is a loose association between pain and depression . . . mixed up with frustration and other emotions"*
>
> (48 year old man)

Several of the other components of standard pain management can be expected to mitigate depressed mood: education can overcome misapprehensions about pain, quality of life improves with functional gains, and elements of behavioural therapy for depression, such as scheduling of pleasant activities and increasing availability of social reinforcement, are part of behavioural rehabilitation for pain. Exercise may produce mood elevation, although predominantly in those who are not depressed, but is not as powerful as behavioural or cognitive interventions.

There is also an unhelpful historical precedent for taking a behavioural approach to aspects of the cognitive domain. For instance, Morley et al. (2000) commented that: "what professionals may see as unhelpful 'pain talk' may serve a critical function in maintaining the sufferer's self-esteem", and the meaning and emotional impact of spouse behaviours cannot be incorporated in operant terms (Newton-John and Williams, 2000). The risks of overapplication by health professionals of 'pain behaviour' labels to patients' attempts to cope with pain, and lack of comprehension of spouse and family members' beliefs about pain and appropriate treatment, have particular relevance to primary and secondary prevention.

Group treatment, as is common in pain management, is designed to normalise the experience of chronic pain and associated difficulties, and to reduce stigma and isolation (Rudy et al., 1988). Therapist time and skill is needed to elicit and target individuals' relevant cognitions within the format of a standard cognitive teaching component; investment in the group by its members make disclosure easier. Time and skills suffer under the drive to economise, and group cohesion is weaker in brief and poorly facilitated groups.

7. Conclusion

The aim of this chapter has been to broaden the debate about the relationship between chronic pain and depression and to move away from the futile investigation into depression as a simple cause or consequence of chronic pain. We have endeavoured to enhance understanding about the complexity of the relationship by exploring new models and related ways of measuring depression in the context of chronic pain, and by increasing awareness of factors that contribute to distress. This extends opportunities for prevention and mitigation. We hope we have also drawn attention to potential areas for further investigation into the experience of pain sufferers, adopting and testing hypotheses from mainstream psychological research as well as exploring what is unique about depression in the context of pain.

References

Alloy, L.B., Abramson, L.Y., Murray, L.A., Whitehouse, W.G. and Hogan, M.E. (1997) Self-referent information processing in individuals at high and low cognitive risk for depression. Cogn. Emotion, 11: 539–568.

Atkinson, J.H., Slater, M.A., Patterson, T.L., Grant, I. and Garfin, S.R. (1991) Prevalence, onset, and risk of psychiatric disorders in men with chronic low back pain: a controlled study. Pain, 45: 111–121.

Banks, S.M. and Kerns, R.D. (1996) Explaining high rates of depression in chronic pain: a diathesis–stress framework. Psychol. Bull., 199: 95–110.

Barkham, M., Rees, A., Stiles, W.B., Shapiro, D.A., Hardy, G.E. and Reynolds, S. (1996) Dose–effect relations in time-limited psychotherapy for depression. J. Consult. Clin. Psychol., 64: 927–935.

Barton, S.B. (2000) New possibilities in cognitive therapy for depression? Behav. Cogn. Psychother., 28: 1–4.

Barton, S.B. and Morley, S.J. (1999) Specificity of reference patterns in depressive thinking: Agency and object roles in self-representation. J. Abnorm. Psychol., 108: 655–661.

Beck, A.T. (1976) Cognitive Therapy and the Emotional Disorders. Penguin Books, London.

Bradley, B.P. and Matthews, A. (1988) Memory bias in recovered clinical depressives. Cogn. Emotion, 2: 235–245.

Brewin, C. (1988) Cognitive Foundations of Clinical Psychology. Lawrence Erlbaum, London.

Brown, G.K. (1990) A causal analysis of chronic pain and depression. J. Abnorm. Psychol., 99: 127–137.

Brown, G.W., Harris, T.O. and Hepworth, C. (1995) Loss, humiliation and entrapment among women developing depression: a patient and non-patient comparison. Psychol. Med., 25: 7–21.

Calfas, K.J., Ingram, R.E. and Kaplan, R.M. (1997) Information processing and affective distress in osteoarthritis patients. J. Consult. Clin. Psychol., 65: 576–581.

Chapman, C.R. and Gavrin, J. (1999) Suffering: the contributions of persistent pain. Lancet, 353: 2233–2237.

Clark, D.A. and Steer, R.A. (1996) Empirical status of the cognitive model of anxiety and depression. In: P.M. Salkovskis (Ed.), Frontiers of Cognitive Therapy. Guildford Press, New York, NY, pp. 75–96.

Clemmy, P.A. and Nicassio, P.M. (1997) Illness self-schemas in depressed and nondepressed rheumatoid arthritis patients. J. Behav. Med., 20: 273–290.

Clyde, Z.K. (2000) Subtypes of Depression in Chronic Pain: A Study of Cognitive Content. Unpublished Doctoral Thesis, University of Leeds.

Costello, C.G. (1993) From symptoms of depression to syndromes of depression. In: C.G. Costello (Ed.), Symptoms of Depression. Wiley, New York, NY, pp. 291–302.

Derry, P.A. and Kuiper, N.A. (1981) Schematic processing and self-reference in clinical depression. J. Abnorm. Psychol., 90: 286–297.

Dohrenwend, B.P., Raphael, K.G., Marbach, J.J. and Gallagher, R.M. (1999) Why is depression comorbid with chronic myofacial face pain? A family test of alternative hypotheses. Pain, 83: 183–192.

Eccleston, C. and Crombez, G. (1999) Pain demands attention: a cognitive–affective model of the interruptive function of pain. Psychol. Bull., 125: 356–366.

Edwards, L., Pearce, S., Collett, B.-J. and Pugh, R. (1992) Selective memory for sensory and affective information in chronic pain and depression. Br. J. Clin. Psychol., 31: 239–248.

Feldman, L.A. and Gotlib, I.H. (1993) Social dysfunction. In: C.G. Costello (Ed.), Symptoms of Depression. Wiley, New York, NY, pp. 85–112.

Fishbain, D.A., Cutler, R., Rosomoff, H.L. and Rosomoff, R.S. (1997) Chronic pain-associated depression: antecedent or consequence of chronic pain? A review. Clin. J. Pain, 3: 116–137.

Fitzpatrick, R., Newman, S., Archer, R. and Shipley, M. (1991) Social support, disability and depression: a longitudinal study of rheumatoid arthritis. Soc. Sci. Med., 33: 605–611.

Flor, H., Turk, D.C. and Scholz, O.B. (1987) Impact of chronic pain on the spouse: marital, emotional and physical consequences. J. Psychosom. Res., 31: 63–71.

Gamsa, A. (1990) Is emotional disturbance a precipitator or a consequence of chronic pain? Pain, 42: 183–195.

Geisser, M.E. and Roth, R.S. (1998) Knowledge of and agreement with chronic pain diagnosis: relation to affective distress, pain beliefs and coping, pain intensity and disability. J. Occup. Rehabil., 8: 73–88.

Geisser, M.E., Roth, R.S. and Robinson, M.E. (1997) Assessing depression among persons with chronic pain using the Center for Epidemiological Studies-Depression Scale and the Beck Depression Inventory: a comparative analysis. Clin. J. Pain, 13: 163–170.

Gilbert, P. (1992) Depression: the Evolution of Powerlessness. Lawrence Erlbaum, London.

Gotham, A.-M., Brown, R.G. and Marsden, C.D. (1986) Depression in Parkinson's disease: a quantitative and qualitative analysis. J. Neurol. Neurosurg. Psychiatry, 49: 381–389.

Gotlib, I.H. and Hammen, C.L. (1996) Psychological Aspects of Depression. Wiley, Chichester.

Higgins, E.T. (1987) Self-discrepancy: A theory relating self and affect. Psychol. Rev., 94: 319–340.

Hilbert, R.A. (1984) The acultural dimensions of chronic pain: flawed reality construction and the problem of meaning. Soc. Probl., 31: 365–378.

Ingram, R.E., Miranda, J. and Segal, Z.V. (1998) Cognitive Vulnerability to Depression. Guildford Press, New York, NY.

James, F.R. and Large, R.G. (1992) Chronic pain, relationships and illness self-construct. Pain, 50: 263–271.

Klinger, E. (1993) Loss of interest. In: C.G. Costello (Ed.), Symptoms of Depression. Wiley, New York, NY, pp. 43–62.

Magni, G., Moreschi, C., Rigatti-Luchini, S. and Merskey, H. (1994) Prospective study on the relationship between depressive symptoms and chronic musculoskeletal pain. Pain, 56: 289–297.

Maruta, T., Vatterott, M.K. and McHardy, M.J. (1989) Pain management as an anti-depressant: long-term resolution of pain-associated depression. Pain, 26: 335–337.

Matthews, A.M. and MacLeod, C. (1985) Selective processing of threat cues in anxiety states. Behav. Res. Ther., 23: 563–569.

McCracken, L.M. (1998) Learning to live with the pain: acceptance of pain predicts adjustment in persons with chronic pain. Pain, 74: 21–27.

Melzack, R. (1996) Agreement on the value of theories of pain. Pain Forum, 5: 150–153.

Melzack, R. and Wall, P. (1988) The Challenge of Pain. Penguin, London.

Mineka, S. and Sutton, S.K. (1992) Cognitive biases and the emotional disorders. Psychol. Sci., 3: 65–69.

Moorey, S. (1996) When bad things happen to rational people: cognitive therapy in adverse life circumstances. In: P.M. Salkovskis (Ed.), Frontiers of Cognitive Therapy. Guildford Press, New York, NY, pp. 450–469.

Morley, S.J., Eccleston, C. and Williams, A.C.deC. (1999) Systematic review and meta-analysis of randomised controlled trials of cognitive behaviour therapy and behaviour therapy for chronic pain in adults, excluding headache. Pain, 80: 1–13.

Morley, S., Doyle, K. and Beese, A. (2000) Talking to others about pain: suffering in silence. In: M. Devor, M. Rowbotham and Z. Wiesenfeld-Hallin (Eds.), Proceedings of the 9th World Congress in Pain. IASP Press, Seattle, WA, pp. 1123–1129.

Nesse, R.M. and Lloyd, A.T. (1992) The evolution of psychodynamic mechanisms. In: J.H. Barkow, L. Cosmides and J. Tooby (Eds.), The Adapted Mind: Evolutionary Psychology and the Generation of Culture. Oxford University Press, Oxford, pp. 601–624.

Newton-John, T.O. and Williams, A.C.deC. (2000) Solicitousness revisited: a qualitative analysis of spouse responses to pain behaviours. In: M. Devor, M. Rowbotham and Z. Wiesenfeld-Hallin (Eds.), Proceedings of the 9th World Congress in Pain. IASP Press, Seattle, WA, pp. 1113–1122.

Novy, D.M., Nelson, D.V., Berry, L.A. and Averill, P.M. (1995) What does the Beck Depression Inventory measure in chronic pain?: a reappraisal. Pain, 61: 261–270.

Paulsen, J.S. and Altmaier, E.M. (1995) The effects of perceived versus enacted social support on the discriminative cue function of spouses for pain behaviors. Pain, 60: 103–110.

Pincus, T. and Morley, S. (2001) Cognitive processing bias in chronic pain: a review and integration. Psychol. Bull., 127(5): 599–617.

Pincus, T. and Williams, A.C.deC. (1999) Models and measurements of depression in chronic pain. J. Psychosom. Res., 47: 211–219.

Pincus, T., Pearce, S., McClelland, A. and Turner-Stokes, L. (1993) Self-referential selective memory in pain patients. Br. J. Clin. Psychol., 32: 365–374.

Pincus, T., Pearce, S. and McClelland, A. (1995) Endorsement and memory bias of self-referential pain stimuli in depressed pain patients. Br. J. Clin. Psychol., 34: 267–277.

Pincus, T., Fraser, L. and Pearce, S. (1998) Do chronic pain patients stroop on pain stimuli? Br. J. Clin. Psychol., 37: 49–58.

Polatin, P.B., Kinney, R.K., Gatchel, R.J., Lillo, E. and Mayer, T.G. (1993) Psychiatric illness and chronic low back pain. Spine, 18: 66–71.

Price, D.D. (1999) Psychological Mechanisms of Pain and Analgesia. IASP Press, Seattle, WA.

Reid, J., Ewan, C. and Lowy, E. (1991) Pilgrimage of pain: The illness experiences of women with repetition strain injury and the search for credibility. Soc. Sci. Med., 32: 601–612.

Revenson, T.A., Schiaffino, K.M., Majerovitz, S.D. and Gibofsky, A. (1991) Social support as a double-edged sword: the relation of positive and problematic support to depression among rheumatoid arthritis patients. Soc. Sci. Med., 33: 807–813.

Romano, J.M. and Turner, J.A. (1985) Chronic pain and depression: does the evidence support a relationship? Psychol. Bull., 97: 18–34.

Rosenstiel, A.K. and Keefe, F.J. (1983) The use of coping strategies in chronic low back pain patients: relationship to patient characteristics and current adjustment. Pain, 17: 33–44.

Roth, A. and Fonagy, P. (1996) What Works for Whom? A Critical Review of Psychotherapy Research. Guilford Press, New York, NY.

Rudy, T.E., Kerns, R.D. and Turk, D.C. (1988) Chronic pain and depression: toward a cognitive-behavioral mediation model. Pain, 35: 129–140.

Schmitz, U., Saile, H. and Nilges, P. (1996) Coping with chronic pain: flexible goal adjustment as an interactive buffer against pain-related distress. Pain, 67: 41–51.

Schwarzer, R. and Leppin, A. (1992) Social support and mental health: a conceptual and empirical overview. In: L. Montada, S.-H. Filipp and M.J. Lerner (Eds.), Life Crises and Experiences of Loss in Adulthood. Lawrence Erlbaum, Hillsdale, NJ, pp. 435–458.

Scott, J. (1995) Psychological treatments for depression: an update. Br. J. Psychiatry, 167: 289–292.

Skevington, S.M. (1995) Psychology of Pain. Wiley, Chichester.

Smith, T.W., O'Keeffe, J.L. and Christensen, A.J. (1994) Cognitive distortion and depression in chronic pain: association with diagnosed disorders. J. Consult. Clin. Psychol., 62: 195–198.

Sullivan, M.J.L., Reesor, K., Mikail, S. and Fisher, R. (1992) The treatment of depression in chronic low back pain: review and recommendations. Pain, 50: 5–13.

Sullivan, M.J.L., Thorn, B., Haythornthwaite, J.A., Keefe, F., Martin, M., Bradley, L.A. and Lefevre, J.C. (2001) Theoretical perspectives on the relation between catastrophizing and pain. Clin. J. Pain, 17: 53–61.

Tota-Faucette, M.E., Gil, K.M., Williams, D.A., Keefe, F.J. and Goli, V. (1993) Predictors of response to pain management treatment: the role of family environment and changes in cognitive process. Clin. J. Pain, 9: 115–123.

Turk, D.C. and Salovey, P. (1984) 'Chronic pain as a variant of depressive disease': a critical reappraisal. J. Nerv. Ment. Dis., 172: 398–404.

Van Praag, H.M. (1993) Diagnosis, the rate-limiting factor of biological depression research. Neuropsychobiology, 28: 197–206.

Vlaeyen, J.W.S. and Linton, S.J. (2000) Fear-avoidance and its consequences in chronic musculoskeletal pain: a state of the art. Pain, 85: 317–332.

Von Korff, M., Le Resche, L. and Dworkin, S.F. (1993) First onset of common pain symptoms: a prospective study of depression as a risk factor. Pain, 55: 251–258.

Walker, J., Holloway, I. and Sofaer, B. (1999) In the system: the lived experience of chronic back pain from the perspectives of those seeking help from pain clinics. Pain, 80: 621–628.

Wall, P.D. (1979) On the relation of injury to pain. Pain, 6: 253–264.

Williams, A.C.deC. (1998) Depression in chronic pain: mistaken models, missed opportunities. Scand. J. Behav. Ther., 27: 61–80.

Williams, A.C.deC. and Richardson, P.H. (1993) What does the BDI measure in chronic pain? Pain, 55: 259–266.

Williams, A.C.deC., Morley, S.J. and Black, S. (2000) Empirical evaluation of best practice in chronic pain management: influence of patient characteristics and treatment type on outcome. Report to the S Thames NHS Executive, SPGS 558.

Williams, J.M.G. (1992) The Psychological Treatment of Depression: A Guide to the Theory and Practice of Cognitive Behavioural Therapy. Routledge, London.

Williams, J.M.G., Watts, F.N., MacLeod, C. and Matthews, A. (1988) Cognitive Psychology and Emotional Disorders. Wiley, Chichester.

Wilson, K.G., Mikail, S.F., D'Eon, J.L. and Minns, J.E. (2001) Alternative diagnostic criteria for major depressive disorder in patients with chronic pain. Pain, 91: 227–234.

New Avenues for the Prevention of Chronic Musculoskeletal Pain and Disability
Pain Research and Clinical Management, Vol. 12
Edited by S.J. Linton

CHAPTER 9

Cognitive appraisal

Tamar Pincus [1,*] and Stephen Morley [2]

[1] *Department of Psychology, Royal Holloway, University of London, Egham TW20 0EX, UK*
[2] *Academic Unit, Psychiatry and Behavioural Sciences, School of Medicine, University of Leeds, Leeds LS2 9JT, UK*

Abstract: In this chapter we briefly discuss some of the methodological problems that occur in studying the relationship between cognitive factors and the development of chronic pain. We review evidence available from prospective studies that have attempted to measure cognition using questionnaire methods. The application of methods developed to explore information processing approaches to cognition is discussed and a model of schema enmeshment that seeks to relate cognitive processing to the poor adjustment to pain is outlined.

1. Introduction

Without doubt the presence of pain has a profound influence on the behavior, emotional state and the cognitive processes and content of the sufferer. But to what extent do these factors influence the development of chronic pain? In this chapter we will review the evidence for the influence of cognition on the development of chronic pain. Evidence for the direct influence of cognition would be most compelling if it could be shown that some aspect of cognition measured before the onset of pain determined whether or not the pain became chronic or determined the course of psychological adaptation to the experience of chronic pain. The ideal study would assess a random sample of the population at known periods before the onset of pain, which itself would be constrained between set parameters (mode of onset, location, intensity, etc.), and then followed up for an agreed minimum period, say 6 months, in which all other conditions were held constant. The

cognitive factor might reasonably be regarded as a vulnerability factor if only those possessing it developed chronic pain or followed a particular course of adaptation. It is unlikely that a study such as this could ever be performed and the evidence for cognitive factors in the development of chronic pain will necessarily be accrued via more circuitous means.

This chapter will describe and discuss the evidence concerning cognitive factors affecting pain experience and its outcomes (disability, care-seeking and distress) and outline models relating cognition to pain. Although the models described are not specific to musculoskeletal conditions, a significant proportion of the research has taken place in populations with musculoskeletal pain. Despite the attractiveness of the idea, the causal link between poor outcome and cognitive factors as risk factors remains speculative at present. A recent systematic review (Truchon and Fillion, 2000) identified more than 30 psychological variables that might be related to chronicity but lack of clarity in defining the constructs under-

* Correspondence to: T. Pincus, Department of Psychology, Royal Holloway, University of London, Egham TW20 0EX, UK. E-mail: t.pincus@rhul.ac.uk

lying the measures and the scarcity of prospective studies made it impossible for the authors to draw causal conclusions.

This chapter has two major purposes: to review the evidence for the influence of cognitive factors in the development of chronic pain experience and behavior; and to discuss, albeit briefly, some of the methodological and conceptual problems in this field of study. The emergent body of knowledge is generating new, testable models, that have implications for screening, prevention and treatment. Before discussing the particulars of what is known about cognitive mechanisms in the development of chronic pain we need to discuss a number of issues. (1) What is cognition and how do we identify likely candidates as vulnerability factors? (2) What aspects of chronic pain are we trying to relate to vulnerability factors? (3) What sort of time frame are we concerned with — is it relatively long-term (years), medium-term (months) or short-term? Mapping these features should help us clarify our current state of knowledge and suggest the likely candidates for further investigation and how preventative strategies might be developed.

1.1. What is cognition?

Cognition: "1. the mental act or process by which knowledge is acquired, including perception, intuition and reasoning. 2. the knowledge that results from such an act or process."

(Collins English Dictionary, 1993).

This definition rightly identifies the two main features of cognition as investigated by psychologists. The first part of the definition concerns the process by which knowledge is acquired, is reflected in contemporary studies of information processing. These studies typically use experimental methods to manipulate the way in which information is presented to individuals with the aim of testing whether hypothesized mental events influence some aspect of behavior. For example, participants may be presented with words representing variations in the state of illness or health and asked to classify them as to

whether they describe them self or another person. Subsequent tests of recall invariably reveal that self-descriptive words are more likely to be recalled than other-descriptive words, even when other features of the words known to affect recall are taken into account, e.g. word frequency. This and other experimental methods have been developed to test models of how individuals process knowledge. The techniques have been widely used to study psychopathological states such as anxiety and depression but only recently have they been applied to the study of chronic pain (see Section 2.2). The second part of the definition concerns the content of knowledge or the product of information acquisition. In this context content refers not only to the objective knowledge acquired but also to its emotional and motivational properties reflected in the beliefs and attitudes of a person. This information is frequently collected by self-report questionnaires that are designed to sample attitudes, beliefs and knowledge about health and pain.

It is tempting to equate studies of process with experimental methodology and studies of content with self-report methods but this would be unwarranted. For example, in the field of chronic pain there is a solid body of work on 'catastrophizing': a cognitive style of appraising pain and pain-related information (processing) that has relied exclusively on questionnaire measurement. However, in contrast we cannot think of an example of the use of experimental methods to assess the content of cognition, although in principle it is possible. For example, the development of an experimental method to assess implicit attitudes (Greenwald and Farnham, 2000) could, in principle, be applied to measuring cognition associated with pain. The example of implicit attitudes introduces a third feature of cognition not noted in the dictionary definition that concerns whether cognitive processes and content are available to consciousness. We assume that much cognitive activity occurs outside of awareness and is determined by relatively automatic processes that are not available to introspection or available for self-report. Even when cognitive content and processes are available to introspection and self-report an individual may dissimulate in order to present them self in a way that they perceive to be advantageous in a given situation, e.g. to preserve their self-esteem. Material that is available for self-report may also be biased by factors of which the individual is unaware, e.g. reporting remembered pain (Erskine et al., 1990).

1.1.1. Cognitive appraisal

Cognitive appraisal is usually described as two interactive processes that take place in response to a threatening stressful event (Lazarus and Folkman, 1984). Primary appraisal refers to the perception and evaluation of a perceived threat, and has been measured in musculoskeletal conditions through fear of pain, fear avoidance (see Chapter 20), or simply number of symptoms reported (Klenerman et al., 1995). Secondary appraisal involves the individual's appraisal of his ability to cope with the threat and its consequences, and has often been measured through self-efficacy, coping, catastrophizing, and health beliefs.

The relationship between primary and secondary appraisal in health and illness is complex but the model developed by Leventhal and his associates is a widely used framework that facilitates understanding. Their model (Leventhal et al., 1999) of illness representation comprises several components. The *Identity* of the disease, including symptoms and labels, is particularly important in musculoskeletal chronic pain, where chronic patients are often given vague labels like "chronic intractable benign pain syndrome" (Crue, 1985), "non specific low back pain" (Coste et al., 1992). Disagreement with diagnosis is related to high pain and distress levels, a belief in pain being a signal of harm, and overall disability (Geisser and Roth, 1998). The *Time-line* refers to the perceived onset, duration and recovery time. The perceived *Cause* is also considered of primary importance in musculoskeletal pain syndromes, because, for example, the belief that activity will further damage one's back will result in inactivity and ultimately increased disability. The illness representation model also includes beliefs about implications or the *Consequences* and beliefs about the *Control* of the illness.

1.2. What aspects of chronic pain?

Contemporary theories of pain recognize the importance of psychological factors and explicitly deny that there is a "hardwired, line dedicated, specialized pain system" (Wall, 1999, p. 2) between a stimulus and the observed response which is unmodified by psychological factors. Even reaction to brief, acute experimental pain is influenced by psychological characteristics of the stimulus and emotional states (Eccleston and Crombez, 1999; Price, 1999). There is general agreement in the psychological community that a variety of cognitive factors must be considered in developing a full understanding of both acute and chronic pain (Keefe et al., 1992; Turk and Rudy, 1992; Eccleston and Crombez, 1999; Robinson and Riley, 1999) and the dominant cognitive-behavioral paradigm provides a framework for most contemporary research. The cognitive-behavioral approach to chronic pain is based on several propositions (Keefe et al., 1992; Turk and Rudy, 1992), the central one being that an individual's emotions and behavioral activity in response to an event are influenced by the cognitive appraisal and interpretation of that event. Turk and Rudy (1992) summarize the perspective on chronic pain patients as being "viewed as active processors of information. They have negative expectations about their own ability and responsibility to exert any control over their pain. Moreover they often view themselves as helpless. Such negative, maladaptive appraisals about their situation and their personal efficacy may reinforce the experience of demoralization, inactivity, and over reaction to nociceptive stimulation. Such cognitive appraisals and expectations are postulated as having an effect on behavior, leading to reduced effort and activity and increased psychological distress." (Turk and Rudy, 1992, p. 103).

While this summary encapsulates many features of chronic pain patients it may unwittingly imply that patients with chronic pain form a homogeneous group characterized by overwhelmingly negative appraisals, negative motivational states and reduced behavioral repertoire. While this may represent a significant proportion of people, especially those attending tertiary referral centers, it does not capture the variability between people. For example, Turk and his colleagues have used multivariate methods to identify three sub-groups of patients, dysfunctional, interpersonally distress and adaptive copers (Turk and Rudy, 1988; Jamison et al., 1994; Rudy et al., 1995; Bergström et al., 1998). The adaptive copers are characterized by lower affective distress, higher activity level and higher ratings of life control than the other groups and they are more likely to be in employment (Bergström et al., 2001).

In considering whether cognitive appraisal is related to pain we need to separate three possible relationships. (1) Are cognitive factors influential in the persistence of pain, i.e. the experience of the sensory-intensity component of pain? (2) Do cognitive factors influence the likelihood that a person will develop the negative emotional and behavioral adaptations to chronic pain? (3) Do cognitive factors influence the likelihood that despite persistent pain the person will *not* show maladaptive responses i.e. do cognitive factors play a role in determining resilience? The significant point is that there are a variety of outcomes and that a cognitive vulnerability factor may relate to one or more of them. As chronic pain is not indexed by a single measure we need to distinguish between those who become heavy service users, those with high levels of disability and distress and those who apparently adapt to coexisting with a level of pain and perhaps some impairment but no related disability (psychological or physical). The presence of pain per se, therefore, is seldom considered an adequate end point in studies of musculoskeletal pain. In fact, in a recent study in the United Kingdom, researchers found that despite the fact that 60% of patients stopped consulting with their general practitioners about their back pain after only one consultation, only 25% of them reported that they were free of pain at 12 months (Thomas et al., 1999). One prominent consequence of chronic pain is depression. In a major review of the topic Banks and Kerns (1996, p. 99) concluded that major depressive disorder "is a common sequelae to the psychological experience of living with chronic pain". They proposed a stress–diathesis model in which the experience of pain elicits a set

of cognitions and behaviors that evolve into clinical depression. We shall return to this suggestion that subtle differences in cognitive appraisal might account for who becomes depressed and who becomes distressed without being depressed.

The difference between these three questions is mirrored in the choice of population and outcomes studied. In healthy populations, risk is associated with developing back pain. In acute conditions, risk is associated with developing chronic pain and disability, increased care-seeking or long-term absenteeism from work. In chronic conditions risk has also been associated with pain, disability, care-seeking and absenteeism, but in addition includes the risk of doing less well in interventions (predicting poor treatment outcome). Cognitive factors have been investigated in all three areas, but this chapter will focus primarily on the latter two. Within this framework a cognitive vulnerability factor might be related to one or more of a variety of outcomes but we need to be mindful that there are important non-cognitive factors that influence outcome, e.g. family and social dynamics and employment opportunities.

1.3. What is the time frame?

Our framework for this chapter is diagrammatically represented in Fig. 1. At the center of this figure is the onset of pain (the index event) from which chronicity may develop. To the left of the index event is the long-term past; to the right is long-term future. Evidence about the cognitive factors in the long-term past, before the first onset of pain, can only come from population-based studies. We will consider whether there are any data indicating that cognitive factors can predict which individuals are likely to develop chronic pain as the result of an episode of acute pain. We note that this question must be distinguished from the issue of whether cognitive factors carry a predictive role for the occurrence of acute pain, e.g. a cognitive style of sensation seeking may lead a person to expose himself to a behavioral risk (dangerous sports) which may increase the risk of episodes of acute back pain. We do not consider this issue here.

TABLE I

Cognitive predictors of long-term musculoskeletal problems

Reference	Outcomes investigated	Cognitive concept	Sample	Measurements used	Reported findings
Bigos et al. (1991)	Time to report of back pain injury	Controllability	Workers, free of pain at baseline	Health Locus of Control (MHLC)	No significant relationship
Burton et al. (1995)	Functional status (disability) at 12 months	Coping style, controllability	Patients, acute and sub-acute low back pain	Coping Strategy Questionnaire (CSQ), Health Locus of Control (MHLC)	CSQ catastrophizing, hoping and praying, significantly predicted 47% variance of disability, MHLC not significant
Estlander et al. (1998)	Persistent pain (days over 12 months)	Self efficacy	Patients, acute and sub-acute low back pain	Self Efficacy Questionnaire (SEQ)	Not significant
Gallagher et al. (1989)	Return to work	Controllability	Not reported	Health Locus of Control (MHLC)	Not significant
Haldorsen et al. (1998)	Non-return to work	Controllability	Patients, 8–12 weeks low back pain	Health Locus of Control (MHLC)	Significantly predicted 77% of cases
Klaber Moffett et al. (1993)	Report of back pain days over year	Controllability	Nurses, free of pain at baseline	Health Locus of Control (MHLC)	High external locus of control is a risk for developing back pain
Lancourt and Kettelhut (1992)	Absence from work	Coping	Patients, acute and chronic low back pain	Not reported	Not significant
Linton and Halldén (1998)	Accumulated sick leave	Coping style	Patients, acute and sub-acute back and neck pain	Single item from Coping Strategy Questionnaire (CSQ)	Not significant
Linton et al. (1999)	New episode of spinal pain	Coping style	Pain-free general population	Fear avoidance (FAB), catastrophizing (PCS)	Fear avoidance significant, increased risk for back pain at 12 months
Mannion et al. (1996)	First time serious low back pain	Controllability	Workers, free of pain at baseline	Health Locus of Control (MHLC)	High chance locus of control predicted first time serious LBP
Van der Weide et al. (1999)	Time to return to work, functional status	Coping style	Workers, off work for at least 10 days for back pain	??	Avoidant coping style predicted disability at 3 months

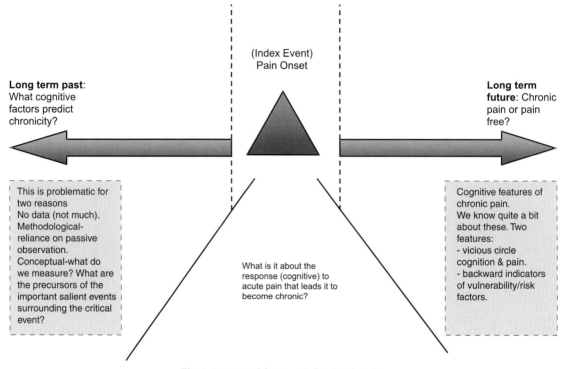

Fig. 1. A temporal framework for chronic pain.

Table I summarizes all the prospective and population-based studies that have measured cognitive factors at baseline and have focused on incidence of new cases of chronic pain as their primary outcome. This research, despite its intrinsic value for understanding population-based health patterns, is not very useful when examining the problem of developing long-term musculoskeletal problems. The limited use is due to several reasons.

First, only a fraction of the population of new cases of musculoskeletal cases can be explained by cognitive variables. The lifetime prevalence of an episode of acute low back pain, for example, is between 60% and 80% (Waddell, 1998, p. 72). In other words, most of us will suffer from acute low back pain at some stage in our lives, but we have a spread and breadth of cognitive responses. It is unlikely that our back pain can be explained, except in a few cases, by cognitive vulnerability alone or even primarily.

Second, only a fraction of acute low back pain sufferers go on to develop chronic disability (which should be considered separately from long-term pain; see below). Therefore, the sample size needed to establish the link from the population to the chronic stage (through the acute stage) would have to be impracticably high. It is not surprising that such data are scarce (see Table I). Despite the fact that most people with acute pain recover swiftly, up to 40% of them report further episodes on a regular basis. However, only 6% report serious disabling low back pain during the 12 months following onset (Papageorgiou et al., 1998).

Third, it is questionable whether cognitive vulnerability can be measured, through self-report before it has been 'activated' through an adverse event, such as the onset of a pain episode. The stress–diathesis model (Banks and Kerns, 1996) hypothesizes that such vulnerability could lie dormant until the interaction with the stress event (in this case, the experience of pain) 'switches it on', at which point it can be observed. There is evidence to support this suggestion from populations with depression. While many researchers now agree that depression is, at least to some extent, the result of a stable tendency to process and interpret information in a negative fashion, this tendency is difficult to demonstrate without the conjunction with the emotional response (i.e. sadness, loss, shame and guilt).

Fourth, currently research in population-based health studies mostly involves passive observation endorsement methods (i.e. questionnaires). These methods are non-experimental, so if the cognitive vulnerability factors are 'silent', they will not be activated or measured. We need to devise the right measures and the right challenges. The concept of vulnerability has been mostly explored in psychopathology (Zubin and Banks, 1977; Ingram et al., 1998). In their important discussion of cognitive vulnerability Ingram et al. (1998) characterize vulnerability as being relatively stable and trait-like and endogenous: it resides in the person not in the environment. The broad swath of vulnerability factors includes genetic factors, including behavioral genetics, as well as acquired biological and psychological traits. It is presumed that most cognitive factors are acquired, probably relatively early in life, and an important feature is that they may be latent until such times when the appropriate conditions activate them. One additional feature of vulnerability that distinguishes it from risk is that vulnerability includes a causal mechanism relating it to the pathological state. This account contrasts vulnerability with risk: risk factors are associated with the increased likelihood of pathology but do not point to what caused the disorder. Ingram and his colleagues discuss the complexities of this analysis of vulnerability with particular reference to depression. Dworkin et al. (1992), Banks and Kerns (1996) and Kerns and Payne (1996) and Dworkin and Banks (1999) have begun to explore vulnerability models for chronic pain and list a range of possible cognitive and psychological factors (somatization, somatic amplification, hypervigilance).

2. The evidence — review

Several recent systematic reviews have examined psychosocial factors as risk for the development of long-term disability in musculoskeletal groups (Truchon and Fillion, 2000; Linton, 2001; Pincus et al., 2002). The most stringent of these (Pincus et al., 2002) applied methodological criteria for appraisal and added two further sets of criteria: the second set focused on the quality of psychological measurement, and the third set including statistical considerations, such as sample size and use of appropriate multivariable tests together with provision of information enabling the calculation of effect size. The reviews found good evidence for depression/distress as a risk factor for the transition from acute to chronic pain. A multitude of cognitive factors have also been measured, but the evidence for increased risk is weaker. The following section outlines the most commonly investigated cognitive factors in prospective studies, and combined evidence from these with other design methodologies, including retrospective studies.

We suggest that with our present state of knowledge we are most likely to benefit from detailed examination of the acute pain (the index event). The question to be asked is: "What is it about the response to acute pain that increases the likelihood of the pain becoming chronic?" However, since the evidence relating this stage to outcome is scarce (see Table I), we will use the evidence from relationships in 'far future' stage, i.e. evidence for correlations at the chronic stage, to suggest theories and inform future research.

2.1. Self-reported cognitive factors

Most of the time people can provide accounts for their behavior. They can explain their reasoning and their beliefs, which have become a focus for investigation. Explicit behaviors, such as care-seeking, medication consumption, compliance and absence from work have been investigated in relation to such cognitions, with less emphasis on implicit behavior by which we mean the experience of pain, including its affective components such as distress, fear and anger. Specific questionnaires have been developed to measure cognitive factors. Despite the shortcomings associated with self-report, to which we will return at the end of this section, most of these questionnaires have excellent psychometric properties and have been used extensively in research.

2.1.1. Health beliefs

General beliefs about one's health and knowledge of a range of illnesses are well established by young adulthood. Health beliefs, and especially the belief that clinicians should be able to correctly and specifically diagnose and treat musculoskeletal conditions have long been considered a hindrance to recovery: strongly held beliefs in the responsibility and power of the medical profession can result in repeated and varied care-seeking, frustration, and passivity on the part of the patient. These beliefs are also in direct contradiction with current guidelines, which emphasize self-management, avoiding giving specific diagnosis and patients remaining active (Royal College of General Practitioners, 1999). However, the evidence on health beliefs as predictors of health care utilization, long-term disability and absenteeism is contradictory (see Table I). Health beliefs are frequently measured with the Multidimensional Health Locus of Control scale, MHLC (Wallston et al., 1978), which includes three subscales: Internal Locus of Control, where a high score indicates that individuals feel they are primarily responsible for their own health; External Locus of Control (also known as Powerful Others), where a high score indicates that an individual believes that the responsibility for their health lies primarily with clinicians; and Chance, where a high score indicates that the individual believes that very little control over health is possible. While this questionnaire has been extensively used in research of pain patients, the interpretation of the results obtained is often difficult and the implications for intervention sometimes obscure. Three prospective cohort studies have examined health locus of control as a risk factor for long-term disability in back pain, and three other studies investigated their role in population which were pain-free at baseline. A Norwegian study examined 260 individuals with sub-acute low back pain (8–12 weeks in duration) in relation to return to work, and established that non-returnees to work

could be predicted through the MHLC, above and beyond reported symptoms (Haldorsen et al., 1998). This finding is supported by North American research (Gallagher et al., 1989), but both studies have been criticized for recruiting individuals at too late a stage to establish a clear causal path (Pincus et al., 2002). In contrast, a smaller study of acute back pain sufferers found no predictive value in the MHLC, when entered with other cognitive and psychological variables (catastrophizing and depression) to predict disability scores at 12 months (Burton et al., 1995). Less specific beliefs about the role of clinicians have also been found to relate to pain, disability and care-seeking. In a large retrospective study, consulting a health professional for back pain was associated with the belief that clinicians are responsible for pain management (Waxman et al., 1998). In contrast, a recent study found that beliefs that physicians should find a definitive cause and permanent cure for back pain predicted neither medication consumption nor visits to clinicians (Saunders et al., 1999). Agreement with the clinical diagnosis provided has also been investigated in relation to pain and distress. A retrospective study of chronic neck and back pain found that patients who disagreed with their diagnosis reported the highest levels of pain, and the greatest level of distress (Geisser and Roth, 1998).

2.1.2. Self-efficacy

Closely related to the concept of locus of control is the concept of self-efficacy, defined by Bandura (1977) as the confidence one has that a desired behavior can be carried out. Recent reviews of health behavior have placed a great emphasis on self-efficacy as a predictor of behavior intentions, and behavior change (Schwarzer, 1992). This is meaningful for clinicians intervening in chronic musculoskeletal conditions, because although it may prove difficult to reduce pain per se, targeting behaviors such as health care utilization, medication consumption and inactivity can result in reducing both suffering and the extent of the disease burden. Self-efficacy is considered to be amenable to change, thus, evidence for low self-efficacy as potential risk has important clinical implications. Despite this, there are very few prospective studies that have included self-efficacy as a potential risk, or mediating factor. A large Finnish study of people over the age of 54 failed to find evidence for self-efficacy as a predictor of health status at 12 months (Estlander et al., 1998). However, individuals were not recruited at early stages of pain. In related populations, and especially in individuals with rheumatoid arthritis, measures of self-efficacy at early stages of diagnosis have been shown to predict functional disability and distress later (Schiaffino et al., 1991; Shifren et al., 1999; Brekke et al., 2001). Retrospective studies have found a relationship between self-efficacy and disability in musculoskeletal groups (Watson et al., 1997; Johansson and Lindberg, 2000), and current psychosocial interventions emphasize treatments that increase a person's sense of efficacy over problem situations.

2.1.3. Catastrophizing

Coping strategies have been extensively investigated in chronic pain populations and specific pain-relevant scales of coping have been developed of which the most frequently used is the Coping Strategies Questionnaire, CSQ (Rosensteil and Keefe, 1983). The CSQ contains several sub-scales to tap the behavioral and cognitive strategies used to cope with pain. It also contains a sub-scale to assess thoughts of catastrophizing about the pain, e.g. "It's terrible and I feel it's never going to get any better" and "I feel I can't stand it any more". These items appear to reflect the secondary appraisal function described by Lazarus and Folkman (1984) rather than a coping strategy per se. Nevertheless catastrophizing as measured by the CSQ and the more recently developed Pain Catastrophizing Scale (Sullivan et al., 1995) is a reliable correlate of adjustment to chronic pain as measured by depression, employment status and perceived disability (Sullivan et al., 1998; Tan et al., 2001).

Catastrophizing is broadly described as an exaggerated orientation towards pain stimuli and pain experience (Sullivan et al., 1995), and has been described as an explanatory construct for variations in pain and depression in chronic pain patients (Keefe

et al., 1989). A well-constructed prospective study, albeit with a small sample size, measured catastrophizing in patients with acute back pain at baseline and 12 months later, using disability as a primary outcome (Burton et al., 1995). Catastrophizing was a significant predictor of adjustment with a large effect size.

Recently, researchers have questioned whether catastrophizing is simply a sub-set of depressive symptoms, constituting the cognitive and affective components of negative mood (Sullivan and D'Eon, 1990). At least two of the theoretical components of catastrophizing (Sullivan et al., 1995), namely rumination and helplessness, are also integral components of distress and depression. Unfortunately, the majority of research suggesting the catastrophizing 'predicts' disability and pain independently of depression, is based on cross-sectional studies (e.g. Sullivan et al., 1998). Future research should focus on clarifying the independent properties of the concept of catastrophizing from those that overlap with negative mood or distress. Although the causal path remains unclear, there is some evidence from research in chronic pain to suggest that targeting catastrophizing could reduce subsequent distress/depression (Turner et al., 2000a,b).

2.1.4. Comment

All of the evidence reviewed is based on self-report questionnaire measurements and while this method provides some evidence it is limited by problems of response bias. Individuals completing the questionnaires are often aware that there are favorable responses indicating socially desirable attitudes. In addition, self-report measures sample the products of cognitive processing rather than cognitive processes. People are sometimes unaware of their beliefs and attitudes especially in relation to threat (and pain is always a threat) where mechanisms such as denial or exaggeration act to obscure the true state of affairs.

A highly influential model of processing emotional information, including pain and illness, separates conceptual processing, which is conscious and controllable by the individual, from schematic processing, which is automatic, non-volitional and often unnoticed (Leventhal and Everhart, 1979). Experimental studies of cognitive bias enable researchers and clinicians to gain access to levels of cognitive structure not accessible through interviews and questionnaires. The following section describes recent research that attempts to account for schematic processing biases in chronic pain patients.

2.2. Automatic cognitive processes

It has been known for years that human processing of information from the world around us is neither an accurate nor a passive behavior. Nonetheless, it is intrinsically surprising that our senses might deceive us, and that our mind, including our beliefs, memories and expectations, might be directly responsible for this deception. General inaccuracies are perhaps best demonstrated by perceptual illusions that are almost universally misinterpreted (Robinson, 1972; Sekuler and Blake, 1994). The Cocktail Party Effect in which the individual's attention is drawn to the sound of his own name even across a crowded noisy room illustrates the interactive relationship between mental processing and the environment. This is an example of the environmental features — the sound of the name — 'grabbing' attention away from current activity. The shift of attention is automatic, and the person involved has little control over it. The converse can also occur: people can 'scan' a crowd for a familiar face, blocking out irrelevant information. This is an active behavior, almost completely controlled by the individual. People spend their lives interacting with the world, and constantly processing information, which is stored in memory, and can be retrieved to assist reasoning and affect behavior. While general distortions in perception have helped clarify perceptual mechanisms, it is individual distortions in perception that are the focus of this chapter, because these distortions have been related to various mental states, such as depression and anxiety.

Pertinent to this chapter is the observation that emotion plays a major part in selective processing. People tend to selectively process information that is congruent to their current mood. When people are happy, they tend to notice and recall more positive words, and when they are sad they tend to notice and recall more negative words (Williams et al., 1997). On the whole, the majority of people tend be in a state of constant flux in terms of their moods, with a decided preference towards happy or neutral moods. Being in a constant state of negative mood for long periods of time is considered unhealthy. Evidence for cognitive bias has been found in many mood disorders, and is especially strong for depression and anxiety. The role these biases play in maintaining and even causing mood disturbance is described as a vicious cycle. In depression, for example, people have been shown to remember more negative events than healthy controls, which results in individuals ruminating on loss and guilt and becoming more distressed and depressed (Teasdale, 1985), which as a consequence maintains their rumination. In anxiety, and especially in phobia, individuals have been found to pay more attention to information associated with their fear. It has been argued that these biases are not just a by-product of emotional disorders but that they play a significant role in their causation and maintenance (Williams et al., 1997; Ingram et al., 1998; Segal et al., 1999). There is evidence that similar cognitive processes occur in patients with pain, and we speculate how they might affect pain, distress and disability. Researchers in the field of chronic pain adapted the experimental methodology used in groups with anxiety and depression and applied them to pain patients. They hypothesized that if people with pain pay more attention to pain-related information they would become more fearful, disabled and distressed, they might impose pain-related interpretations on ambiguous stimuli, and they might selectively recall events associated with pain. Each of these biases will exacerbate a preoccupation with pain, thereby limiting active coping and enhancing distress, helplessness and hopelessness. Cognitive bias is therefore conceptualized as increased risk. The evidence for the existence of this bias is reviewed briefly below. [1]

---

[1] Pincus and Morley (2001) provide an extensive review of the literature.

2.2.1. Schema theory

There are various ways of conceptualizing how selective processes happen. One of the more common explanations uses the concept of a schema to describe the mechanism. Schemata contain a stored body of knowledge that interacts with the demands of the environment. In experimental situations the demands can be carefully controlled to explore various aspects of cognition. The most frequent tasks involve attention to particular information and ignoring other salient information, responding to information that has more than one potential meaning, and memory task where people are presented with different ways of encoding and retrieving information (Segal, 1988; Williams et al., 1997). These tasks are viewed as ways to explore the content and processing of the hypothesized schema that acts as a template for interpreting information. Information that matches the template receives preferential processing. So in addition to the environmental features dictating processing, e.g. complex information takes longer to process, our own previous experiences together with the emotions attached to them play a role in what we notice, how we interpret it, and how we remember it.

Individuals have multiple schemas ranging from those representing relatively objective classes of objects such as birds and animals to more abstract ones related to class or race. We are concerned with three particular ones: pain, illness and self. The pain schema represents the immediate properties of pain experience such its intensity and sensory intensity. It is associated with the interruption of ongoing behavior, escape from the source of pain and engagement in self-protective behaviors and recuperation. While the pain schema is closely related to the illness schema they must be considered as independent because there are illnesses that do not necessarily include pain as a symptom, e.g. hypertension and diabetes, and occasions when pain does not imply illness, as in acute experimental pain. The illness schema contains information about the affective and behavioral consequences of illnesses, and contains information about the identity, time-line, perceived causes, consequences and control of a particular illness. Individuals have separate schemas for partic-ular disease entities (e.g. influenza) which are structured in a similar way as the general illness representation framework (Leventhal, 1984). The self-schema has received considerable attention in recent years. Mathews and Bradley (1983, p. 174) simply describe it as "an organized cognitive structure within long-term memory, which may incorporate both general trait-like information about the self, as well as specific behavioral episodes". As with all schemas the content is not fixed, is acquired and discarded as new experiences are processed (Markus and Wurf, 1987). A salient property of the self-schema is to give information pertinent to the self priority over other more general information. At the hub of the self is a system that evaluates behavior, feelings and thought and generates a sense of self-worth.

Schemas are individual and unique. The elements within a schema are inter-related and structured so that the activation of one element will preferentially activate others close to it within the schema. The information contained within schemas is acquired through experience, and the complexity, size and activation of them depends on many factors. One factor is simply familiarity (frequency effect): the more an individual is exposed to certain information, the more the schema associated with this information will be prominent in processing. It is reasonable to assume that people with chronic pain are exposed to, and use, more pain words than other groups and that they have well developed schemas for processing information relating to pain and illness. This assumption underpins the research but it also means that it is necessary to control for the effects of mere frequency. For example, studies that have compared selective processing of pain words between pain patients and control groups made of students or other healthy individuals are considered inferior to studies that have used control groups that include people who use pain language often (such as physiotherapists, or nurses).

While it is reasonable to propose that people with substantial experience of pain may develop schemas representing specialized knowledge of pain, the suggestion that pain schemas may be present in non-patients and influence the development of chronic pain is harder to sustain. There is, however, good evidence of individual differences in cognitive biases for anxiety and depression-related material in non-clinical groups that may reflect vulnerability (Ingram et al., 1998; MacLeod, 1999). Within the field of pain there is recent evidence that variation in self-reported fear of pain in a student population without pain is associated with an attentional bias towards pain-related information (Keogh et al., 2001) and biases have also been shown to be activated by acute experimental pain (Pearce et al., 1990; Seltzer and Yarczower, 1991). Singer (1995) has shown how individuals with strong motivational desire to avoid pain are more likely to recall autobiographical memories of painful events. These studies suggest that schemas for processing pain-related information might be generally present in the non-pain population. The following three sections briefly review the available evidence for cognitive biases in chronic pain.

Attention bias. Attention bias towards pain-related information has been investigated using the emotional Stroop task. In this task individuals are asked to name the color in which words are printed, while ignoring the content of the words. The time taken to name the color of pain words such as sore, aching, and hurting, is compared with the time taken to name the color of neutral or emotional words. Although this paradigm has been criticized on the grounds that it is impossible to discern exactly where the bias takes place, it has been shown to produce a robust effect in a range of conditions, including anxiety states, phobias, eating disorders, PTSD, panic and depression (Williams et al., 1996). The general finding is that people take longer to name the color of words that have special significance for them, e.g. people with a specific fear of spiders are slower to name the color of words associated with spiders. It is hypothesized that the threatening information contained in significant words is selectively attended to and as a consequence it interferes with the simple task of color naming.

By analogy one might expect people with chronic pain or an activated pain schema to show interference in color naming pain-related words. However,

the effect appears to be more fragile in chronic pain. Two studies (Pearce and Morley, 1989; Snider et al., 2000) provide evidence for the hypothesis that the state of chronic pain biases attention towards pain-related stimuli. Another study (Boissevan, 1994) found slower color naming of pain-sensory words in pain patients but no group difference in color naming pain-affect words. [2] Other studies have failed to find the expected effect (Pincus et al., 1998; Crombez et al., 2000). One explanation for this contradiction suggests that it is not pain per se that results in selective attention towards pain stimuli, but an interaction between pain and fear, and specifically fear of pain. We have also suggested that paradoxically patients with chronic pain may be better at performing the Stroop task than 'new' pain patients because they have acquired strategies for managing the concurrent cognitive demand that is presented by pain. As a consequence we have predicted that people with recent onset of pain would be more likely to show the interference effect in the Stroop task (Pincus and Morley, 2001). This hypothesis has yet to be tested.

In addition to the Stroop test the dot-probe task has also been used to explore attention bias in pain patients. In this task two words are presented, one above the other, on a computer screen for a very brief period. At the offset of the words a dot is displayed in one of the locations and the participant is asked to press a key as soon as the dot is detected. Studies on people with anxiety have shown that faster responses occur when the dot is presented in the same spatial location as an anxiety cue (Williams et al., 1996). If pain patients do have a bias toward pain-related information they should show faster responses to probes presented at the same spatial location as pain-related cues. Asmundson et al. (1997) showed that people with chronic pain showed the predicted effect but only when they were classified as having high

---

[2] Many studies of cognitive bias have used pain descriptors selected from the McGill Pain Questionnaire (MPQ; Melzack and Katz, 1992) that includes words chosen to reflect the sensory and affective components of pain. We refer to these as pain-sensory and pain-affect words.

fear of pain. In contrast patients with low fear of pain showed evidence of attention away from pain words towards neutral words. As noted above, a study by Keogh and his colleagues (Keogh et al., 2001) showed that bias towards pain words was present in students with a high fear of pain. Keogh et al. also demonstrated that the bias was specific to pain-related words and not words conveying social threat.

Interpretation bias. Several studies have used tasks that require the individual to respond to ambiguous information. In the homophone task words that have two distinct meanings, depending on their written form, are presented aurally, for example pane/pain, flew/flu, groan/grown. Participants are simply required to write down the word that they hear. Under these conditions of ambiguity an individual must call on additional resources to respond and one such source of information is the salient active schema. When people with chronic pain are asked to perform this and similar tasks they typically provide significantly more pain- and illness-related words than the control group (Edwards and Pearce, 1994; Pincus et al., 1994, 1996; Griffith et al., 1996). However, these findings may reflect a simple frequency effect or participants may be aware of the ambiguity and deliberately bias their responses. Methods for controlling for these alternative explanation suggest that the results are not attributable to these alternative explanations and there is consistent evidence for bias across three experimental methods for illness- and health-related material, and where words describing the sensory component of pain have been included there is evidence that bias is related to the presence and intensity of current pain (Pincus and Morley, 2001).

Memory bias. There is strong evidence for a recall bias of pain-related information in people with chronic pain. The basic experimental method is to present the individual with a list of words that includes pain and neutral words and subsequently and unexpectedly asking them to recall as many words as they can. Pain patients have been shown to recall more pain words than other groups (Pearce et al., 1990; Edwards et al., 1992; Pincus et al., 1993,

1995; Johnson and Spence, 1994; Koutantji et al., 1999). This effect is particularly strong if participants are asked to make an initial judgment as to whether words describe themselves (Pincus et al., 1993, 1995; Clemmey and Nicassio, 1997; Koutantji et al., 1999). Another important finding has been that despite scoring high on depression questionnaires, depressed pain patients do not show the same bias as other depressed groups. Typically, recall bias in depressed groups has been towards words associated with low self-worth, such as guilty, unlovable, and shameful (Williams et al., 1997). In contrast, depressed pain patients show a marked bias towards illness-related words (Pincus et al., 1995). Preliminary findings have also suggested that this bias may be related to care-seeking. In a small study of chronic low back patients attending a general practice, Pincus and colleagues (Pincus et al., 2001) found a correlation between the degree of recall bias towards pain-related information, and the health costs for back pain treatment for each patient in the previous 12 months.

Summary of cognitive bias in pain patients. The studies reviewed represent a novel approach to studying cognitive factors in chronic pain. Previous work in the field has been strongly dependent on measurement via questionnaires. The approach to cognitive biases represented in the studies reported here offers potential to overcome these methodological constraints. In addition, some the more robust findings have important clinical implications. These include the dominant role of self-schema in cognitive bias, and the differentiation between the content of bias between pain patients who are depressed, and other depressed groups. Nevertheless, as with studies that have used questionnaires there is a paucity of longitudinal observations and in the absence of such data one can only speculate about the relationship between cognitive factors an the course of chronic pain. We have conjectured on how biases in appraisal of pain-related information might lead to the poor adaptation in the presence of continuing pain with particular emphasis on the occurrence of depression in chronic pain. A central feature of the model is that people who show poor adaptation to the presence of chronic pain do so because features of the pain and illness schemas become enmeshed with their self-schema.

3. Enmeshment and chronic pain

A major psychological property of acute pain is its ability to interrupt ongoing activity (Eccleston and Crombez, 1999). The interruption may be quite transitory such as that experienced in laboratory settings and in many everyday accidents: a cut while shaving merely interrupts the process of shaving but has no further consequences. Other acute pain may be more interruptive, e.g. menstrual cramps, because it lasts longer, nevertheless with most experiences of acute pain one is able to complete the ongoing activity. If a pain is repeated or continuous then it is more likely to have the effect of interfering with the task, so that one is either unable to complete it, or, if it is completed, one's performance is degraded to such an extent that it is regarded as personally unsatisfactory. Interruption and interference have unwanted consequences both in terms of task performance and emotional arousal, often experienced as frustration and irritation, but these are likely to dissipate when a pain abates and normal functioning is restored. If, however, pain and the associated interference persist, more deleterious consequences may follow in that a person may begin to experience a threat and change to their identity. We surmise that this is most likely when key aspects of a person's view of himself or herself are interfered with by pain. For example, a person who derives his major source of satisfaction from his ability to work to provide for his family is threatened not just by the interference with his ability to work but by the fact that the meaning of his work lost, even when he is provided for financially. If the person has no other source of self-esteem the interference with work is likely to have a devastating impact on his self-appraisal and identity (Leventhal et al., 1999).

We surmise that the poor adaptation to chronic pain is the consequence of marked changes in how people appraise and process information about pain,

health and the self. The schema enmeshment model proposes that the particular aspects of a person's self-schemas that are disrupted by pain determine the focus of enmeshment, and the cognitive and emotional consequences of it. Most importantly the model distinguishes between enmeshment where core elements of self-worth are involved and enmeshment where other aspects of the self are a focus. The pain, illness and self-schemas overlap to varying degrees. Fig. 2 shows four possible positions. In panel A the three partly overlap and it is unlikely that the pain schema is ever completely dissociated from either the illness or self-schemas. In panel B the pain and illness schemas are partly enmeshed but crucial elements of the self-schema remain relatively separate. We consider this to represent the state of chronic pain patients classified as adaptive copers (Turk and Rudy, 1990; Jamison et al., 1994). Their pain may interfere with their daily activity but crucially it does not impinge upon their core sense of self-worth. Such patients may have possessed a very resilient sense of self-worth and been relatively unaffected by the pain or as time has passed they may have forged a new self-identity in which pain and illness do not impact upon their sense of self-worth. There are also occasions where the pain and self-schema are enmeshed but where illness is not involved. For example an acute but transiently painful injury may have implications for a professional athlete's sense of self-worth. The most psychologically taxing situation arises when all three schemas become enmeshed and pain and illness become incorporated into the self. The significant feature is the degree to which the chronically activated pain schema becomes associated with the dominant content of the self-schema. Of particular concern is the development of depression and distress in chronic pain. People are most vulnerable when the content of their self-schema contains information that is congruent with dependence and distress. There is variation in the extent to which the self-schema is vulnerable with at least three possibilities. First there will be a small percentage of patients that have had a prior episode of depression. Even if they are not depressed at the onset of chronic pain it is likely that they will be

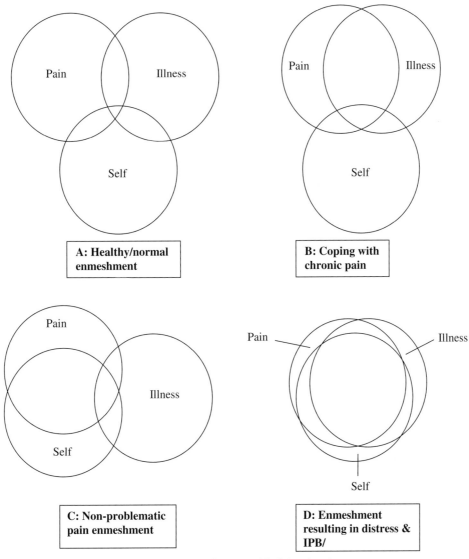

Fig. 2. The enmeshment model of chronic pain.

vulnerable to the development of chronic distress because they have a previously established cognitive vulnerability. In principle this vulnerability could be detected by the sort of experimental tasks we have described but simply enquiring about episodes of previous mood disorder will be easier. The second group of people vulnerable to depression following the onset of chronic pain comprises those who, although they have not experienced a previous episode of depression, have been exposed to events that have

compromised their sense of self-worth. They have been rendered vulnerable by prior experiences. Even without the onset of pain, people in this group are more likely to experience a depressive episode, and pain acts as a 'trigger' event. Both these groups of patients should exhibit their vulnerability to depression by showing bias towards stimuli incorporating self-denigration when their self-schema is activated. The final group of patients is those for whom vulnerabilities have not been established by earlier adverse experiences. They are less likely to become depressed as a result of chronic pain but they may become distressed. Pain appears to have a unique ability to "to pervade consciousness and interfere with cognitive functioning" (Banks and Kerns, 1996, p. 102), and as a consequence to interfere with many aspects of life. These patients will not show biases towards material reflecting negative self-worth but they will show biases towards negative references to negative aspects of illness and pain. At the level of self-report they refer to their situation as distressing but do not regard themselves in a self-denigratory light. The difference between those who are distressed and those who are depressed is reflected in the content of the cognitive biases observed, and especially by the extent to which negative views of the self are exhibited.

4. Conclusion

Cognitive appraisal of the pain experience in its complexity clearly plays a major role in decisions about behavior, and impacts on pain distress and suffering. Theoretically, it should be possible to research and model individual cognitive processes and test their impact on pain and health. This impact should include positive processes, resulting in resilience and successful coping, as well as negative processes, resulting in increased distress, and perhaps maintenance of pain. We have outlined several theories that explain how cognitive processing might impact on pain at several different levels, both conscious and preconscious. To date, there is only partial evidence for the models. Although there is sufficient evidence to conclude that cognitive appraisal in pain is varied (i.e. that individual differences exist in terms of content and process), and that these differences are related to pain and suffering, there is almost no evidence to suggest causal paths. This means that the models at present are limited in terms of their clinical application.

Further research is indicated. The most gaping hole in the evidence is the lack of prospective studies, to clarify issues of risk and vulnerability. There

are now methodologies to carry out the complex analysis necessary to test for multiple variables both at baseline and outcome, and to develop, test and compare the explanatory quality of different models. Self-report of cognitive processes needs refining, and combining experimental approaches with qualitative in-depth self-report could inform about patients' level of awareness of their cognitions, and especially their biases. This information is necessary if we aim to change cognitive processing, since co-operation and empowerment of patients is a key element for success, or even a pre-requisite for participation in treatment.

Finally, the review of the evidence for cognitive appraisal and its impact on pain reveals that despite the scarcity of data, the variability of methodologies and the contradictory findings, there appears to be a repeating element common to positive findings. The strongest evidence is for catastrophizing as a strategy for maladaptive coping, and for preconscious processing biases towards pain and distress stimuli. The uniting element is the concept of the self.

References

Asmundson, G.J., Kuperos, J.L. and Norton, G.R. (1997) Do patients with chronic pain selectively attend to pain-related information? Preliminary evidence for the mediating role of fear. Pain, 72: 27–32.
Bandura, A. (1977) Self-efficacy: toward a unifying theory of behavioral change. Psychol. Rev., 84: 191–215.
Banks, S.M. and Kerns, R.D. (1996) Explaining high rates of depression in chronic pain: a diathesis stress framework. Psychol. Bull., 119: 95–110.
Bergström, G., Jensen, I.B., Bodin, L., Linton, S.J., Nygren, A.L. and Carlsson, S.G. (1998) Reliability and factor structure of the Multidimensional Pain Inventory — Swedish Language Version (MPI-S). Pain, 75: 101–110.
Bergström, G., Jensen, I.B., Bodin, L., Linton, S.J. and Nygren, A. (2001) The impact of psychologically different patient groups on outcome after a vocational rehabilitation program for long-term spinal pain patients. Pain, 93: 209–237.
Bigos, S.J., Battie, M.C. and Spengler, D.M. et al. (1991) A prospective study of work perceptions and psychosocial factors affecting the report of back injury. Spine, 16: 688–696.
Boissevan, M. (1994) Information processing in chronic pain. Unpublished doctoral dissertation. University of Western Ontario, London, Ontario, Canada.
Brekke, M., Hjortdahl, P. and Kvien, T.K. (2001) Self efficacy

and health status in rheumatoid arthritis: a two year longitudinal observational study. Rheumatology, 40: 387–392.

Burton, A.K., Tillotson, K.M., Main, C. and Hollis, S. (1995) Psychosocial predictors of outcome in acute and sub chronic low back trouble. Spine, 20(6): 722–728.

Clemmey, P.A. and Nicassio, P.M. (1997) Illness self-schema in depressed and nondepressed rheumatoid arthritis patients. J. Behav. Med., 20: 273–290.

Coste, J., Paolaggi, J.B. and Spira, A. (1992) Classification of non-specific low back pain. Psychological involvement in low back pain. Spine, 17: 1028–1037.

Crombez, G., Hermans, D. and Adriaensen, H. (2000) The emotional stroop task and chronic pain: what is threatening for chronic pain sufferers? Eur. J. Pain, 4: 37–44.

Crue, B.L. (1985) Multidisciplinary pain treatment programs: current status. Clin. J. Pain, 1: 31–38.

Dworkin, R.H. and Banks, S.M. (1999) A vulnerability-diathesis-stress model of chronic pain: herpes zoster and the development of postherpetic neuralgia. In: R.J. Gatchel and D.C. Turk (Eds.), Psychosocial Factors in Pain: Critical Perspectives. Guilford Press, New York, NY, pp. 247–269.

Dworkin, S.F., von Korff, M.R. and LeResche, L. (1992) Epidemiologic studies of chronic pain: a dynamic–ecologic perspective. Ann. Behav. Med., 14: 3–11.

Eccleston, C. and Crombez, G. (1999) Pain demands attention: a cognitive–affective model of the interruptive function of pain. Psychol. Bull., 125: 356–366.

Edwards, L. and Pearce, S. (1994) Word completion in chronic pain: Evidence for schematic representation of pain. J. Abnormal Psychol., 103: 379–382.

Edwards, L., Pearce, S., Collett, B.-J. and Pugh, R. (1992) Selective memory for sensory and affective information in chronic pain and depression. Br. J. Clin. Psychol., 31: 239–248.

Erskine, A., Morley, S. and Pearce, S. (1990) Memory for pain: a review. Pain, 41: 255–265.

Estlander, A.M., Tkala, E.P. and Viikari-Juntura, E. (1998) Do psychological factors predict changes in musculoskeletal pain? A prospective, two year follow-up study of the working population. J. Occup. Environ. Med., 40: 445–453.

Gallagher, R.M., Rauh, V. and Haugh, L.D. (1989) Determinants of return to work among low back pain patients. Pain, 39: 55–67.

Geisser, M.E. and Roth, R.S. (1998) Knowledge of and agreement with chronic pain diagnosis: relation to affective distress, pain beliefs and coping, pain intensity and disability. J. Occup. Rehabil., 8: 73–88.

Greenwald, A.G. and Farnham, S.D. (2000) Using the Implicit Association Test to measure self-esteem and self-concept. J. Pers. Soc. Psychol., 79: 1022–1038.

Griffith, J., McLean, M. and Pearce, S.A. (1996) Information processing across three chronic pain groups. In: abstracts of 7th World Congress on Pain. Seattle, WA. International Association for the Study of Pain, p. 75.

Haldorsen, E.M., Indahl, A. and Ursin, H. (1998) Patients with low back pain not returning to work. A 12 month follow up study. Spine, 23: 1202–1208.

Ingram, R.E., Miranda, J. and Segal, Z.V. (1998) Cognitive Vulnerability to Depression. Guilford Press, New York, NY.

Jamison, R.N., Rudy, T.E., Penzien, D.B. and Mosley Jr., T.H. (1994) Cognitive-behavioral classifications of chronic pain: replication and extension of empirically derived patient profiles. Pain, 57: 277–292.

Johansson, E. and Lindberg, P. (2000) Low back pain patients in primary care: subgroups based on the multidimensional pain inventory. Int. J. Behav. Med., 7: 340–352.

Johnson, R. and Spence, S. (1994) Pain affect and cognition in children: Recall bias associated with pain. In: G.F. Gebhart, D.L. Hammond and T.S. Jensen (Eds.), Progress in pain research and management, vol . Proceedings of the 7th World Congress On Pain. International Association for the Study of Pain, Seattle, WA, pp. 877–884.

Keefe, F.J., Brown, G.K., Wallston, K.A. and Caldwell, D.S. (1989) Coping with rheumatoid arthritis pain: catastrophizing as a maladaptive strategy. Pain, 37: 51–56.

Keefe, F.J., Dunsmore, J. and Burnett, R. (1992) Behavioral and cognitive-behavioral approaches to chronic pain: recent advances and future directions. J. Consult. Clin. Psychol., 60: 528–536.

Keogh, E., Ellery, D., Hunt, C. and Hannent, I. (2001) Selective attentional bias for pain-related stimuli amongst pain fearful individuals. Pain, 91: 91–100.

Kerns, R.D. and Payne, A. (1996) Treating families of chronic pain patients. In: R.J. Gatchel and D.C. Turk (Eds.), Psychological Approaches to Pain Management: A Practitioner's Handbook. Guilford Press, New York, NY, pp. 283–304.

Klaber Moffett, J.A., Hughes, G.I. and Griffiths, P. (1993) A longitudinal study of low back pain in student nurses. Int. J. Nurs. Stud., 30: 197–212.

Klenerman, L., Slade, P.D. and Stanley, M. et al. (1995) The prediction of chronicity in patients with an acute attack of low back pain in a general practice setting. Spine, 20: 478–484.

Koutantji, M., Pearce, S.A., Oakley, D.A. and Feinmann, C. (1999). Children in pain: An investigation of selective memory for pain and psychological adjustment. Pain, 81: 237–244.

Lancourt, J. and Kettelhut, M. (1992) Predicting return to work for low back pain patients receiving workers compensation. Spine, 17: 629–640.

Lazarus, R. and Folkman, S. (1984) Stress Appraisal and Coping. Springer, New York, NY.

Leventhal, H. (1984) Perceptual motor theory of emotion. Adv. Exp. Soc. Psychol., 17: 117–182.

Leventhal, H. and Everhart, D. (1979) Emotion, pain and physical illness. In: C.E. Izard (Ed.), Emotions in Personality and Psychopathology. Plenum Press, New York, NY, pp. 263–299.

Leventhal, H., Idler, E.L. and Leventhal, E.A. (1999) The impact of chronic illness on the self system. In: R.J. Contrada and R.D. Ashmore (Eds.), Self, Social Identity, and Physical Health: Interdisciplinary Explorations. Rutgers Series on Self and Social Identity, Vol. 2, Oxford University Press, New York, NY, pp. 185–208.

Linton, S.J. (2001) Occupational psychological factors increase the risk for back pain: a systematic review. J. Occup. Rehabil., 11: 53–66.

Linton, S.J. and Halldén, K. (1998) Can we screen for problematic back pain? A screening questionnaire for predicting outcome in acute and subacute back pain. Clin. J. Pain, 14: 209–215.

Linton, S.J., Buer, N., Vlaeyen, J. and Hellsing, A.L. (1999) Are fear-avoidance beliefs related to a new episode of back pain? A prospective study. Psychol. Health, 14: 1051–10519.

MacLeod, C. (1999) Anxiety and anxiety disorders. In: T. Dalgleish and M.J. Power (Eds.), Handbook of Cognition and Emotion. Wiley, Chichester, pp. 447–477.

Mannion, A.F., Dolan, P. and Adams, M.A. (1996) Psychological questionnaires: do 'abnormal' scores precede or follow first-time low back pain? Spine, 21: 2603–2611.

Markus, H. and Wurf, E. (1987) The dynamic self-concept: a social psychological approach. Annu. Rev. Psychol., 38: 299–337.

Mathews, A. and Bradley, B. (1983) Mood and the self-referential bias in recall. Behav. Res. Ther., 21: 233–239.

Melzack, R. and Katz, J. (1992) The McGill Pain Questionnaire: appraisal and current status. In: D.C. Turk and R. Melzack (Eds.), Handbook of Pain Assessment. Guilford Press, New York, NY, pp. 152–168.

Papageorgiou, A.C., Croft, P.R., Thomas, E., Ferry, S., Jayson, M.I.V. and Silman, A.J. (1996) Influence of previous pain experience on the episode incidence of low back pain: results from the South Manchester Back Pain Study. Pain, 66: 181–185.

Papageorgiou, A.C., Croft, P.R., Thomas, E., Silman, A.J. and Macfarlane, G.J. (1998) Psychosocial risks for low back pain: are these related to work? Ann. Rheum. Dis., 57: 500–502.

Pearce, J. and Morley, S. (1989) An experimental investigation of the construct validity of the McGill Pain Questionnaire. Pain, 39: 115–121.

Pearce, S.A., Isherwood, S., Hrouda, D., Richardson, P.H., Erskine, A. and Skinner, J. (1990) Memory and pain: tests of mood congruity and state dependent learning in experimentally and clinically induced pain. Pain, 43: 187–193.

Pincus, T. and Morley, S. (2001) Cognitive processing bias in chronic pain: a review and integration. Psychol. Bull., 127: 599–617.

Pincus, T., Pearce, S., McClelland, A. and Turner-Stokes, L. (1993) Self-referential selective memory in pain patients. Br. J. Clin. Psychol., 32: 365–375.

Pincus, T., Pearce, S., McClelland, A., Farley, S. and Vogel, S. (1994) Interpretation bias in responses to ambiguous cues in pain patients. J. Psychosom. Res., 38: 347–353.

Pincus, T., Pearce, S., McClelland, A. and Isenberg, D. (1995) Endorsement and memory bias of self-referential pain stimuli in depressed pain patients. Br. J. Clin. Psychol., 34: 267–277.

Pincus, T., Pearce, S. and Perrott, A. (1996) Pain patients' bias in the interpretation of ambiguous homophones. Br. J. Med. Psychol., 69: 259–266.

Pincus, T., Fraser, L. and Pearce, S. (1998) Do chronic pain patients 'Stroop' on pain stimuli? Br. J. Clin. Psychol., 37: 48–59.

Pincus, T. and Newman, S. (2001). Recall bias, pain, depression

and cost in back pain patients. Br. J. Clin. Psychol., 40: 143–156.

Pincus, T., Burton, A.K., Field, A. and Vogel, S. (2002) A systematic review of psychological factors as predictors of chronicity/disability in prospective cohorts of low back pain. Spine, 27(5): E109–120.

Price, D.D. (1999) Psychological Mechanisms of Pain and Analgesia. IASP Press, Seattle, WA.

Robinson, J.O. (1972) The Psychology of Visual Illusion. Hutchinson University Library, London.

Robinson, M.E. and Riley, J.L. III (1999) The role of emotion in pain. In: R.J. Gatchel and D.C. Turk (Eds.), Psychosocial Factors in Pain: Critical Perspectives. Guilford Press, New York, NY, pp. 74–88.

Rosensteil, A.K. and Keefe, F.J. (1983) The use of coping strategies in chronic low back pain. Pain, 17: 33–40.

Royal College of General Practitioners (1999) Clinical Guidelines for the Management of Acute Low Back Pain. Royal College of General Practitioners (www.rcgp.org.uk), London.

Rudy, T.E., Turk, D.C., Kubinski, J.A. and Zaki, H.S. (1995) Differential treatment responses of TMD patients as a function of psychological characteristics. Pain, 61: 103–112.

Saunders, K.W., von Korff, M., Pruitt, S.D. and Moore, J.E. (1999) Prediction of physician visits and prescription medicine use for back pain. Pain, 83: 369–377.

Schiaffino, K.M., Revenson, T.A. and Gibofsky, A. (1991) Assessing the impact of self-efficacy beliefs on adaptation to rheumatoid arthritis. Arthritis Care Res., 4: 150–157.

Schwarzer, R. (1992) Self-efficacy in the adoption and maintenance of health behaviors: theoretical approaches and a new model. In: R. Schwarzer (Ed.), Self-efficacy: Thought Control of Action. Hemisphere, Washington, DC, pp. 217–43.

Segal, Z.V. (1988) Appraisal of the self-schema construct in cognitive models of depression. Psychol. Bull., 103: 147–162.

Segal, Z.V., Lau, M.A. and Rokke, P.D. (1999) Cognition and emotion research and the practice of cognitive-behavioural therapy. In: T. Dalgleish and M.J. Power (Eds.), Handbook of Cognition and Emotion. Wiley, Chichester, pp. 705–726.

Sekuler, R. and Blake, R. (1994) Perception, 3rd edn. McGraw-Hill, New York, NY.

Seltzer, S.F. and Yarczower, M. (1991) Selective encoding and retrieval of affective words during exposure to aversive stimulation. Pain, 47: 47–51.

Shifren, K., Park, D.C., Bennett, J.M. and Morrell, R.W. (1999) Do cognitive processes predict mental health in individuals with rheumatoid arthritis? J. Behav. Med., 22: 529–547.

Singer, J.A. (1995) Seeing one's self: locating narrative memory in a framework of personality. J. Pers., 63: 429–457.

Snider, B.S., Asmundson, G.J.G. and Wiese, K.C. (2000) Automatic and strategic processing of threat cues in patients with chronic pain: a modified Stroop evaluation. Clin. J. Pain, 16: 144–154.

Sullivan, M.J. and D'Eon, J.L. (1990) Relation between catastrophizing and depression in chronic pain patients. J. Abnorm. Psychol., 99: 260–263.

Sullivan, M.J.L., Bishop, S.R. and Pivik, J. (1995) The Pain

Catastrophizing Scale: development and validation. Psychol. Assess., 7: 524–532.

Sullivan, M.J.L., Stanish, W., Waite, H., Sullivan, M. and Tripp, D.A. (1998) Catastrophizing, pain, and disability in patient with soft-tissue injuries. Pain, 77: 253–260.

Tan, G., Jensen, M.P., Robinson-Whelen, S., Thornby, J.I. and Monga, T.N. (2001) Coping with chronic pain: a comparison of two measures. Pain, 90: 27–33.

Teasdale, J.D. (1985) Psychological treatments for depression: how do they work? Behav. Res. Ther., 23: 157–165.

Thomas, E., Silman, A.J., Croft, P.R., Papageorgiou, A.C., Jayson, M.I. and Macfarlane, G.J. (1999) Predicting who develops chronic low back pain in primary care: a prospective study. BMJ, 318: 1662–1667.

Truchon, M. and Fillion, L. (2000) Biopsychosocial determinants of chronic disability and low-back pain: a review. J. Occup. Rehabil., 10: 117–142.

Turk, D.C. and Rudy, T.E. (1988) Toward an empirically derived taxonomy of chronic pain patients: integration of psychological assessment data. J. Consult. Clin. Psychol., 56: 233–238.

Turk, D.C. and Rudy, T.E. (1990) The robustness of an empirically derived taxonomy of chronic pain patients. Pain, 43: 27–43.

Turk, D.C. and Rudy, T.E. (1992) Cognitive factors and persistent pain: a glimpse into Pandora's box. Cogn. Ther. Res., 16: 99–122.

Turner, J.A., Franklin, G. and Turk, D.C. (2000a) Predictors of chronic disability in injured workers: a systematic literature synthesis. Am. J. Ind. Med., 38: 707–722.

Turner, J.A., Jensen, M.P. and Romano, J.M. (2000b) Do beliefs, coping, and catastrophizing independently predict functioning in patients with chronic pain? Pain, 85: 115–125.

Van der Weide, W.E., Verbeek, J.H.A.M., Salle, H.J.A. and van Dijk, F.J.H. (1999) Prognostic factors for chronic disability from acute low-back pain in occupational health care. Scand. J. Work Environ. Health, 25: 50–56.

Waddell, G. (1998) The Back Pain Revolution. Churchill Livingstone, Edinburgh.

Wall, P.D. (1999) Pain the Science of Suffering. Weidenfeld and Nicholson, London.

Wallston, K.A., Wallston, B.S. and DeVellis, R. (1978) Development of Multidimensional Health Locus of Control (MHLC) scales. Health Educ. Monogr., 6: 161–170.

Watson, P.J., Booker, C.K. and Main, C.J. (1997) Evidence for the role of psychological factors in abnormal paraspinal activity in patients with chronic low back pain. J. Musculoskeletal Pain, 5: 41–56.

Waxman, R., Tennant, A. and Helliwell, P. (1998) Community survey of factors associated with consulting for low back pain. BMJ, 317: 1564–1567.

Williams, J.M.G., Mathews, A. and MacLeod, C. (1996) The emotional Stroop task and psychopathology. Psychol. Bull., 120: 3–24.

Williams, J.M.G., Watts, F.N., MacLeod, C. and Mathews, A. (1997) Cognitive Psychology and Emotional Disorders, 2nd. edn. Wiley, Chichester.

Zubin, J. and Banks, S.M. (1977) Vulnerability: a new view of schizophrenia. J. Abnorm. Psychol., 86: 103–126.

New Avenues for the Prevention of Chronic Musculoskeletal Pain and Disability
Pain Research and Clinical Management, Vol. 12
Edited by S.J. Linton

On occupational ergonomic risk factors for musculoskeletal disorders and related intervention practice

Rolf H. Westgaard [1,*] and Jørgen Winkel [2]

[1] *Division of Industrial Economics and Technology Management, Norwegian University of Science and Technology, N-7491 Trondheim, Norway*
[2] *National Institute for Working Life West, Stockholm, Sweden*

Abstract: The first part of this chapter reviews work-related ergonomic risk factors for musculoskeletal complaints. This is the knowledge base for intervention measures to improve the musculoskeletal health of workers at the workplace. On this basis, as well as a recent review by R.H. Westgaard and J. Winkel (Int. J. Ind. Ergon. 20: 463–500, 1997), the second part summarises current experiences of ergonomic workplace intervention studies. We point to some explanatory factors for the intervention results, and indicate possible alternatives to the traditional approaches to workplace interventions. Finally, practical approaches to ergonomic risk assessment and strategies for managing ergonomic interventions are suggested.

1. Ergonomic exposure as a risk factor for musculoskeletal complaints

1.1. General considerations

Work-related biomechanical exposures are, together with sports activities, predominant physical risk factors for musculoskeletal complaints. In this chapter we first discuss some potential physiological mechanisms in the development of occupational musculoskeletal disorders and thereafter the quantification and risk assessment of work-related biomechanical exposures. Some issues regarding psychosocial factors relating to musculoskeletal disorders at work are also considered. More comprehensive discussions of psychosocial factors are found elsewhere in this book.

Much effort is put into ergonomic research dealing with musculoskeletal injury mechanisms, exposure classification issues, etiological epidemiology of risk factors, and workplace interventions, with the common aim of improving the musculoskeletal health of workers. The results can be summarised in two grounded theories on risk factors for musculoskeletal complaints:

- Work demands can generate a biomechanical loading on the musculoskeletal system (biomechanical exposure) that causes pain. Conceptually, there are three dimensions to exposure: amplitude (e.g., due to external loads and/or posture), the time-variation pattern of exposure ('repetitiveness'), and exposure duration. Harmful exposures can be avoided by appropriate measures at the workplace or directed towards the indi-

* Correspondence to: R.H. Westgaard, Division of Industrial Economics and Technology Management, Norwegian University of Science and Technology, N-7491 Trondheim, Norway. Tel.: +47 7359-3496; Fax: +47 7359-3107; E-mail: rolf.westgaard@iot.ntnu.no

vidual worker (e.g., Bernard, 1997; Buckle and Devereux, 1999; Commission on behavioral and social sciences and education, National Research Council and Institute of Medicine, 2001).

• Stress at the workplace (conceptualised in, e.g., psychological demands, job autonomy, effort–reward balance, supervisor, fellow worker or customer relationships) may cause health effects independently or interactively with biomechanical exposure (Bongers et al., 1993; Cox et al., 2000; Ariëns et al., 2001).

The scientific basis is field studies relating work exposures to musculoskeletal health. Laboratory studies complement this work by providing insight in physiological effects of exposures and possible pathophysiological pathways, which are poorly understood for most musculoskeletal disorders (cf. Keyserling, 2000a,b for reviews of laboratory studies). The general formulation of the grounded theories is therefore on purpose: research reports and scientific reviews tend to identify generic risk factors for biomechanical exposure and stress.

There are several reasons for this less than satisfying situation. Firstly, our understanding of physiological limitations and thereby potentially harmful exposures and corrective intervention measures has changed over the years. Fig. 1 shows the approximate timing of new concepts for musculoskeletal problems ('physiological models of work-related musculoskeletal problems') that have influenced research and professional advice on ergonomic exposure intervention ('intervention concerns and measures'). The physiological models and associated intervention measures introduced over the years have not invalidated earlier concepts, which remain operative to the extent they are relevant, and are often further refined. As an example, tissue damage was a popular injury concept for 'occupational cervicobrachial disorders' in the 1970s (Itani et al., 1983), but ran into difficulties explaining pain development at very low exposure levels (e.g., Westgaard, 1988). Tissue damage remains, however, a viable injury model for, e.g., carpal tunnel injury and research has added further refinement to this model (Armstrong et al., 1994).

The time line in Fig. 1 can also be viewed as an illustration of the dynamic interaction between the stakeholders who shape work life on the basis of business considerations, and those who attend to worker concerns. It can be interpreted to partly document the *success* of ergonomic workplace interventions: exposure problems of the past are to a considerable extent eliminated in current work life. Unfortunately, new problems have emerged that often make the old ergonomic solutions, still valid in their original context, less relevant. The ergonomist may furthermore not claim credit for the improvements there are, e.g., heavy manual labour is in many cases eliminated not because of ergonomic considerations, but because it is cost-effective to substitute human labour by machines. Table I presents a summary of common musculoskeletal disorders implicated in work-related musculoskeletal complaints. This topic is extensively discussed by Hagberg et al. (1995) and in more recent reports, e.g., Sluiter et al. (2000). In this chapter a focus is maintained on trapezius myalgia, as both biomechanical and psychosocial exposures are confirmed risk factors for this health outcome and the condition relates to our own research experience.

1.2. Recent physiological injury models

In the last half century there has been an accelerated mechanisation of the manufacturing industry. This has created jobs with low-level biomechanical exposure of long duration, as well as new psychosocial demands. At the same time the service sector has expanded, presenting a similar mix of low-level, long-duration biomechanical exposure and psychosocial demands. Under these circumstances shoulder and neck complaints seem to become an increasing problem. Ergonomic scientists are therefore looking for valid injury models to be used as a basis for risk assessment of such exposures.

The recently most popular physiological injury model valid at low force levels is the "Cinderella" hypothesis (Hägg, 1991). It proposes that musculoskeletal pain developing under low-force conditions be due to overexertion of low-threshold motor

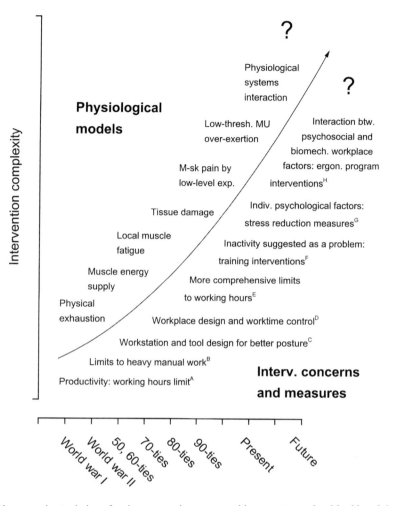

Fig. 1. An overview of the approximate timing of major ergonomic concerns with respect to workers' health and the associated corrective measures conceptualised by the line indicating increasing intervention complexity with time. Intervention concerns and measures (below the line) and the corresponding physiological models to explain musculoskeletal problems (above the line) are indicated. Letters in uppercase refers to scientific papers representative of a period and concern. A: Vernon, 1921; B: Åstrand, 1960; C: Grandjean, 1969; D: Ohara et al., 1976; E: Arendt, 2001; F: Silverstein et al., 1988; G: Bigos et al., 2001; H: Westin, 1990.

units. If proven correct, such an injury mechanism can be a common path of pain induction for low-amplitude, long-duration mechanical exposures and stress-associated pain (Melin and Lundberg, 1997; Westgaard, 1999). The model does not consider how the situation with overexertion of motor units is established, or the link between motor activity and pain (Edwards, 1988; Johansson and Sojka, 1991). There are extensive research efforts to unravel the chain of physiological events from muscle activity

to pain, which is particularly important to identify methods for the *treatment* of pain (e.g., Sjøgaard et al., 2000). Conditions that influence motor activity are of interest in a *prevention* and thereby *ergonomic intervention* perspective. Such conditions are studied both in the laboratory and the field.

Laboratory studies have shown that sustained motor unit activity is a common response to stress and that trapezius is one of the most responsive muscles in this respect (Wærsted and Westgaard, 1996). It is fur-

TABLE I

Common musculoskeletal disorders relating to ergonomic exposures at work

Condition	Major body locations	Comment
Tendon disorders (tendonitis, tenosynovitis)	Rotator cuff muscles Long head biceps brachii Tendons at the elbow Tendons at the wrist Achilles tendon	Tendons move long distances and participate in wide range of movements
Peripheral nerve disorders	Carpal tunnel Thoracic outlet (motor nerves in spinal cord)	Nerve compression in tight anatomical space
Tension neck	Trapezius Other stabilisers of scapula, neck muscles	Myofascial syndrome localised to shoulder and neck
Joint disorders (osteoarthrosis)	Joints active in weight-bearing and/or frequent movement	Degeneration of cartilage
Low back disorders (sciatica, lumbago)	Low back	Radiating or local pain in the back, due to the previous listed conditions

ther shown that trapezius muscle activity during sustained mental exposure is elevated for patients with pain of putative musculoskeletal origin (e.g., Bansevicius et al., 1999) and for normally pain-free subjects who develop shoulder pain during the experiment relative to those who do not develop pain (Bansevicius et al., 1997). If a combination of biomechanical and psychosocial exposure exists, the muscle activity level is higher than for biomechanical exposure alone (Weber et al., 1980; Lundberg et al., 1994).

An example of a work task that induces a particular motor unit response is double clicking on a computer mouse. This task does not appear very different from single click by observation. However, the double click promotes motor unit 'doublet' firing, a distinct physiological response that elevates the intramuscular free calcium level and thereby force generation (Søgaard et al., 2001). This exemplifies the difficulties in the interpretation of the physiological effects of the motor unit activity pattern. It should furthermore be kept in mind that these results from laboratory studies do not by themselves prove the Cinderella hypothesis correct. And even if the hypothesis is true under some circumstances, this may not be an exclusive mechanism of pain generation at low exposure levels.

The Cinderella hypothesis is examined indirectly in field studies by examining whether there is evidence of higher trapezius muscle activity levels for workers with shoulder pain relative to those pain-free in work situations with low biomechanical exposure. The results have so far been inconsistent; some studies of low-exposure work situations show elevated muscle activity and/or sustained activity pattern for workers with pain (Vasseljen and Westgaard, 1995; Hägg and Åström, 1997), or a non-significant tendency in this direction (Sandsjö et al., 2000). Other studies do not find this difference (Westgaard et al., 2001). It is suggested that there is a tendency of such differences to appear in work situations where low-level biomechanical exposure is likely to dominate as a risk factor (Westgaard, 1999).

In a recent study the temporal relationship between muscle activity and pain was examined in long-duration recordings, first over the full workday and thereafter in recordings over 24 h. The study groups were service workers (shop assistants and health care workers) with low biomechanical exposure and work stress induced by customer/client contact and time pressure. The workers reported high prevalence of shoulder pain, despite low trapezius muscle activity. The static and median electromyo-

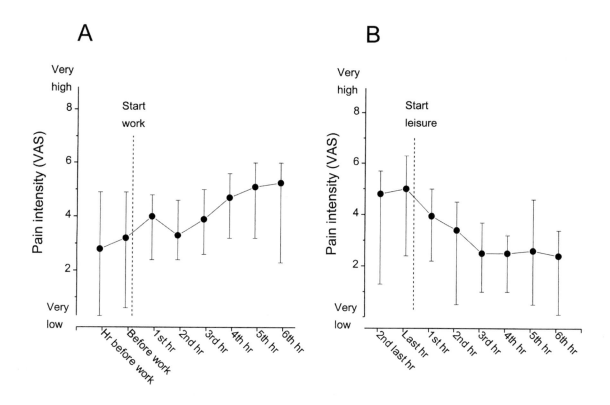

Fig. 2. Development of shoulder pain over the workday and in leisure time for service workers who have reported incidences of shoulder-neck pain the last six months. The panels show mean hourly pain scores with 95% confidence intervals. (A) Hourly pain scores are aligned by start of work. (B) Hourly pain scores are aligned by start of leisure time. (From Holte and Westgaard, 2002)

graphic (EMG) activity level over the workday was measured to only 0.2% and 3% EMG_{max}, respectively. The fraction of work time with the trapezius in a state of rest (defined as muscle activity < 0.5% EMG_{max}) was 10–20% of the work period (Westgaard et al., 2001), which is much less muscle activity than measured for industrial workers (Westgaard et al., 1996). Workers with pain in the shoulder–neck region were not distinguished from pain-free workers by muscle activity level or rest time. In the follow-up study the hourly pain scores for shoulder and neck (including the trapezius) augmented during work and reversed to lower pain score in leisure time, demonstrating that an exposure situation with pain induction existed at work (Fig. 2). The EMG activity level was unchanged from work to leisure time for the pain-afflicted workers, but a small reduction was observed for the pain-free group (Holte and

Westgaard, 2002). Subjectively scored indicators of stress did not correlate with the muscle activity level or pattern. We concluded that pain, presumably due to psychosocial risk factors such as customer/client contact and pressure on performance, developed in work situations where biomechanical exposure is unlikely to be a risk factor. The fact that psychosocial risk factors were not detected in the surface EMG recorded muscle activity can be due to methodological limitations, including individual motor units not monitored, critical muscle activity patterns not observed, or data reduction techniques insensitive to critical aspects of the muscle activity pattern. Alternatively, pain induction in response to psychosocial stress may develop by physiological responses other than muscle activity and presumably involving the sympathetic nervous system. The very low EMG activity levels in the study of service workers, which furthermore are mostly unchanged from work to leisure, may argue in favour of the last alternative.

Some studies convincingly point to sustained low-level muscle activity as a risk factor for muscle pain, e.g., healthy workers who carry out repetitive work tasks with short breaks in the trapezius activity pattern ('EMG gaps') are less inclined to develop shoulder pain (Veiersted et al., 1993). It is therefore prudent to examine measures that can be taken to break up a sustained motor unit activity pattern. Laboratory studies with single motor unit recording have demonstrated the phenomenon of motor unit substitution, i.e., motor units stop firing and other units of initially higher threshold substitute their force contribution during a sustained contraction (Westgaard and De Luca, 1999). EMG gaps appear to promote substitution. After a period of inactivity, typically of a few minutes duration, the motor unit is re-recruited. The substitution phenomenon may serve as a protection mechanism against overexertion of single motor units.

Recent studies have shown that also brief periods of *increased* muscle activity promote motor unit substitution (Westad and Westgaard, 2001). This result supports the traditional ergonomic recommendation of designing work tasks to promote variation in muscle usage.

2. Ergonomic perspective on work-related risk factors for musculoskeletal pain

2.1. Ergonomic exposure models for intervention

Fig. 3 shows a model to illustrate the association between work-related mechanical exposure and musculoskeletal health effects. It furthermore illustrates work life and community factors that determine the mechanical exposure of individuals. In the lower part of the model, considering the worker, a causal relationship is indicated between physical work demands and work-related health effects. Forces generated within the body ('internal' or 'biomechanical' exposure) are needed to meet the demands specified by the work situation ('external' or 'mechanical' exposure).

Internal exposure requires a number of physiological responses from micro-level (e.g., elevated calcium levels in muscle cells) to systems-level (e.g., elevated heart rate) to support force generation. The physiological responses are normal reactions that in the longer term and under unfortunate circumstances may cause deteriorating musculoskeletal health. The relationship between the different levels in the model chain is subject to considerable individual variation, determined by environmental and personal factors (modifiers). Fig. 3 furthermore illustrates that work demands, i.e., mechanical exposure, is a consequence of production system characteristics, determined by the technology level and rationalisation strategy. For the purpose of intervention classification, discussed later, the figure shows the production system divided into two parts, *rationalisation strategy*, reflecting the material production system design, and *organisational culture*, representing systematic company-wide health and safety activities. Fig. 3 finally illustrates that the production system and thereby working conditions are influenced by the company's position in the international marketplace, and that community stakeholders may attempt to influence working conditions and thereby workers' health through, e.g., legislation (community interventions). The model does not consider psychosocial exposure, which may share common pathophysiological pathways with some forms of harmful biomechanical exposure or take effect through physiologically independent pathways, as already discussed.

The influence of the production system on worker exposure is illustrated by two examples previously published. The first example concerns the mechanisation of forestry work (Attebrant et al., 1995). This industry developed from heavy manual work and energy expenditure of about 40 kJ/min in the first part of the last century to highly mechanised work and low biomechanical exposure today. This development took place in stages, with the introduction of the power-saw in the 1950s and increasingly sophisticated forestry machines in the 1960s and 1970s. Productivity increased from 1.4 m^3/man-day in the 1940s to 10.6 m^3/man-day in 1985. As part of the running rationalisation the operators became

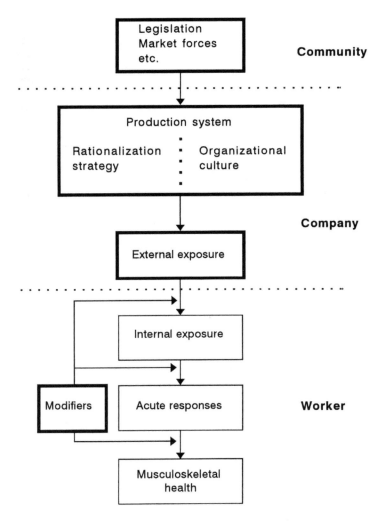

Fig. 3. A model illustrating significant factors determining occupational musculoskeletal health. With respect to the worker, the model shows that physical work demands (external exposure) cause the generation of forces in the body (internal exposure). Associated physiological responses take place that may influence health. Modifiers influence the outcome of this chain of events. Workload is influenced by decisions increasingly removed from the worker. The heavy-framed boxes are potential targets for ergonomic interventions. See text for further detail. (From Westgaard and Winkel, 1997.)

contractors owning the machines themselves. Due to their high capital investments they often had to run their machines for 12–15 h a day with obvious exposure implications. Accordingly, the prevalence of shoulder and neck disorders increased from 50 to 80% from the 1960s to 1980s while low back disorders remained at the same magnitude, but were possibly less severe. The example illustrates how rationalisation of an industry through increases in technological level and organisational changes implies comprehensive ergonomic effects that are not easily addressed by the ergonomist. A further example is the comparison of assembly work in China and Sweden (Bao et al., 1997).

Another illustration of the effect of production system design on exposures and workers' health is the situation of dentists in Sweden (Fig. 4). Dentists have traditionally suffered from poor work posture.

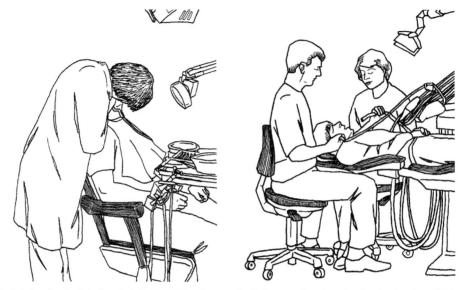

Fig. 4. Left: Workstation for dentists from late 1950s. Right: Ergonomically improved workstation for dentists from 1970s. (From Winkel and Westgaard, 1999.)

New and ergonomically much better workstations were developed in the 1960s. Standing, twisted and forward bending postures were replaced by comfortable seated postures. The patient was placed in a supine resting position with the mouth a little higher than the elbow height of the dentist. Tools were redesigned according to ergonomic guidelines and put in optimal positions. Despite these efforts, high prevalence of musculoskeletal complaints among dentists was documented 10 years later, particularly in the shoulder–neck region. Presumably this was due to their work situation, which at the same time was reorganised by principles of Tayloristic rationalisation. The traditional work situation of dentists was to perform different tasks of short duration. But for the purpose of salary saving, lower-paid support staff was introduced. A new work situation was created whereby the dentist was expected to work in the mouth of his patients in an ergonomically improved posture for the major part of the workday, promoted by the concurrent introduction of piece-rate salary payment. The exposure amplitude in, e.g., upper trapezius was reduced, but the exposure duration was at the same time substantially prolonged. This interaction between ergonomic improvement of the workstation design and organisational changes

with negative ergonomic implications is named "the ergonomic pitfall" (Winkel and Westgaard, 1996). The two examples (forestry, dentistry) illustrate how business decisions further upstream in the model of Fig. 3 determine whether potential risk factors at the individual level become manifest or not.

Fig. 5 shows a proposed U-shaped association between mechanical exposure amplitude and musculoskeletal complaints (Winkel and Westgaard, 1992). We suggested that proper risk evaluation should consider the three conceptual exposure dimensions *amplitude*, *time-variation pattern* ('repetitiveness') and *duration* for quantification of mechanical exposure. One purpose of the model was to emphasise the importance of time variables in the risk evaluation and not just equate high biomechanical exposure with high force amplitude, which was common practice at the time. Here the model is used as basis for a discussion of risk factors at high and low biomechanical exposure amplitude.

Additional to the increased complexity in the evaluation of biomechanical exposure, other considerations have emerged. Low amplitude of long duration accentuates the considerable individual variation in the capacity of workers to tolerate biomechanical exposure. Workers are presumed to have more vari-

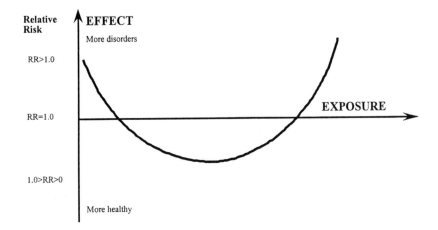

Fig. 5. Suggested conceptual exposure amplitude–musculoskeletal health association for biomechanical exposures, illustrating the relative risk of contracting musculoskeletal disorders. (From Winkel and Westgaard, 1992.)

able and possibly lower tolerance for physical strain today due to more sedentary lifestyles. This is exemplified by forestry workers in the early part of last century, who had resting heart rate of about 50 beats per minute, suggesting very high fitness level. The variation in exposure tolerance is the basis of 'modifier' interventions aimed at 'work hardening'. Low-amplitude physical work may furthermore allow psychosocial risk factors to become a more dominant influence with respect to health outcome (Westgaard et al., 1996). Since psychosocial risk factors operate in an interaction between the worker and his/her surroundings, exemplified by the effort–reward imbalance model (Siegrist et al., 1997) or by way of "coping" (Ursin et al., 1993), the effect of psychosocial exposure is also individually determined. Finally, risk factors outside working hours may interact with those at work. Altogether, this makes the evaluation of exposures and selection of appropriate intervention measures increasingly difficult.

2.2. High biomechanical exposure

High exposure amplitude is a recognised risk factor for musculoskeletal pain due to the relatively rapid onset of health effects, temporal relationship, and some well-known injury mechanisms such as spinal disk generation (e.g., Marras et al., 1995; Bernard, 1997). Very high exposure amplitude on the right-hand side of the U-curve in Fig. 5 corresponds to situations where amplitude alone causes tissue damage. The time element becomes increasingly important in determining health risks as exposure amplitude is reduced, manifest as exposure duration, time pattern of exposure amplitude variation, and recovery time. Operative definitions of high biomechanical exposure and specific examples of risk situations are available from the literature, including the European Union ergonomic standards for safety in the design of machinery (CEN standards) and guidelines published in ergonomic journals and handbooks (Woodson et al., 1992; Salvendy, 1997). A collection of articles on this (and other) subjects, published on a CD by the International Journal of Industrial Ergonomics, the 'Industrial and Occupational Ergonomics Users' Encyclopedia' is available from the publisher (Elsevier). Examples of ergonomic reference manuals and databases can be found (e.g., Human Scale, published by MIT Press). Finally, the amount of web-based information is growing rapidly (cf. ergonomics information on web-addresses *http://osha.eu.int* and *http://www.osha-slc.gov/SLTC/ergonomics/*).

The time-dependent risk factors, their interrelation and the relationship to exposure amplitude are difficult to handle in terms of exposure guidelines.

This is due to the delayed onset of health problems for low-amplitude, relative to high-amplitude exposures, the many different time scales (seconds to years) relevant for risk assessment of exposure, the cyclic nature of the pain, which makes the risk factors difficult to assess by epidemiological methods, and the interaction with productivity (cf. Winkel and Westgaard, 1996). Kilbom (1994) presented a guideline on exposure repetitiveness as risk factor for musculoskeletal health. However, many factors are listed that may modify the recommendations. Thus, these guidelines for time-based exposure variables are at present preliminary due to inadequate scientific basis.

Ergonomic guidelines vary by body location of the injury and depend on the injury model and exposure measurement used. As an example, speed of movement is not considered in the NIOSH model for evaluation of risk of back injury (Waters et al., 1993), but is a significant risk factor in the similar equation by Marras and co-workers (Marras et al., 1995). Risk factors for arm, hand and shoulder–neck include force (e.g., weight handled), posture (e.g., arm elevation or neck flexion), and repetition, quantified by observation.

Alternatively, electromyographic (EMG) recording of muscle activity can be used to indicate force. The most common risk indicators are median and static force level (Jonsson, 1978), but also the time variation pattern of exposure amplitude can be determined ("EMG gaps", Veiersted et al., 1990; "exposure variation analysis", Mathiassen and Winkel, 1991). Jonsson (1978) suggested that the static muscle force level should not exceed 2–5% of maximal force during continuous work. The guideline has been criticised on the basis of observed high pain prevalence for workers with much lower activity levels (Westgaard, 1988). However, psychosocial stress may not be represented in the surface EMG recording despite being a risk factor for some musculoskeletal disorders (cf. discussion of mechanisms relating to Fig. 2). The above guideline may thus be reformulated as a criterion for biomechanical exposure quantified by surface EMG: static activity levels higher than 2% in continuous work represent a clear biomechanical risk. A modification of the guideline is that lower activity levels does not protect against all musculoskeletal health risks, due to the independent effects of sustained very-low-level muscle activity and also psychosocial exposure.

In recent research projects where surface EMG is used as an exposure indicator, it has become accepted practice to calibrate the EMG activity by the EMG level recorded in maximal voluntary contraction (% EMG_{max}), and not use the EMG-force calibration procedure. This considerably simplifies surface EMG as an exposure assessment method. Even so, there are many sources of error in the recording and evaluation of surface EMG. Therefore we do not recommend electromyography as an exposure assessment method for the ergonomics practitioner not trained in this methodology.

2.3. Low biomechanical exposures

In Fig. 5 an increased risk of musculoskeletal complaints at low biomechanical exposure amplitude is indicated. During the eighties inactivity was discussed and experimentally supported as a specific risk factor for complaints, by observations of impaired circulation under conditions of inactivity (Winkel, 1985). Harmful effects of extreme inactivity, e.g., bed rest, were documented (Greenleaf, 1984), and physical training was (and is) acknowledged as health promoting. The inactivity observed in work life is, however, less extreme than the above example.

In reconsidering the hypothetical exposure amplitude–health effect curve in Fig. 5, we find that there are still indications of elevated work-related musculoskeletal health risk at low exposure amplitude, beyond those associated with a sedentary lifestyle. This relates to long periods with invariant posture in ergonomically well designed work places, coined by the term "postural fixity" (Grieco, 1986). Specific work situations are work by visual display terminals (VDT) or repetitive monotonous work performed in a good posture. Hypotheses regarding the physiological basis for increased risk at low biomechanical exposure amplitude are discussed in the first section of this chapter.

Guidelines on how to counteract musculoskeletal health risks at low exposure amplitude focus on time rather than amplitude. Planned breaks in continuous work pattern have been investigated (Henning et al., 1989, 1997). Typically, breaks of 5–10 minutes every hour in sustained VDT work are recommended (e.g., Labour Standards Bureau, Ministry of Labour, 1985). A general recommendation is to design the work situation for variation, i.e., include tasks that require varied body usage.

2.4. Exposure modifiers

Exposure modifiers are defined as factors that influence the relationship between the different levels relating to the worker in the model in Fig. 3, which adopts a work exposure–health effect perspective. Individual variables are considered to buffer the effects of work-related biomechanical and psychosocial exposures, but may also be risk factors in their own right, i.e., they have an association with musculoskeletal health. Examples of individual variables include smoking, age, gender and general health variables, which are studied to a considerable extent in epidemiological surveys of different occupational groups.

Individual risk factors were tabulated in a review of epidemiological studies on the association between work-related exposures and shoulder and neck disorders (Winkel and Westgaard, 1992). Gender and previous experience of musculoskeletal complaints are consistent risk factors, but of little interest in the context of ergonomic intervention strategy since these variables can only be modified by administrative decisions, not at the individual level. The insight is, however, useful to identify populations at risk that can be targeted by specific intervention measures. A higher prevalence of musculoskeletal disorders for female workers compared to males with same job title may, at least in part, be due to gender difference in actual exposures (Mergler et al., 1987). Age is not a consistent risk factor, but the interpretation of this finding is not clear due to selection bias. In a physiological perspective, it is expected that physical load tolerance is reduced with increasing age. Finally, a

stressed personality, indicated by the feeling of high bodily tension level or type A personality, has shown up as risk factor for shoulder and neck disorder in several studies (e.g., Hägg et al., 1990; Westgaard, 1999).

3. Implementing ergonomic interventions

3.1. General considerations

The primary aim of an ergonomic intervention to improve musculoskeletal health is to optimise biomechanical and psychosocial exposure, and modifiers, based on knowledge of risk factors as detailed in the previous section. The ergonomist must know whether a biomechanical exposure represents a risk of musculoskeletal complaint and how to eliminate this risk or turn it into a health-promoting exposure. He/she must further discriminate between biomechanical and psychosocial exposures at work and recognise other risk factors relevant for the worker and his/her environment, even including leisure time activities.

Thereafter the ergonomist must sufficiently impact the dominant risk factors for musculoskeletal complaints to eliminate health risks in a situation where constraints of technical, organisational, cultural and economic nature operate. Such constraints include, e.g., choice of production technology and allocation of tasks between the workers, management attitudes and the requirement to stay competitive in a marketplace. Business decisions are the overriding consideration of management. If the ergonomist can promote an intervention as positive also in a business perspective, management support for the intervention is likely secured. The support and active participation of the workers are also essential. The anchoring of the intervention effort with the main stakeholders is equally important to the success of an ergonomic intervention to proper assessment of ergonomic exposures.

Ergonomic intervention effectiveness is conceptualised in Fig. 6 (Westgaard and Winkel, 1997). The figure is based on the assumption of a well-

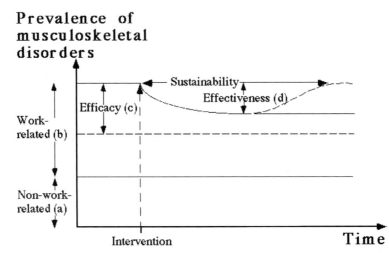

Fig. 6. Graphic presentation of some important terms in ergonomic intervention research. Ergonomic preventable fraction is computed as b/(a + b), ergonomic intervention impact is d/c. (From Westgaard and Winkel, 1997.)

defined change at a given time and does not reflect the 'continuous improvement process' that is an aim in many companies today. The ergonomic workplace intervention is assumed to remedy only musculo-skeletal complaints that are work-related and usually only a subset of the relevant work-related risk factors is addressed. If the intervention targets many of the existing risk factors for work-related disorders, the intervention *efficacy* is high. The intervention should furthermore solve the ergonomic problems targeted, i.e., have high *impact*. Finally, the intervention should be *sustainable*. The conceptualisation of ergonomic intervention effectiveness in the triple aims of high efficacy, high impact and high sustainability highlights the different concerns in achieving a successful intervention. A prerequisite in achieving intervention impact is *intervention latitude*: constraints of organisational, economic, and/or technical nature are barriers that prevent us from achieving the desired exposure condition. Important production system variables are often determined before the ergonomist becomes involved. Other stakeholders, who focus rationalisation strategy, product and production system design for purposes other than health and safety, make decisions with ergonomic implications continuously and independently of the ergonomist, as illustrated by the forestry and dentistry examples in Section 2.1 'Ergonomic exposure

models for intervention'. This is further discussed in the later sections on production system interventions.

There is little documented knowledge on how an intervention is best sustained. It seems clear that an effort that purely relies on the enthusiasm of individuals likely fails sooner or later. The effort to secure good working conditions must be put in an organisational context. A question on how to sustain interventions was put to health care personnel in Norway in an informal survey. One response was the importance of documenting the results. Management expects results, as they do for any other investment decision. If an ergonomic intervention is shown to have positive health effects or even better, contribute to the company balance sheet, it will get a sustained high priority.

Fig. 3 shows the different possibilities for targeting the intervention (heavy framed boxes). The most common intervention strategy is possibly measures directed towards the individual worker ('modifier intervention'). Alternatively, the workstations or even the full production system can be targeted. The last approach allows for more latitude in promoting healthy biomechanical exposures, by considering both technology level (e.g., degree of automation), work organisation (e.g., distribution of work tasks between the workers), and organisational culture (defined as systematic health and safety activities independent of the primary production system). 'Rationalisation strategy interventions' aim to improve workers' health by designing the material production system so that it furthers the dual aims of workers' health, productivity and quality issues. However, these rationalisation strategy interventions are only a small subset of the many similar interventions that aim to improve production without consideration of potential health effects. 'Organisational culture' interventions attempt to improve workers' health through systematic, company-wide health and safety efforts that have organisational implications.

3.2. Modifier interventions

In the chain of events illustrated in Fig. 3, modifier interventions try to tip the association between the chain elements for the individual worker towards a positive health outcome. The modifier intervention approach is criticised on the basis that the intervention does not eliminate harmful exposures. This is a valid criticism if there is evidence of harmful exposures. However, any intervention with documented positive health effects should be considered.

Westgaard and Winkel (1997) concluded, "modifier interventions that target the individual worker, especially those focusing workers at risk and using measures that actively involve the worker, have a good chance of success". Physical exercise and stress management are popular examples of modifier interventions. In addition, intervention measures reviewed included pain management, health education, physical therapy and massage, instruction in work technique, and different combinations of these measures. Passive measures, such as health education, showed little evidence of success. A common feature of the interventions with a positive health outcome is active interest and participation of the workers involved.

This class of interventions can be difficult to sustain, and to motivate those most in need of attention. Modifier intervention should be included as part of the overall ergonomic intervention strategy, but not to the exclusion of interventions that target mechanical and psychosocial exposures at work.

3.3. Workstation interventions

In workstation interventions the ergonomics expert focuses the individual worker and modifies the workstations accordingly, without consideration of the overall production system. The rationale, according to Fig. 3, is that workplace and work duties define the biomechanical exposure of the worker. If the exposure represents a risk of musculoskeletal complaints, modifications to workstation design and work duties best remedy this. A problem with this approach is that intervention latitude, i.e., the scope for modification of exposure, is usually limited. A repetitive work task remains repetitive for most work situations even though posture is improved. The successful intervention may reduce exposure amplitude, but exposure time variables are not sufficiently improved to eliminate health risk and may even be worsened if productivity considerations dictate higher work pace (cf. dentist example). The production systems are furthermore rapidly changing in many industries: the original intervention may be less relevant after a short period.

Stand-alone workstation interventions are typical of the early intervention literature. Most intervention studies using this approach took place in the 1970s and early 1980s. Unfortunately, the documentation of the results is mostly of poor scientific quality and thus does not allow positive conclusions. However, some examples of apparent successful interventions with reduction of high exposure amplitude and subsequent improved musculoskeletal health were reported (Westgaard and Aarås, 1985).

3.4. Production system interventions: rationalisation strategy

Choices made with respect to production model affect the mechanical exposures of the workers by determining, e.g., weights, postures, and time pattern of exposure. A rationalisation goal is to increase productivity by minimising lost time, i.e., eliminate pauses in the exposure pattern. This is not always easy in line production, but the last decades have seen alternative strategies to achieve this goal

(Björkman, 1996). Prevalent examples are Lean Production, Time-Based Management and Business Process Reengineering. The common denominator of these is downsizing, which has been shown to be strongly associated with medically certified sick leave (Vahtera et al., 1997). Other studies illustrate that effective production engineering of assembly line production may reduce the exposure porosity (i.e., reduce the occurrence of short pauses due to technical/organisational reasons; Bao et al., 1997; Neumann et al., 2002) The new production systems emphasise flexibility, multiple skills, integrated quality control, increased responsibility of workers etc. One of the prevalent new 'success factors' is 'flexibility'. This concept may have considerable ergonomic implications and we therefore examine it in some detail.

Organisations try to improve their flexibility to meet rapidly changing market demands. New conditions of work are analysed from a flexibility perspective (Howard, 1995). One aspect of flexibility is the context of integrated information technology that facilitates the location of paid work to times and sites other than those traditionally assumed (Andriessen and Roe, 1994). Another is the new organisational patterns that emerge (horizontal, vertical, network-based etc.), also facilitated by new production technology (Ashkenas et al., 1995). A third aspect is the changing character of labour markets with an increase in temporary contracts and decreasing frequency of long-term relations between employer and employee (Felstead and Jewson, 1999). Research into the flexibility concept has identified at least five aspects of flexibility (e.g., Atkinson, 1984; Felstead and Jewson, 1999):

- *Numerical*. The number of employees in permanent positions is reduced and the number of contingent jobs and workers from hire agencies increased. It becomes increasingly difficult to identify workplaces and individuals at risk.
- *Functional*. Increased competence of the employees makes the production systems more flexible. Multi-skilled workers may imply ergonomic improvement, but also increased demands on each worker.

- *Time*. Work becomes goal directed rather than regulated through working hours. This may create increased control over work, but also increased mental stress. There are many examples of the elimination of the border between working hours and leisure time, which tends to increase working hours.
- *Spatial*. Mobile working/telecommuting has increased considerably in recent years. Another aspect is the increasing amount of outsourcing to smaller companies. Ergonomic issues often receive less attention in small companies and when workplaces are dispersed.
- *Financial*. Wages and benefits are increasingly differentiated to increase performance. Team goals are encouraged rather than an optimal work pace for the individual. The workers with the lowest wages may need more than one job with obvious exposure implications.

All these elements emphasise the time aspect of exposure and may thus have considerable ergonomic implications. Elevated psychosocial exposures may be indicated due to the increased performance demands. This shows the need to move upstream from the individual to the production system level to influence the source of the risk factors. Ergonomic consequences of rationalisation decisions should be investigated to find the appropriate balance between productivity and ergonomics.

'Rationalisation strategy interventions' in the context of ergonomic intervention aim to achieve both high productivity and good musculoskeletal health of the workforce through modifications to the material production system. A few studies that examined health effect of production systems designed with such dual aims were identified in our intervention review (Westgaard and Winkel, 1997). These studies did not find a positive health effect of this intervention approach. Possible reasons for the negative results can be less than optimal design of the new production systems from a health perspective, improvement in exposure is negated by increased productivity (work pace), and/or an increase in psychosocial exposure, all causes that can be amended by better-designed production systems.

Interventions that attempt to merge the two aims of health and productivity are attractive in a company perspective and therefore more likely sustained. Research to clarify the potential of this intervention approach, both for new and traditional production systems, is needed.

3.5. Production system intervention: the organisational culture approach

The other subgroup of production system interventions is organisational culture interventions, i.e., promoting health and safety through company-wide organisational means. Examples are systems to identify and correct ergonomic problems, educational programs to increase awareness of health issues among major stakeholders, efforts to influence management attitudes towards health and safety, and participative ergonomics by focus groups. Many different risk factors exist in large organisations, with jobs spanning from, e.g., manual assembly to office environments. In most cases this requires a working environment program with systems for proper identification of risk factors and implementation of targeted intervention measures.

This group of studies was the second largest in our intervention review (Westgaard and Winkel, 1997). The interventions were heterogeneous with respect to focus, approaches, and size of organisation. The starting point of all interventions was an awareness of ergonomic problems and willingness to deal with these in an organisational manner, without significantly changing the material production system. The results ranged from complete failures to reportedly successful interventions. Reporting bias is expected, there would be a tendency to over-represent the success stories. Also, the scientific quality of many of the papers is in doubt. However, it was concluded on the basis of studies with reasonable quality (e.g., including a control group) that this intervention approach has a reasonable chance of success, provided the intervention carries high commitment from stakeholders, who utilise multiple intervention measures to reduce identified risk factors. Further scrutinising the results

did not establish any single factor as critical to the success.

The distinction between organisational culture and workstation interventions may not be apparent for the individual worker, who in either case will experience the intervention as modifications to workstation and/or work duties. The distinction is the intervention setting and the organisational systems supporting the intervention effort.

Organisational culture in a company reflects community values and varies throughout the world. Examples from countries with traditional good labour relations may not be achievable elsewhere. However, legislative initiatives, particularly in Europe and North America tend to move in the direction of mandatory ergonomics programs, as part of a systematic work environment effort. International quality and environmental standards, the ISO 9000 and 14000 series, recognises the work environment and can be built upon to create a concerted effort that merges considerations of quality, external environment and work environment.

4. Practical considerations in ergonomic interventions

4.1. Assessing mechanical and psychosocial exposure in interventions

The ergonomics practitioner needs to identify exposures that are potentially harmful by methods relevant in an intervention perspective. He/she is subject to cost and time constraints and needs to minimise the cost of exposure assessment. At the same time, the exposure assessment must be interpretable in terms of the results of scientific studies of risk factors. Considerable efforts have been made to establish convenient methods for objective assessment of biomechanical exposure. One line of research has been to evaluate reliability and validity of objective indicators of exposure, such as percent time with arm elevated or back flexed, collected by subjective scoring. Such variables have low validity (Wiktorin et al., 1993). However, time variables that are easier

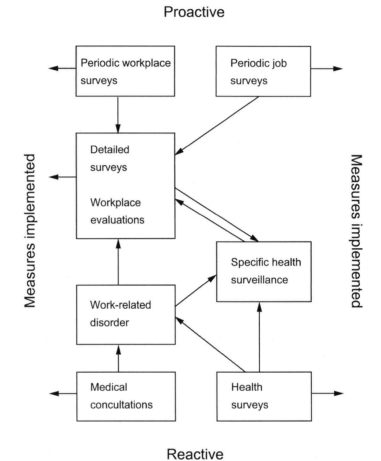

Proactive

Fig. 7. Flow diagram of a surveillance system to detect work-related musculoskeletal disorders. The system is part proactive, part reactive. See text for further details. (From Westgaard, 2000.)

to conceptualise, such as time performing a specific work task, have shown better validity (Winkel et al., 1995). A modified approach is therefore to use a combination of subjective and objective methods. In task-based job exposure assessment the exposure amplitude is quantified by observation or technical measurements while task distribution is quantified by self-assessment (Winkel and Mathiassen, 1994).

Management systems that utilise different types of flexibility introduce combinations of biomechanical and psychosocial work stress. The time variables of traditional biomechanical exposure assessment methods may detect a change in work routines indi-

cating a change in health risk, but should be supplemented by instruments like the questionnaire used to determine variables in the demand–control–support theory of psychosocial work stress (Karasek and Theorell, 1990). Unfortunately, this and other questionnaires intended for epidemiological studies may not provide sufficient specific information needed to initiate targeted intervention measures. This comment is valid also for studies of biomechanical risk factors.

A Danish group has suggested an alternative approach that merges the need for psychosocial exposure evaluation of both the researcher and the practitioner. From a questionnaire with 150 items, used by researchers, a short version with the most relevant questions is put together for use by the practitioners (Kristensen, 2001). In the study of service workers discussed in the section 'Recent physiological injury models' a qualitative approach was used with interviews structured on the basis of open questions, e.g., "What do you feel is the most demanding psychosocial factor in your work environment?" Such questions provided detailed and diverse information about workplace exposure factors and can be a useful method also for the ergonomic practitioner.

It is important to include the worker in the biomechanical exposure evaluation. Worker opinion of own workload is a check on the professional exposure evaluation and may identify specific, person-related problem exposures, helpful in assessing borderline exposures. Two prospective studies support the use of worker assessment of own workload by way of an impact scale (Veiersted and Westgaard, 1994; Balogh et al., 2001). Both studies showed high incidence of musculoskeletal complaints over a one-year observation period for pain-free workers who at baseline perceived current exposure as heavy or demanding.

In large companies many different exposure situations must be evaluated. Simple observation or walk-through allows a crude classification of exposures as acceptable, borderline or clearly unacceptable. If a problem is obvious, intervention measures should be initiated right away. Borderline exposures require more sophisticated analyses. A two-stage procedure for exposure assessment is thus indicated, using a simple screening system in combination with more detailed follow-up analyses when required. Fig. 7 shows a block diagram of a detection and evaluation system according to these principles that has had success in some Norwegian companies (Westgaard, 2000). The guiding principle is to detect and rectify problem exposures with as little effort and costs as possible. It is recognised that many ergonomic problems can be identified through simple inspection, thus periodic workplace surveys is carried out by representatives from management and labour together with an ergonomics specialist. Detailed exposure assessment is done when needed. The system

also responds to cases of work-related disorder or other indications of too-strenuous work situations. A wide array of exposure factors can be considered by such a system.

The ergonomic practitioner must allow for practical considerations in using reference literature for exposure evaluation. As an example, CEN standards on workplace design give specific criteria for construction of machinery (i.e., workplaces) and have legal status in that new machinery must comply with the standards to be certified for sale within the European Community. However, the standards are intended for designers of new machinery: a stooped posture is unacceptable in the design of a new piece of machinery. But the health effects of a stooped posture ('high amplitude') further depend on its repetitiveness and duration. The ergonomist must consider the combined effects of all exposure variables when evaluating an existing work situation.

4.2. Implementing ergonomic interventions

A system to ensure implementation of the ergonomic solutions is equally important to the success of ergonomic interventions. Fig. 8 shows a form used in a total quality management (TQM)-type approach to secure compliance, implemented by another Norwegian company. Important determinants, such as a description of the intervention measure, the person in charge of implementation and deadlines for completion, are recorded and distributed to those involved. The work environment implementation systems have similar status to other organisational systems in the company.

Health and safety systems such as those exemplified in Figs. 7 and 8 must be tailored to the company to not represent an unreasonable burden. Smaller companies may use scaled-down versions operating on the same general principles. Alternative approaches to ergonomic problem solving are found in the proposed OSHA ergonomics standard (*http://www.osha-slc.gov*) and in the detection and handling of 'caution zone jobs' detailed in Washington State health and safety regulations (*http://www.lni.wa.gov/rules/*).

Revision carried out (date):	**H&S ACTIVITIES** **Summary Report**		Mailed to:		
Participants:	Dept./unit:...............		(Survey participants, maintenance, upper-level manager etc.)		
	Signatures:				
	(department leader) (worker representative)				

Status/follow-up cases	Suggestions for intervention measures	Responsible	Deadline	Implemented	Longer-term measures
Training, attitudes Management issues Safety measures Machines, technical equipment Transport, warehouse Maintenance, repairs Order, cleanliness Communication, experience transfer Procedures, activities etc. (A mix of headlines tailored to the local situation. Each headline may be backed up with checklists where the different points are marked as satisfactory or not.)	(If problems are identified, measures to rectify the situation are listed here.)	(Person responsible)	(Date to finish impleme ntation)	(Date when implemented)	(Measures that cannot be implemented locally are carried upwards in the organisation to plant or company level)

Fig. 8. Form used to secure implementation of ergonomic interventions. A complete stakeholder representation is documented. Project responsibility and time period are highlighted. The company experience is that most cases are resolved at a low (department) organisational level. The cases that remain are handled at higher organisational level. Similar systems for implementation exist at plant and company level. (From Westgaard, 2000.)

The ergonomic practitioner is an important stakeholder and is often the one responsible for maintaining an ergonomically acceptable working environment. However, this is not the case in the Scandinavian countries where the line manager is the person immediately responsible and overall responsibility rests with the company executive director. To the extent the ergonomics practitioner has responsibility, he/she must clarify his/her organisational perspective in dealing with interventions; perhaps another person is better suited to carry the responsibility of implementation. Whatever role is given to the ergonomist, an important task is to ensure that other stakeholders act according to their responsibilities. If the ergonomist ends up with executive responsibility for managing the intervention, he/she must clarify his/her mandate and try to expand it if too restricted. He/she must further secure good relationship with other stakeholders, enlist their support and clarify their expectations. Documentation of intervention re-

sults is recommended. Although health effects are the ultimate aim, the many risk factors potentially operating make health measures uncertain indicators of intervention success. Exposure variables may therefore be a better choice.

Much good can be achieved by specific intervention towards individuals and their workstations, but most likely many more workers are not reached by this approach. There is furthermore the risk that other stakeholders, who influence working environment conditions, relax in their attitude to work environment matters with substantial negative exposure effects. We advice to adopt a production system perspective using both organisational culture and rationalisation strategy principles. Even modifier interventions should be considered, as discussed before. Rationalisation strategy interventions are only efficient if the ergonomist is actively involved in the planning of new production systems. A working relationship with production engineers and other decision-makers is therefore necessary.

Finally, the issue of intervention sustainability must be considered. Unfortunately, the intervention literature does not offer much advice on this point. Anchoring the intervention effort in the organisational structure of the company is already mentioned. It is common experience that work environment is among the priorities that first suffer if a company falls on hard times. A strong company culture may resist such a development. Even times of rapid expansion in production can be a challenge. Proven positive effects of ergonomic interventions is an important contribution to build this culture.

5. Conclusions

The complexities of ergonomic interventions including exposure assessment and intervention implementation are highlighted. The main points in our discussion of these issues can be summarised as follows.

General:

- establish an organisational structure for your work and clarify your own perspective in dealing with ergonomic interventions;
- aim for organisational efficiency;
- establish working relationships with other stakeholders;
- work proactively, preferably by influencing and improving the production system design, but show also concern for the individual worker.

Exposure assessment:

- establish a structured, comprehensive and cost-effective system for identification of harmful exposures;
- combine objective and subjective indicators for the most flexibility in the exposure assessment;
- include the worker and allow for individual variation.

Intervention implementation:

- clarify responsibilities of other stakeholders and ensure they are aware of their duties;

- try to achieve equal priority for the implementation of accepted ergonomic interventions to other investment decisions;
- establish formal systems to monitor progress in intervention implementation, scaled to match the company resources;
- document results.

References

Andriessen, E. and Roe, R.A. (1994) Telematics and Work. Lawrence Erlbaum, Howe.

Arendt, R. (2001) Work posture and musculoskeletal problems of video display terminal operators — review and reappraisal. Am. Ind. Hyg. Assoc. J., 44: 437–446.

Ariëns, G.A.M., van Mechelen, W., Bongers, P.M., Bouter, L.M. and van der Wal, G. (2001) Psychosocial risk factors for neck pain: a systematic review. Am. J. Ind. Med., 39: 180–193.

Armstrong, T.J., Foulke, J.A., Martin, B.J., Gerson, J. and Rempel, D.M. (1994) Investigation of applied forces in alphanumeric keyboard work. Am. Ind. Hyg. Assoc. J., 55: 30–35.

Ashkenas, R., Ulrich, D., Jick, D. and Kerr, S. (1995) The boundaryless organization. Breaking the chains of organizational structure. Jossey Bass, San Francisco, CA.

Åstrand, I. (1960) Aerobic work capacity in men and women with special reference to age. Acta Physiol. Scand., 49(Suppl. 169): 1–92.

Atkinson, J. (1984) Flexibility, uncertainty and manpower management. Institute of Manpower Studies, Brighton, Report 89.

Attebrant, M., Winkel, J. and Mathiassen, S.E. (1995) Forestry rationalization in Sweden. Implications for physical work load and musculoskeletal disorders. Second International Scientific Conference on Prevention of Work-Related Musculoskeletal Disorders. Institut de recherche en santé et en sécurité du travail du Québec, Montreal, pp. 205–207.

Balogh, I., Ørbaek, P., Winkel, J., Nordander, C., Ohlsson, K., Ektor-Andersen, J. and Malmö Shoulder–Neck Study Group (2001) Questionnaire-based mechanical exposure indices for large population studies — reliability, internal consistency and predictive validity. Scand. J. Work Environ. Health, 27: 41–48.

Bansevicius, D., Westgaard, R.H. and Jensen, C. (1997) Mental stress of long duration: EMG activity, perceived tension, fatigue, and pain development in pain-free subjects. Headache, 37: 499–510.

Bansevicius, D., Westgaard, R.H. and Sjaastad, O.M. (1999) Tension-type headache: pain, fatigue, tension and EMG responses to mental activation. Headache, 39: 417–425.

Bao, S., Winkel, J., Mathiassen, S.E. and Shahnavaz, H. (1997) Interactive effect of ergonomics and production engineering on shoulder–neck exposure — A case study of assembly work in China and Sweden. Int. J. Ind. Ergon., 20: 75–85.

Bernard, B.P. (1997) Musculoskeletal disorders and workplace factors. DHHS (NIOSH) Publication No. 97-141, Cincinnati, OH.

Bigos, S.J., Battié, M.C., Spengler, D.M., Fisher, L.D., Fordyce, W.E., Hansson, T.H., Nachemson, A. and Wortley, M.D. (2001) A prospective study of work perceptions and psychosocial factors affecting the report of back injury. Spine, 16: 1–6.

Björkman, T. (1996) The rationalisation movement in perspective and some ergonomic implications. Appl. Ergon., 27: 111–117.

Bongers, P.M., de Winter, C.R., Kompier, M.A.J. and Hildebrandt, V.H. (1993) Psychosocial factors at work and muskeletal disease. Scand. J. Work Environ. Health, 19: 297–312.

Buckle, P. and Devereux, J. (1999) Work-related neck and upper limb musculoskeletal disorders. Office for Official Publications of the European Communities, Luxembourg.

Commission on behavioral and social sciences and education, National Research Council and Institute of Medicine (2001) Musculoskeletal Disorders and the Workplace: Low Back and Upper Extremities. National Academy Press, Washington, DC.

Cox, T., Griffiths, A. and Rial-González, E. (2000) Research on Work-Related Stress. Office for Official Publications of the European Communities, Luxembourg.

Edwards, R.H.T. (1988) Hypotheses of peripheral and central mechanisms underlying occupational muscle pain and injury. Eur. J. Appl. Physiol., 57: 275–281.

Felstead, A. and Jewson, N. (1999) Global Trends in Flexible Labour. Mac Millan Business, London.

Grandjean, E. (1969) Fitting the Task to the Man. Taylor and Francis, London.

Greenleaf, J.E. (1984) Physiological responses to prolonged bed rest and fluid immersion in humans. J. Appl. Physiol., 57: 619–633.

Grieco, A. (1986) Sitting posture: an old problem and a new one. Ergonomics, 29: 345–362.

Hagberg, M., Silverstein, B., Wells, R., Smith, M.J., Hendrick, H.W., Carayon, P. and Pérusse, M. (1995) Work Related Musculoskeletal Disorders (WMSDs): a Reference Book for Prevention. Taylor and Francis, London.

Hägg, G.M. (1991) Static work loads and occupational myalgia — a new explanation model. In: P.A. Anderson, D.J. Hobart and J.V. Danoff (Eds.), Electromyographical Kinesiology. Elsevier, Amsterdam, pp. 141–143.

Hägg, G.M. and Åström, A. (1997) Load pattern and pressure pain threshold in the upper trapezius muscle and psychosocial factors in medical secretaries with and without shoulder/neck disorders. Int. Arch. Occup. Environ. Health, 69: 423–432.

Hägg, G.M., Suurküla, J. and Kilbom, Å. (1990) Prediktorer för belastningsbesvär i skuldra/nacke. En longitudinell studie på kvinnliga montörer. Arbete och Hälsa, H/O. National Institute for Working Life, Stockholm, pp. 1–78.

Henning, R.A., Sauter, S.L., Salvendy, G. and Krieg, E.F. (1989) Microbreak length, performance, and stress in a data entry task. Ergonomics, 32: 855–864.

Henning, R.A., Bopp, M.I., Tucker, K.M., Knoph, R.D. and Ahlgren, J. (1997) Team-managed rest breaks during computer-supported cooperative work. Int. J. Ind. Ergon., 20: 19–29.

Holte, K.A. and Westgaard, R.H. (2002) Daytime trapezius muscle activity and shoulder–neck pain of service workers with work stress and low biomechanical exposure. Am. J. Ind. Med., 41: 393–405.

Howard, A. (1995) The Changing Nature of Work. Jossey Bass, San Francisco, CA.

Itani, T., Kondo, T., Matsubayashi, S., Oze, Y., Watanabe, A., Ohara, H. and Aoyama, H. (1983) Occupational cervicobrachial disorder and the effect of improved work condition on prevention. J. Sci. Stress Rest, 2: 15–23.

Johansson, H. and Sojka, P. (1991) Pathophysiological mechanisms involved in genesis and spread of muscular tension in occupational muscle pain and in chronic musculoskeletal pain syndromes: A hypothesis. Med. Hypotheses, 35: 196–203.

Jonsson, B. (1978) Kinesiology. With special reference to electromyographic kinesiology. In: W.A. Cobb and H. Van Duijn (Eds.), Contemporary Clinical Neurophysiology. EEG Suppl. 34, pp. 417–428.

Karasek, R. and Theorell, T. (1990) Healthy Work. Basic Books, New York, NY.

Keyserling, W.M. (2000a) Workplace risk factors and occupational musculoskeletal disorders, part 1: A review of biomechanical and psychophysical research on risk factors associated with low-back pain. Am. Ind. Hyg. Assoc. J., 61: 39–50.

Keyserling, W.M. (2000b) Workplace risk factors and occupational musculoskeletal disorders, part 2: A review of biomechanical and psychophysical research on risk factors associated with upper extremity disorders. Am. Ind. Hyg. Assoc. J., 61: 231–243.

Kilbom, Å. (1994) Repetitive work for the upper extremity, Part I. Guidelines for the practitioner. Int. J. Ind. Ergon., 14: 51–57.

Kristensen, T.S. (2001) A new tool for assessing psychosocial work environment factors: The Copenhagen Psychosocial Questionnaire. In: M. Hagberg, B. Knave, L. Lillienberg and H. Westberg (Eds.), Arbete och Hälsa 10. National Institute for Working Life, Stockholm, pp. 210–213.

Labour Standards Bureau, Ministry of Labour (1985) Guidelines to occupational health in VDT operation. Japan Industrial Safety and Health Association (JISHA) 5-35-1 Shiba Minato-ku, Tokyo.

Lundberg, U., Kadefors, R., Melin, B., Palmerud, G., Hassmén, P., Engström, M. and Elfsberg Dohns, I. (1994) Psychophysiological stress and EMG activity of the trapezius muscle. Int. J. Behav. Med., 1: 354–370.

Marras, W.S., Lavender, S.A., Leurgans, S.E., Fathallah, F.A., Ferguson, S.A., Allread, W.G. and Rajulu, S.L. (1995) Biomechanical risk factors for occupationally related low back disorders. Ergonomics, 38: 377–410.

Mathiassen, S.E. and Winkel, J. (1991) Quantifying variation in physical load using exposure-vs-time data. Ergonomics, 34: 1455–1468.

Melin, B. and Lundberg, U. (1997) A biopsychosocial approach to work-stress and musculoskeletal disorders. J. Psychophysiol., 11: 238–247.

Mergler, D.M., Brabant, C., Vézina, N. and Messing, K. (1987) The weaker sex? Men in women's working conditions report similar health symptoms. J. Occup. Med., 25: 417–421.

Nuemann, P., Kihlberg, S., Medbo, P., Mathiassen, S.E. and Winkel, J. (2002) A case study evaluating the ergonomic and productivity consequences of partial automation strategies in the electronic industry. Int. J. Prod. Res., in press.

Ohara, H., Aoyama, H. and Itani, T. (1976) Health hazard among cash register operators and the effect of improved working conditions. J. Hum. Ergol., 5: 31–40.

Salvendy, G. (1997) Handbook of Human Factors and Ergonomics. Wiley, New York, NY.

Sandsjö, L., Melin, B., Rissén, D., Dohns, I. and Lundberg, U. (2000) Trapezius muscle activity, neck and shoulder pain, and subjective experiences during monotonous work in women. Eur. J. Appl. Physiol., 83: 235–238.

Siegrist, J., Klein, D. and Voigt, K.-H. (1997) Linking sociological with physiological data: the model of effort–reward imbalance at work. Acta Physiol. Scand., 161(Suppl. 640): 1–5.

Silverstein, B.A., Armstrong, T.J., Longmate, A. and Woody, D. (1988) Can in-plant exercise control musculoskeletal symptoms? J. Occup. Med., 30: 922–927.

Sjøgaard, G., Lundberg, U. and Kadefors, R. (2000) The role of muscle activity and mental load in the development of pain and degenerative processes at the muscle cell level during computer work. Eur. J. Appl. Physiol., 83: 99–105.

Sluiter, J.K., Rest, K.M. and Frings-Dresen, M.H.W. (2000) Criteria document for evaluation of the work-relatedness of upper extremity musculoskeletal disorders. Coronel Institute for Occupational and Environmental Health, University of Amsterdam, Amsterdam.

Søgaard, K., Sjøgaard, G., Finsen, L., Olsen, H.B. and Christensen, H. (2001) Motor unit activity during stereotyped finger tasks and computer mouse work. J. Electromyogr. Kinesiol., 11: 197–206.

Ursin, H., Endresen, I.M., Svebak, S., Tellnes, G. and Mykletun, R. (1993) Muscle pain and coping with working life in Norway: a review. Work Stress, 7: 247–258.

Vahtera, J., Kivimäki, M. and Pentti, J. (1997) Effect of organisational downsizing on health of employees. Lancet, 350: 1124–1128.

Vasseljen, O. and Westgaard, R.H. (1995) A case-control study of trapezius muscle activity in office and manual workers with shoulder and neck pain and symptom-free controls. Int. Arch. Occup. Environ. Health, 67: 11–18.

Veiersted, K.B. and Westgaard, R.H. (1994) Subjectively assessed occupational and individual parameters as risk factors for trapezius myalgia. Int. J. Ind. Ergon., 13: 235–245.

Veiersted, K.B., Westgaard, R.H. and Andersen, P. (1990) Pattern of muscle activity during stereotyped work and its relation to muscle pain. Int. Arch. Occup. Environ. Health, 62: 31–41.

Veiersted, K.B., Westgaard, R.H. and Andersen, P. (1993) Electromyographic evaluation of muscular work pattern as a predictor of trapezius myalgia. Scand. J. Work Environ. Health, 19: 284–290.

Vernon, H.M. (1921) Industrial Fatigue and Efficiency. Dutton, New York, NY.

Wærsted, M. and Westgaard, R.H. (1996) Attention-related mus-

cle activity in different body regions during VDU work with minimal physical activity. Ergonomics, 39: 661–676.

Waters, T.R., Putz-Anderson, V., Garg, A. and Fine, L.J. (1993) Revised NIOSH equation for the design and evaluation of manual lifting tasks. Ergonomics, 36: 749–776.

Weber, A., Fussler, C., O'Hanlon, J.F., Grierer, R. and Grandjean, E. (1980) Psychophysiological effects of repetitive tasks. Ergonomics, 23: 1033–1046.

Westad, C. and Westgaard, R.H. (2001) Reducing the risk of motor unit overexertion: methods of inducing motor unit substitution. Fourth International Scientific Conference on Prevention of Work-Related Musculoskeletal Disorders. Coronel Institute, Univ. of Amsterdam, Amsterdam, p. 61.

Westgaard, R.H. (1988) Measurement and evaluation of postural load in occupational work situations. Eur. J. Appl. Physiol., 57: 291–304.

Westgaard, R.H. (1999) Effects of physical and mental stressors on muscle pain. Scand. J. Work Environ. Health, 25(suppl 4): 19–24.

Westgaard, R.H. (2000) Work-related musculoskeletal complaints: some ergonomics challenges upon the start of a new century. Appl. Ergon., 31: 569–580.

Westgaard, R.H. and Aarås, A. (1985) The effect of improved workplace design on the development of work-related musculo-skeletal illnesses. Appl. Ergon., 160: 91–97.

Westgaard, R.H. and De Luca, C.J. (1999) Motor unit substitution in long-duration contractions of the human trapezius muscle. J. Neurophysiol., 82: 501–504.

Westgaard, R.H. and Winkel, J. (1997) Ergonomic intervention research for improved musculoskeletal health: a critical review. Int. J. Ind. Ergon., 20: 463–500.

Westgaard, R.H., Jansen, T. and Jensen, C. (1996) EMG of neck and shoulder muscles: the relationship between muscle activity and muscle pain in occupational settings. In: S. Kumar and A. Mital (Eds.), Electromyography in Ergonomics. Taylor and Francis, London, pp. 227–258.

Westgaard, R.H., Vasseljen, O. and Holte, K.A. (2001) Trapezius muscle activity as a risk indicator for shoulder and neck pain in female service workers with low biomechanical exposure. Ergonomics, 44: 339–353.

Westin, A.F. (1990) Organizational culture and VDT policies: a case study of the federal express corporation. In: S. Sauter, M. Dainoff and M. Smith (Eds.), Promoting Health and Productivity in the Computerized Office. Taylor and Francis, London, pp. 147–162.

Wiktorin, C., Karlqvist, L. and Winkel, J. (1993) Validity of self-reported exposures to work postures and manual materials handling. Scand. J. Work Environ. Health, 19: 208–214.

Winkel, J. (1985) On foot swelling during prolonged sedentary work and the significance of leg activity. Arbete och Hälsa 35. National Institute for Working Life, Stockholm, pp. 1–84.

Winkel, J. and Mathiassen, S.E. (1994) Assessment of physical wok load in epidemiologic studies: concepts, issues and operational considerations. Ergonomics, 37: 979–988.

Winkel, J. and Westgaard, R.H. (1992) Occupational and individual risk factors for shoulder–neck complaints, Part II. The scientific basis (literature review) for the guide. Int. J. Ind. Ergon., 10: 85–104.

Winkel, J. and Westgaard, R.H. (1996) Editorial: a model for solving work related musculoskeletal problems in a profitable way. Appl. Ergon., 27: 71–77.

Winkel, J. and Westgaard, R.H. (1999) Belastningsergonomiska förändringsstrategier In: E. Holmström, M. Eklundh and K. Ohlsson (Eds.), Människan i arbetslivet. Studentlitteratur, Lund, pp. 107–127.

Winkel, J., Asterland, P., Balogh, I., Byström, J., Granqvist, L., Hansson, G.-Å., Isacsson, S.-O., Larsson, B., Ohlsson, K., Pålsson, B. et al. (1995) A research program on assessment of mechanical exposure in epidemiologic studies. Second International Scientific Conference on Prevention of Work-Related Musculoskeletal Disorders. Institut de recherche en santé et en sécurité du travail du Québec, Montreal, pp. 280–282.

Woodson, W.E., Tillman, B. and Tillman, P. (1992) Human Factors Design Handbook. McGraw-Hill, New York, NY.

New Avenues for the Prevention of Chronic Musculoskeletal Pain and Disability
Pain Research and Clinical Management, Vol. 12
Edited by S.J. Linton
© *2002 Elsevier Science B.V. All rights reserved*

CHAPTER 11

Stress in the development of musculoskeletal pain

Ulf Lundberg [1,*] and Bo Melin [2]

[1] *Department of Psychology and Centre for Health Equity Studies (CHESS), Stockholm University, S-106 91 Stockholm,*
Sweden
[2] *National Institute for Working Life, Stockholm, Sweden*

Abstract: Stress has often been suggested to be a critical mechanism for the development of musculoskeletal pain. Indeed, many studies demonstrate a relationship between stress and such symptoms. However, in order to be able to treat and prevent these disorders, it is important to understand the possible psychobiological mechanisms involved in these relationships. This chapter therefore emphasizes the role of stress in musculoskeletal pain from a psychobiological perspective. One of the most interesting ideas is the Cinderella hypothesis which purports that sustained activation of low-threshold motor units causes muscle pain. While this low-level activation is important, the Allostatic Load Model suggests that this becomes problematic when the balance between activation and rest is disturbed. A normal adaptive response to stress means activation of various allostatic systems in order to increase the individual's resources to cope with the stressor and then shut off the response as soon as the stress terminates. This activation is necessary for survival and for protection of the body. However, health problems may be caused by over- or under-activation of the allostatic systems. These findings are considered in relation to gender differences and modern work organizations. It is concluded that the importance of rest and recovery are particularly important for preventing stress-related pain in modern society.

1. Introduction

Today, a large body of evidence shows that physical conditions alone cannot explain the development of musculoskeletal pain in the modern work environment. For example, despite considerable ergonomic improvements of the work environment during the last few decades and attempts to eliminate as much heavy lifting and pushing as possible, the incidence of musculoskeletal disorders (MSD) has remained high and still constitutes a major health problem in the industrialized part of the world. Improvements in the physical work environment were particularly noticeable during the 1980s and, at the same time, there was a surprisingly marked increase in MSD. In Europe today, 20–30% of the workers report that they are suffering from work-related backache and muscular pains. In Sweden, where physical work conditions are considered to be particularly good, about 40% of the employees are suffering from neck and shoulder pain. This pattern is difficult to explain by traditional models according to which biomechanical load and awkward working positions are the dominating causes of MSD. Thus, influence from other factors seems likely.

The decrease in physical work demands during

---

* Correspondence to: U. Lundberg, Department of Psychology and Centre for Health Equity Studies (CHESS), Stockholm University,
S-106 91 Stockholm, Sweden. E-mail: ul@psychology.su.se

the 1980s and 1990s has been accompanied by an increase in mental demands. In order to increase productivity and efficiency and to become competitive on a global market, workload and work pace have increased considerably in most companies. Buffers in the production line and storage of product components have been replaced by 'just-in-time' production, which has forced the workers to become constantly active in order to meet several deadlines every day. In recent years, this trend is not only prevailing in private companies but also in the public service sector. In Sweden, for example, an economic crisis in the early 1990s resulted in increased demands for efficiency and productivity also in education and health care. In the late 1990s, the pronounced cut down of personnel was followed by a successive increase in the number of work-related health problems and in long-term absenteeism from work among teachers, nurses, medical doctors, administrators etc., an increase which is still going on. Also, conditions outside the occupational area have undergone rapid changes, such as political, economic, technological, and social conditions, which have contributed to a more rapid pace of life and constant demands for adjustment to new conditions. The allostatic load caused by repeated or sustained exposure to psychosocial stress is considered to be an important health risk (McEwen, 1998).

MSD are common not only in physically demanding jobs, but also in light physical work, such as data entry at video display units and assembly work in the electronic industry, where only a very small fraction (<1–2%) of the worker's physical capacity is used. This is difficult to explain on the basis of traditional models of MSD and suggests that other factors may contribute to these disorders. Women generally report more neck and shoulder pain problems than men. Among white-collar workers, the prevalence of MSD is more than twice as high among women as among men. In view of the small amount of muscular strength necessary in most white-collar jobs, this gender difference is not likely to be explained by gender differences in physical capacity. Additional support for this conclusion is obtained by the fact that physical strength per se

does not protect against the development of MSD (Battié, 1989).

A great number of studies show an association between psychosocial stress at work and a high incidence of MSD (Bongers et al., 1993; Moon and Sauter, 1996). Most of them are cross-sectional (e.g., Johansson, 1994), which makes conclusions regarding causality difficult or impossible. It seems reasonable that workers who are suffering from neck, shoulder or back pain problems would be more prone to report negative work conditions and a low job satisfaction, than workers without such symptoms. However, a causal relationship between psychosocial work stress and MSD is supported by prospective studies. Bigos et al. (1991) found that workers with a low job satisfaction were more likely to develop back pain problems during a 4-year follow-up period, compared with workers who enjoyed going to work. Leino and Magni (1993) found that workers in the metal industry who reported high distress at work had significantly elevated risk of MSD 10 years later.

In summary, evidence from several sources supports the conclusion that psychosocial factors such as stress play a role in the development of MSD. In the modern work environment, where physical demands have been reduced considerably and the ergonomic conditions have been improved, factors other than biomechanical load may have become more important for musculoskeletal pain. Thus, in order to be able to treat and prevent these disorders, it is of importance to learn about the possible psychobiological mechanisms involved in these relationships today.

2. Stress responses in jobs with a high prevalence of MSD

If psychosocial stress contributes to MSD in light physical work, then occupations with a high prevalence of neck, shoulder, and back pain problems should be associated with high stress levels. Examples of jobs with a high incidence of MSD are traditional assembly line work and work at checkout counters at supermarkets (Lundberg et al., 1989, 1999; Melin et al., 1999). These jobs are characterized by conditions such as monotonous and repetitive work tasks, machine (or customer) paced work, lack of influence and control over the content and conditions at work, physical restriction to the work place, low occupational status, and low income. Such conditions are likely to induce stress according to several well-known stress models. Stress or strain is caused by a combination of high demands and low control (Karasek, 1979), by under-stimulation (Frankenhaeuser, 1976), and by high effort combined with low reward (Siegrist, 1996). In keeping with these models, not only self-reports of stress but also objective indicators of stress, such as catecholamines and cardiovascular responses, confirm that assembly line workers (Timio and Gentili, 1976; Timio et al., 1979; Lundberg et al., 1989; Melin et al., 1999) and cashiers at the supermarket (Lundberg et al., 1999; Rissén et al., 2000) have significantly elevated stress levels at work compared with, e.g., white-collar workers (Frankenhaeuser et al., 1989; Lundberg and Frankenhaeuser, 1999). In addition, stress levels in monotonous and repetitive work also seem to remain high after the end of the work shift, compared with more flexible work conditions (Johansson, 1981; Melin et al., 1999).

A review of stress responses in different groups of blue- and white-collar workers shows that white-collar workers increase their epinephrine output at work about 50% compared with their non-work level, whereas blue-collar workers show a corresponding increase of about 100% (Lundberg and Johansson, 2000). For norepinephrine, there is usually an increase of about 50% among blue-collar workers and a very small increase or no increase at all among white-collar workers (Lundberg and Johansson, 2000). This difference in responsiveness between the two catecholamines can be explained by the fact that norepinephrine, which is also a transmitter in the sympathetic nervous system, is influenced by physical demands and body posture, whereas epinephrine, emanating from the adrenal medulla, is mainly sensitive to mental stress (Lundberg, 2000). Thus, the lack of norepinephrine response among white-collar workers is likely to reflect the low physical activity in their job and the fact that they are

spending most of their time sitting at a desk or a computer.

In conclusion, light physical work associated with a high prevalence of musculoskeletal disorders seems to be overrepresented by factors known to induce stress and with elevated psychophysiological stress levels during and after work. Blue-collar workers are generally exposed to a greater allostatic load than white-collar workers.

3. Work conditions and muscular activity

Whereas the effects of physical demands on muscle tension and that of mental demands on physiological stress responses, such as catecholamines, blood pressure and heart rate etc., are well-known, much less is known about the effects of mental stress on muscle activity. In order to identify a causative role of mental stress in the development of MSD, the demonstration of an effect of mental stress on muscle tension seems important, although other psychobiological mechanisms, not involving the muscle cells (Knardahl, 2002), are also possible.

In recent years, a number of experiments have been performed in order to explore the role of mental factors (stress, cognitive demands etc.) on muscle tension. Interest has focused on the trapezius muscle, which covers the upper back, the neck, and the shoulders. The reason for this interest is based on the fact that this is the part of the body where most people contract disorders. However, from a psychological perspective, the trapezius muscle is also of interest for other reasons. Through evolution, this muscle, in addition to the facial muscles, seems to have played an important emotional role for survival and development of many species. For instance, by raising the shoulders, making the hair on the upper back standing on end or spreading the wings, individuals of different species are trying to frighten their enemies and, thus, increase their chances of survival. Human expression of other emotions, such as surprise and fear, also involves raising of the shoulders. In an experimental study, Wærsted (1997) measured electromyographic (EMG) activity in different muscles in response to cognitive demands and found that the facial muscles and the trapezius were more responsive than other muscles to this type of stimulation. This sensitivity of the trapezius muscle to cognitive and emotional stimuli, in addition to its biomechanical role, may help to explain the contribution of emotional stress to the development of trapezius myalgia.

A significant effect of mental stress on trapezius muscle activity has been demonstrated in several experiments, although the individual differences in responsiveness are pronounced. Svebak et al. (1993) found a significant increase in EMG activity of the trapezius muscle in fibromyalgic and in control subjects exposed to a mental task. Wærsted et al. (1991) measured EMG activity in response to a cognitive computer task and found significant increases in a group of 'high responders'. Lundberg et al. (1994a) found a significant increase in trapezius EMG activity in 62 women exposed to mental tasks such as the Stroop Color Word Test and Mental Arithmetic. An additional finding of potential interest was that the effect of mental stress on EMG activity was enhanced when the subject was exposed to a standardized physical demand at the same time (test contraction). This indicates a possible interaction between mental and physical demands on muscle tension (Melin and Lundberg, 1997; Lundberg et al., 2002).

In modern society, where stress is more often caused by psychosocial factors than by physical threats and demands, the trapezius muscle may frequently be activated by mental factors. In the hunter–gatherer societies, in which the modern human evolved, the demands were quite different. It is likely that ancient humans were exposed to occasional periods of mental and physical demands, e.g., when hunting for food, but that life in between could be quite stable and calm for long periods. The effects of mentally induced muscle tension are likely to differ from those caused by physical demands. In heavy physical work, the accumulation of lactic acid signals fatigue to the individual and forces him or her to take a break in order to rest and recover. Under optimal conditions of physical activity, such as aer-

obic exercise, increased vasodilation and blood flow through the muscle may 'wash out' metabolites and inflammatory substances and, thus, serve a protective role against muscle pain. However, muscle tension caused by mental stress, such as time pressure, low job satisfaction, low status, low income, fear of loosing the job, interpersonal conflicts etc., is more likely to be associated with vasoconstriction and reduced blood flow. In addition, psychosocial stress is usually more lasting than exposure to heavy physical work and the energy released during stress in terms of lipids and glucose is excessive in view of the limited biomechanical work being performed. The lack of adequate signals of fatigue during light physical work or during stress-induced muscle tension may keep the individual constantly active, for instance on a data entry task, without noticing that some muscle fibres are overloaded. In order to understand how such low but sustained levels of muscle tension may cause MSD, new explanatory models have been proposed.

4. New explanatory models

In recent years, a number of new models have been proposed in order to explain the high prevalence of MSD in light physical but psychologically stressful jobs (Hägg, 1991; Johansson and Sojka, 1991; Schleifer and Ley, 1994; Knardahl, 2002). These models are not mutually exclusive but may all contribute to the understanding of the psychobiological mechanisms linking different work conditions to MSD in different individuals. As MSD seem to have a very complex and multifactorial etiology, it is reasonable to assume that a number of different mechanisms are involved. However, it is interesting to note that psychological stress is considered to play an important role in all these models and the pain syndromes caused by these mechanisms may then be maintained or become even more severe, and eventually chronic, through additional psychological and biological mechanisms (Linton, 1994).

In the present chapter, we will focus on one of the explanatory models, the 'Cinderella hypothesis', proposed by Hägg (1991) and the empirical evidence in support of this model (Sjøgaard et al., 2000). However, in view of the complexity of these phenomena, three alternative models will first be reviewed briefly.

One model is focused on the important role of breathing under stress. Schleifer and Ley (1994) have noticed that individuals under stress tend to hyperventilate, that is they breathe more heavily than necessary for metabolic reasons, which has significant effects on the blood chemistry. For example, excessive breathing reduces endtidal CO_2 levels, which causes an increase in blood pH-levels. A very high blood pH-level causes alcalosis, which among other things increases muscle tension and reduces parasympathetic activity, which makes the muscles more sensitive to sympathetic activity.

Johansson and Sojka (1991) have noticed that the density of muscle spindles is particularly high in the neck and shoulder region, i.e., in the trapezius muscle, where pain syndromes are most frequent. These sensory organs embedded in the muscles are very important for the coordination of movements, for an optimal allocation of muscle activity and for the regulation of muscle stiffness. Repetitive work and mental stress may cause increased activity in the muscle spindles, which starts a vicious circle where elevated muscle stiffness may cause increased concentrations of inflammatory substances (bradykinin, serotonin etc.) in the muscles. This condition signals back to the muscle spindles to become even more active. The inflammatory substances also affect the pain receptors to become more sensitive and increase pain perception. Elevated sympathetic activity influences the regulation of the muscle spindles and may, under certain conditions, even block their activity, which causes dysfunctional coordination and inadequate muscle activity. Such vicious circles in one muscle may spread to other muscles in the body through nerve signals.

Knardahl (2002) has proposed a model according to which "pain originates from the vessel–nerve interactions of the connective tissue of the muscle, rather than from energy crisis of the muscle cells". Different vessel–nociceptor mechanisms known to cause pain, e.g., in migraine, may be involved, such as vasodilation stretching the vessel wall, release of algogenic substances from the nerves and/or the vessels, such as prostaglandins, and inflammatory processes which may sensitize nociceptors.

The model by Hägg (1991), described below, is based on the assumption of an overuse of low-threshold motor units. It has been called the 'Cinderella hypothesis', which refers to Cinderella in the fairy tale, who was first to rise in the morning and last to go to bed in the evening,

5. The Cinderella hypothesis

The Cinderella hypothesis is based on earlier findings by Henneman et al. (1965), showing an orderly recruitment of motor units — the smallest functional units of the muscle — in response to static muscle load. Small, low-threshold motor units (Type I fibres) are always recruited first, before larger ones, and these low-threshold units are assumed to remain constantly active until complete relaxation of the muscle. Motor units with higher thresholds are activated at higher force levels and are shut off as soon as the force level decreases. This means that the low-threshold or 'Cinderella' motor units are constantly active under sustained physical work, whereas motor units with higher thresholds are activated only during heavy physical work. Even if these Cinderella units are assumed to be fatigue-resistant, there is likely to be an upper limit for constant activation. Overuse may cause exhaustion of these motor units with metabolic disturbances (lack of energy to the muscle cells, accumulation of metabolites etc.), damaged muscle fibres, and the development of pain syndromes. Constant activation of these motor units may also prevent repair of damaged muscle fibres ('red ragged fibres'). Under conditions of low muscular activity, signals of fatigue may be subliminal, which means that the risk of overuse of low-threshold motor units is high if the individual continues to work. Additional factors, which under chronic stress may contribute to these degenerative processes, are impairment of the immune functions and a slow healing process (Kiecolt-Glaser et al., 1994).

6. Empirical support for the Cinderella hypothesis

As the Cinderella hypothesis is based on the assumption that sustained activation of low-threshold motor units may cause muscle pain, it indicates that rest and recovery are factors of significant importance preventing this degenerative process. In keeping with this, Veiersted et al. (1993) found that lack of muscle rest during breaks at work was a risk factor for the development of trapezius myalgia. In this prospective study, Veiersted et al. (1993) followed female workers performing repetitive tasks by successive measurements of trapezius EMG activity during work as well as during breaks at work over a period of about 1 year from the start of their employment. About half of the workers developed trapezius myalgia problems during this period, most of them already after 6 months. The group of workers who developed symptoms was found to have significantly elevated EMG activity during breaks at work, but not significantly so during actual work, compared with workers who remained healthy. This suggests that not only muscle activity during work but also lack of muscle rest during breaks is a risk factor for the development of MSD. In addition, Veiersted (1995) found that among women with more EMG gaps, i.e., very short periods of muscle rest, only about 30% developed myalgia problems, compared with about 70% among women with fewer (below median) EMG gaps. This suggests that short periods of muscle rest may prevent pain syndromes, which is consistent with the implications from the Cinderella hypothesis.

The findings from the prospective study by Veiersted et al. (1993) have been supported by cross-sectional studies. Hägg and Åström (1997) found that female medical secretaries with neck and shoulder pain had more elevated EMG activity during breaks at work compared with women without symptoms and Sandsjö et al. (2000) found that women with neck and shoulder pain working at the supermarket had significantly less muscle rest than women without such symptoms.

Thus, data consistently shows an association between lack of muscle rest and trapezius myalgia.

Lundberg et al. (1999) also found significantly more trapezius EMG activity in female cashiers with symptoms compared to workers without neck and shoulder pain. The elevated EMG activity in individuals with pain are not likely to be caused by pain itself as each individual's EMG activity was compared with her own reference level during a standardized test contraction. In addition, pain is more likely to reduce than to increase EMG activity in the affected muscle (Sjøgaard et al., 2000). Possible reasons for the higher EMG activity among workers with symptoms could be experiences of more stress, a higher workload, and/or a less optimal work technique. Higher stress levels were indicated by self-reports and elevated blood pressure among cashiers with symptoms, but no differences were found in workload or work technique (Lundberg et al., 1999).

These findings are in agreement with the Cinderella hypothesis but they do not exclude other explanatory models. In view of the Cinderella hypothesis and the assumption that mentally induced muscle tension may keep low-threshold motor units active, it is important to find out if the same motor units are activated by mental stress as by physical effort. This question was tested in a recent experiment (Lundberg et al., 2002) by exposing subjects successively to mental and physical stressors. Intramuscular recordings based on techniques developed within the PROCID (Prevention of muscle disorders in operation of computer input devices) project (Colombo et al., 1999; Forsman et al., 1999a,b; Kadefors et al., 1999; Wellig and Moschytz, 1999) were used to identify activity in individual motor units of the trapezius. The results show that in most subjects, one or more motor units were active both during mentally and physically induced muscle tension.

This means that mental stress, which is usually longer lasting than physical activity, may keep low-threshold motor units active also in the absence of physical activity and, thus, contribute to metabolic disturbances. Breaks at work may not necessarily reduce the risk of MSD unless it is accompanied by mental relaxation. Work conditions combining mental and physical demands may constitute a particular risk for MSD.

7. Additional psychological mechanisms relevant to work-related muscular pain

Despite lack of theory, a relationship between the work environment and the risk of developing and/or maintaining MSD has been known for a long time. The very first systematic observations were made by Ramazzini in 1713. He is regarded as the 'father of occupational medicine' and his findings relate to the role of organizational factors in the development of MSD. Early models of pain development, such as the von Frey's specificity and Goldscheider's pattering theories of pain described by Odgen (1997), did not include organizational and psychological factors. However, a significant contribution to pain research was the development of the 'Gate Control Theory' (GCT) (Melzack and Wall, 1965, 1982). This theory has increased our understanding of pain by including descending influences, which suggest a potential role for psychological and work-related psychosocial factors. The GCT proposes a physiological function by which psychological factors can affect the experience of pain through a gating mechanism in the spinal cord. This neural gate can regulate incoming pain signals before activating transmission cells, which send impulses to the brain. The more the gate is opened, the greater the perception of pain. It is assumed that physical (injuries, heat, or cold, which activate large fibres), emotional (anxiety, worry, tension, and depression), and behavioral factors (focusing on the pain or boredom) contribute to opening the gate. Closing the gate reduces the perception of pain, which can also be achieved by physical (medication, which stimulates the small fibres), emotional (happiness, optimism, or relaxation) and behavioral factors (concentration, distraction, or involvement in other activities) (e.g., Odgen, 1997). The GCT has received most attention with regard to work-related neck and shoulder pain.

The multi-factorial etiology of MSD is assumed to involve both physical and psychological factors, which have key roles in the understanding of the development, maintenance, prevention, or even treatment of MSD. The explanatory models described above can be complemented with other relevant psychological theories, such as associative theories and theories of anxiety and cognitive state.

Research suggests that associative learning has an effect on the maintenance and perception of pain. An individual may associate a particular environment with the experience of pain. For example, if an individual associates the dentist with pain due to past experience, the perception of pain may be enhanced when attending the dentist. Because of the association, the individual may experience increased anxiety when attending the dentist, which may also increase the perception of pain. Patients with a long history of pain tend to react with increased anxiety and pain when confronted with words associated with pain. In addition, chronic pain patients are overly sensitive to painful stimulation as well as to non-painful but pain-related stimuli (Flor et al., 1997).

However, associative theories are not only relevant for pain perception, but also for the understanding of more general psychophysiological mechanisms on how pain sustains over time. Magneto-encephalographic recording techniques have been used during an aversive classical conditioning procedure with healthy volunteers (Wik et al., 1996). The reinforced conditioned stimuli (CS) were displayed on a screen for 2 s; as it disappeared, an unconditioned electric shock was presented to the right middle finger (causing some pain). A control stimulus, not paired with shock, was also presented. A conditioned neuromagnetic response elicited by the visual CS was located in the somatic sensory area. The outcome of this experiment implies that an earlier non-pain-related stimulus could become pain-related and elicit a similar neurological response as a real pain stimulus. This might be part of a psychophysiological explanation of why pain is still experienced while the mechanical stimuli originally causing the pain have disappeared. Other psychophysiological studies (e.g., Flor et al., 1995a,b, 1997), based on classical conditioning theory and the Hebbian cell assembly model, imply that stimuli that are associated with the experience of pain may excite pain-related cell assemblies and create a painful experience, even in the absence of stimulation from the periphery. Flor and co-workers have also shown that the primary somatosensory cortex plays a major role in this reorganization process and it is likely that more extensive changes in associative cortex also take place.

On a cognitive level it has been reported (Jamner and Tursky, 1987) that presentation of descriptors relevant to the patient's pain problem increases peripheral physiological activity. Studies also indicate a heightened perceptual sensitivity and increased ability to discriminate pain-related stimuli in individuals suffering from long lasting pain problems. For example, compared to individuals without pain problems chronic pain patients seem to be more perceptive to pain-related words and to do more pain-related associations to ambiguous words. Such outcomes indicate that individuals with a long history of pain are more likely to retrieve pain-associated words from memory. From a stress perspective (e.g., Flor et al., 1997), it can be argued that heightened perceptual sensitivity might be a consequence of the elevated level of chronic stress that patients with long lasting pain seem to experience.

8. Acute and chronic pain in regard to stress

Stress and anxiety per se appear to influence pain perception. Fordyce and Steger (1979) examined the relationship between anxiety and acute and chronic pain. They found that anxiety had different relationships to these two types of pain. When individuals experience acute pain, they also experience increased anxiety. Successful treatment reduces the pain, which subsequently reduces the level of anxiety. Reduced anxiety then causes a further reduction in pain. Because of the relative ease with which acute pain can be treated, anxiety can generally be reduced, which contributes to the cycle of pain reduction (Odgen, 1997). With regard to diffuse and long lasting pain, which often is resistant against treatment, patients' stress and anxiety levels will remain high or even

increase, which further increases pain perception. The heightened stress level is due to the fact that treatment of chronic pain is often ineffective and the patient anticipates continued pain, which increases anxiety. In summary, acute pain signals that this pain will be reduced, whereas lasting pain signals that this pain will stay or even get worse.

At work lasting and diffuse pain sensations can be suppressed by cognitive demands or a high work force. This suppression of the pain signal makes it difficult for the individual to decide when it is time to stop performing specific tasks. When stress is reduced after work, the pain signal may become stronger and interfere with both daily activities and sleep at night.

9. Effect of work-related organizational changes on stress and MSD

A variety of psychosocial factors associated with the individual worker and the work environment have been linked to shoulder, neck, and lower back pain problems (e.g., Bernard, 1997; SBU, 2000; Melin, 2001). The effects of different forms of individual treatment programs on these disorders have recently been evaluated (SBU, 2000), whereas very few work-related stress interventions have been performed. In view of the high incidence of neck, shoulder, and lower back pain problems in light physical work, such as assembly work in the electronic industry, and experimental data (Lundberg et al., 1994a) and the results showing significantly elevated muscular tension during psychological stress, knowledge about the mechanisms linking work-related stress to MSD is important in the planning of treatment and preventive actions on an organizational level.

Traditional assembly line work, characterized by high repetitivity, monotony, little variation, and low personal control, is associated with low job satisfaction, high absenteeism, and elevated psychobiological stress levels (Frankenhaeuser, 1986; Melin et al., 1999). A plausible explanation for these relationships is given by the Karasek Model (Karasek, 1979), according to which a combination of high demands and low control contributes to job strain and increased health risks.

The increased health risks of 'high strain jobs' may also be due to reduced ability to 'unwind' after work. The speed at which a person unwinds, for example, after a day of monotonous work, will influence the total load on the organism. A quick return to neuroendocrine and physiological baseline implies an 'economic' response, in the sense that physiological resources are 'demobilized' as soon as they are no longer needed (Frankenhaeuser, 1986). This mechanism has been investigated only in a few occupational studies, whereas different aspects of deactivation or unwinding have been focused on in more physiological and clinical studies, e.g., studies of blood pressure and heart rate during and after physical performance (e.g., Melin, 1993; Melin and Sandqvist, 1994). Johansson and Aronsson (1984) compared epinephrine levels of females in computerized repetitive data entry work with females in more flexible secretarial work. Five hours after work, the data entry group had still not reached their baseline level (measured during a day at home) in contrast to the secretarial group. Lundberg et al. (1989) compared physiological unwinding after repetitive data entry and a computerized learning task at a video display terminal and found slower deactivation after data entry in five of the six physiological variables measured.

The way of organizing assembly work has gone through dramatic changes since the beginning of the 1970s in many companies (Melin et al., 1999). For example, at the Volvo car engine factory in Skövde, Sweden, the Taylor oriented assembly line was abandoned for a work organization with carriers. At that time this was seen as an ergonomic revolution in comparison to traditional assembly line work with a conveyer belt, which was common in most European car factories in that period. The amount of personal control was enlarged, the work pace became more flexible, and the duration of the work cycle was expanded and the worker could work on an engine that was not moving. However, this still represented a combination of high demands and relatively low control and each worker was depending on the work

pace of his or her co-workers, which according to any stress model accentuates health risks.

Recently, Melin et al. (1999) investigated a far more flexible type of work organization for assembly work introduced at Volvo. The aim was to increase the amount of control and possibilities for social interactions between workers, to decrease the monotony of assembly line work by enlarged work cycles, but at the same time maintain the same production level (external demand). Each group of workers became responsible for the whole final assembly process, including the functional testing of the completed engine. The team worked independently of other groups, i.e., it was not influenced by earlier events in the production process and the members of the team could choose to follow their own engine through the whole process or to collaborate. The general aim of the study was to compare psychological and physiological stress reactions during and after work in the more flexible organization with the more traditional way of organizing assembly line work. From a control perspective, it was hypothesized that the flexible form of organization would elicit a more favorable stress profile than the assembly line. The general pattern of subjective and physiological measures (e.g., catecholamines, blood pressure) confirms this hypothesis and shows lower and more stable stress levels among assembly workers in the flexible form of work organization and a more rapid return to baseline after work, compared to that of the workers at the assembly line. This pattern was particularly pronounced for the female workers. However, no significant differences were found in self-reported strain in neck and shoulders, lower back, or wrists according to type of work organization or gender.

In another study on work organization (Rissén et al., 2000) women cashiers were investigated before, during, and after a work re-organization at four different supermarkets. Data from 72 cashiers were collected before the intervention (Lundberg et al., 1999). Psychobiological stress reactions and trapezius surface electromyography (EMG) were obtained during normal work, during unwinding after work, and during a corresponding period off from work and showed elevated stress reactions and muscle tension during work and a high incidence of MSD.

The aim of the prospective part of the study was to determine the effects of a work re-organization program on 31 female cash register operators from the first study still remaining at work. The intention of the re-organization was to increase influence over work, and to reduce stress and musculoskeletal problems by use of an expanded job rotation model. Cashiers suffering from pain tended to have higher surface EMG and a less favorable mean resting EMG profile than cashiers without pain (Sandsjö et al., 2000), and cashiers with negative emotional reactions showed higher EMG activity compared with their colleagues who reported more positive reactions (Rissén et al., 2000). The outcome of this study showed that extended job rotation seems to produce positive effects on several physiological stress-related health parameters. For example, trapezius EMG and systolic and diastolic blood pressure were significantly lower after implementation of the job rotation model. However, job rotation is not a treatment, since the same proportion of cashiers (70%) suffered from MSD after as before intervention, although the intensity of pain was reported to be significantly lower at follow-up. It should also be noted, that the new work organization might still have had a preventive effect since an increase in the pain prevalence could be expected due to the fact that the cashiers had been exposed to the same work environment almost 3 additional years at follow-up.

In conclusion, the two interventions described above (assembly line workers and cashiers, respectively) had a positive effect on several physiological stress parameters and on the perceived intensity of pain, whereas the proportion of individuals suffering from pain remained unchanged. Nevertheless, preventive effects on MSD cannot be excluded.

10. Gender differences in MSD

In view of the fact that gender differences in MSD are most pronounced among white-collar workers, women's higher prevalence of MSD is not likely to be explained by gender differences in physical strength. Although biological differences between men and women, such as sex hormones and differences in muscle fibre composition, may be of importance for pain syndromes, a primary role is assumed to be played by the fact that women more often than men are holding white-collar jobs where the risks of contracting MSD are high. In most occupational areas, such as administration, service, communication, and manufacturing (Statistics Sweden, 2000), more women than men perform repetitive tasks. Repetitive work, a high work pace, and lack of influence and control are factors that, according to the stress models above, cause job strain and elevated health risks. Another factor that may be of importance for employed women's higher risk is the additional load from unpaid work at home, which may cause stress off the job and reduce women's opportunities for rest and recovery.

With regard to the role of unpaid work for women's total workload, it has been found that full-time employed women below the age of 50, matched for age and type of occupation, spend more time on household work and child care than men (Lundberg et al., 1994b). The difference between the genders was found to increase with the number of children in the family. In families with three children or more women's total workload was almost 20 h greater on a normal week. In addition, more women than men reported having the primary responsibility for almost all unpaid duties at home associated with household chores and child care. This means that even if women do not necessarily have to perform all duties at home, they usually take the primary responsibility for planning ahead, worrying about things in the future, and seeing to it that things get done. Frankenhaeuser et al. (1989) compared physiological stress levels on and off the job for men and women matched for age and occupational status and found that women's stress levels tended to remain high also after work, whereas men usually returned to their baseline level after coming home from work. More recently, Lundberg and Frankenhaeuser (1999) replicated those findings and found that women's elevated stress levels after work were related to the presence of children at home. Only women with children had elevated stress levels after work, whereas men with children did not differ from men without children in this respect. It has also been demonstrated (Lundberg, 1996) that women's stress at work, but not men's, is reflected in stress levels in the evenings and on weekends at home, indicating a greater interaction between stress at work and stress at home in women compared to men.

In conclusion, and without excluding a possible role of biological factors, it is assumed that the most important factors contributing to women's higher risk of MSD are gender differences in type of work tasks and women's greater total workload (paid + unpaid work), which reduces opportunities for rest and recovery.

11. A general model of stress and health, the Allostatic Load Model

McEwen (1998) has proposed a model called the Allostatic Load Model, which predicts under what conditions physiological stress responses are adaptive and when they may cause health problems. An important feature of this model is the balance between activation and rest/recovery. A normal adaptive response to stress means activation of various allostatic systems in order to increase the individual's resources to cope with the stressor and then shut off the response as soon as the stress terminates. This activation is necessary for survival and for protection of the body. However, health problems may be caused by over- or under-activity of the allostatic systems.

Health risks increase in response to frequent or lasting stress. Repeated activation of the stress responses without enough time for rest and recovery as well as constant activation of various physiological systems, without ability to shut off these responses after the end of the stressor, for instance after work, may cause disturbances in various regulatory functions and cause damage to systems and organs. Long-lasting activation of the stress response means overexposure to stress hormones (catecholamines, cortisol) and sustained high blood pressure and heart rate. Eventually, this condition may lead to mental and/or physiological exhaustion and lack of adequate responses to new stressors. Inability to activate one physiological system in response to a new acute stressor may cause compensatory overactivation of other systems and dysregulation of the stress systems.

The importance of an optimal balance between effort and activity on the one hand and rest and recovery on the other, according to the Allostatic Load Model, also seems relevant for the development of MSD and is in agreement with the Cinderella hypothesis.

12. A general model of MSD

The evidence available so far on the development of MSD has been summarized in Fig. 1, which concludes that biomechanical demands and ergonomic conditions at work are of primary importance for muscle tension and the development of MSD, but that psychosocial conditions such as stress, separately, and in addition to physical conditions, may contribute to elevated physiological arousal and muscle tension. Some data indicate an interaction and an enhanced risk when mental and physical demands are combined (Lundberg et al., 1994a; Theorell and Hasselhorn, 2002).

However, conditions at work, such as repetitive tasks, lack of control, and time pressure may contribute to keeping stress levels and muscle tension elevated also after work and thus reduce the time for rest and recuperation. Additional demands from unpaid work responsibilities, such as household chores and child care, which affect women more than men, may further contribute to keep stress levels and muscle tension elevated off work and, consequently, increase the health risks.

13. Conclusions

The Allostatic Load Model and the Cinderella hypothesis emphasize the importance of rest and re-

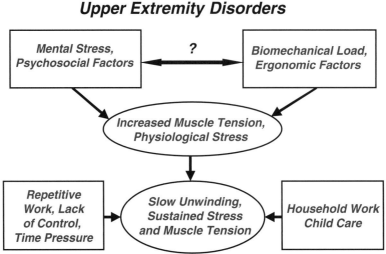

Fig. 1. A model describing factors assumed to influence muscle tension and the risk for musculoskeletal disorders (based on Melin and Lundberg, 1997).

covery for health protection. In modern society, with increasing focus on a high work pace, competitiveness, efficiency, lean production, downsizing etc., lack of time for rest, recovery, and recreation is likely to play an even more important role than the magnitude of stress or physical effort during work. Highly elevated physiological stress levels are necessary for coping and survival under acute intensive stress, for example during child birth (Alehagen et al., 2001), whereas constant exposure to daily stress even on a moderate level may increase the risk of various health problems. Support for this conclusion is also obtained from studies on the health-promoting effects of recreational environments (Hartig et al., 1996). A parallel phenomenon has been observed in sport psychology. Although physical training and exercise generally is assumed to have positive effects on health, well-being and performance, excessive training combined with lack of rest and time for recovery ('overtraining') may cause deteriorating performance ('staleness') and mental and physical health problems (Kentää, 2001).

The dramatic increase in stress-related disorders in Sweden and several other European countries in recent years, such as burnout syndromes, depression,

and MSD, has been linked to changes in the work environment in the mid 1990s. This indicates the important role of economic, political, and structural factors for people's health. The social gradient in health, where individuals with high socioeconomic status are almost always healthier than individuals with lower status, is another example of this. In view of this, it seems reasonable that interventions on a societal level and organizational changes in the work place, aimed at reducing stress and promoting health, should be combined with individual stress management programs influencing cognitive, behavioral, and emotional factors. Measurements of psychobiological mechanisms known to be involved in these processes can then be used as objective indicators of changes in health risks.

Considering the very pronounced gender differences in MSD as well as in many other symptoms, where women consistently report more health problems than men, political actions to create equal opportunities for women and men to combine a stimulating occupational career with a meaningful and creative family life seem necessary. In addition, organizational changes and a new allocation of unpaid work responsibilities seem important to reduce stress and health problems in women. In view of the dramatic costs and individual suffering associated with MSD, actions contributing to reduce these health problems are likely to be particularly cost-effective.

Acknowledgements

Financial support has been obtained from the Bank of Sweden Tercentenary Foundation and from the former Swedish Council for Work Life Research and Swedish Council for Research in the Humanities and Social Sciences.

References

Alehagen, S., Wijma, K., Lundberg, U., Melin, B. and Wijma, B. (2001) Catecholamine and cortisol reaction to child birth. Int. J. Behav. Med., 8: 50–65.

Battié, M. (1989) The Reliability of Physical Factors as Predictors of the Occurrence of Back Pain Reports: A Prospective Study Within Industry. Doctoral Dissertation, Göteborg University.

Bernard, B.P. (1997) Musculoskeletal disorders and workplace factors. A critical review of epidemiologic evidence for work-related musculoskeletal disorders of the neck, upper extremity, and low back. U.S. Department of Health and Human Services, Cincinnati, NIOSH, I-C-59.

Bigos, S., Battié, M., Spengler, D., Fisher, L., Fordyce, W., Hansson, T., Nachemson, A. and Wortley, M. (1991) A prospective study of perceptions and psychosocial factors affecting the report of back injury. Spine, 16: 1–6.

Bongers, P.M., de Winter, C.R., Kompier, M.A.J. and Hildebrandt, V.H. (1993) Psychosocial factors at work and musculoskeletal disease. Scand. J. Work Environ. Health, 19: 297–312.

Colombo, R., Crosetti, A., Farin, D. and Merletti, R. (1999) Evaluation of needle EMG decomposition algorithms with synthetic test signals. In: H. Christensen and G. Sjøgaard (Eds.), PROCID Symposium — Muscular Disorders in Computer Users: Mechanisms and Models. Copenhagen, 25–27 November, 1999. National Institute of Occupational Health, Copenhagen, pp. 73–77.

Flor, H., Breitenstein, C., Birbaumer, N. and Fuerst, M. (1995a) A psychophysiological analysis of spouse solicitousness towards pain behaviors, spouse interaction, and pain perception. Behav. Ther., 26: 255–272.

Flor, H., Elbert, T., Knecht, S., Wienbruch, C., Pantev, C., Birbaumer, N., Larbig, W. and Taub, E. (1995b) Phantom-limb pain as a perceptual correlate of cortical reorganization following arm amputation. Nature, 8: 375 (6531), 482–484.

Flor, H., Knost, B. and Birbaumer, N. (1997) Processing of pain-

and body-related verbal material in chronic pain patients: central and peripheral correlates. Pain, 73: 413–421.

Fordyce, W.E. and Steger, J.C. (1979) Chronic pain. In: O.F. Pomeleau and J.P. Bradely (Eds.), Behavioral Medicine: Theory and Practice. Williams and Wilkins, Baltimore, MD, pp. 125–153.

Forsman, M., Birch, L., Zhang, Q. and Kadefors R. (1999a) Motor-unit recruitment in the trapezius muscle during coarse arm movements. In: H. Christensen and G. Sjøgaard (Eds.), PROCID Symposium — Muscular Disorders in Computer Users: Mechanisms and Models. Copenhagen, 25–27 November, 1999. National Institute of Occupational Health, Copenhagen, pp. 104–108.

Forsman, M., Kadefors, R., Zhang, Q., Birch, L. and Palmerud, G. (1999b) Motor-unit recruitment in the trapezius muscle during arm movements and in VDU precision work. Int. J. Ind. Ergon., 24: 619–630.

Frankenhaeuser, M. (1976) The role of peripheral catecholamines in adaptation to understimulation and overstimulation. In: G. Serban (Ed.), Psychopathology of Human Adaptation. Plenum, New York, NY, pp. 173–191.

Frankenhaeuser, M. (1986) A psychobiological framework for research on human stress and coping. In: M.H. Appley and R. Trumbull (Eds.), Dynamics of Stress. Plenum, New York, NY.

Frankenhaeuser, M., Lundberg, U., Fredrikson, M., Melin, B., Tuomisto, M., Myrsten, A.-L., Hedman, M., Bergman-Losman, B. and Wallin, L. (1989) Stress on and off the job as related to sex and occupational status in white-collar workers. J. Organ. Behav., 10: 321–346.

Hägg, G. (1991) Static work loads and occupational myalgia — a new explanation model. In: P.A. Anderson, D.J. Hobart and J.V. Danhoff (Eds.), Electromyographical Kinesiology. Elsevier, Amsterdam, pp. 141–144.

Hägg, G. and Åström, A. (1997) Load pattern and pressure pain threshold in the upper trapezius muscle and psychosocial factors in medical secretaries with and without shoulder/neck disorders. Int. Arch. Occup. Environ. Health, 69: 423–432.

Hartig, T., Böök, A., Garvill, J., Olsson, T. and Gärling, T. (1996) Environmental influences on psychological restoration. Scand. J. Psychol., 37: 378–393.

Henneman, E., Somjen, G. and Carpenter, D.O. (1965) Excitability and inhibitibility of motoneurons of different sizes. J. Neurophysiol., 28: 599–620.

Jamner, L.D. and Tursky, B. (1987) Syndrome-specific descriptor profiling: a psychophysiological and psychophysical approach. Health Psychol., 6: 417–430.

Johansson, G. (1981) Psychoneuroendocrine correlated of un-paced and paced performance. In: G. Salvendy and M.J. Smith (Eds.), Machine Pacing and Occupational Stress. Taylor and Francis, London, pp. 277–286.

Johansson, G. and Aronsson, G. (1984) Stress reactions in computerized administrative work. J. Occup. Behav., 5: 159–181.

Johansson, H. and Sojka, P. (1991) Pathophysiological mechanisms involved in genesis and spread of muscular tension in occupational muscle pain and in chronic musculoskeletal pain syndromes: a hypothesis. Med. Hypotheses, 35: 196–203.

Johansson, J. (1994) Psychosocial factors at work and their

relation to musculoskeletal symptoms. Doctoral dissertation, Department of Psychology, Göteborg University.

Kadefors, R., Forsman, M., Zoega, B. and Herberts, P. (1999) Recruitment of low threshold motor-units in the trapezius muscle in different static arm positions. Ergonomics, 42(2): 359–375.

Karasek, R.A. (1979) Job demands, job decision latitude and mental strain: implications for job redesign. Adm. Sci. Q., 24: 285–307.

Kentää, G. (2001) Overtraining, Staleness and Burnout in Sports. Doctoral Dissertation, Department of Psychology, Stockholm University.

Kiecolt-Glaser, J.K., Malarkey, W.B., Cacioppo, J.T. and Glaser, R. (1994) Stressful personal relationships; immune and endocrine function. In: R. Glaser and J. Kiecolt-Glaser (Eds.), Handbook of Human Stress and Immunity. Academic, San Diego, CA, pp. 321–339.

Knardahl, S. (2002) Psychophysiological mechanisms of pain in computer work: The blood vessel–nociceptor interaction hypothesis. Work Stress, in press.

Leino, P. and Magni, G. (1993) Depressive and distress symptoms as predictors of low back pain, neck–shoulder pain, and other musculoskeletal morbidity: a 10-year follow-up of metal industry employees. Pain, 53(1): 89–94.

Linton, S.J. (1994) The role of psychological factors in back pain and its remediation. Pain Rev., 1: 231–243.

Lundberg, U. (1996) The influence of paid and unpaid work on psychophysiological stress responses of men and women. J. Occup. Health Psychol., 1: 117–130.

Lundberg, U. (2000) Catecholamines. In: G. Fink (Ed.), Encyclopedia of Stress, Vol. I. Academic Press, San Diego, CA, pp. 408–413.

Lundberg, U. and Frankenhaeuser, M. (1999) Stress and workload of men and women in high ranking positions. J. Occup. Health Psychol., 4: 142–152.

Lundberg, U. and Johansson, G. (2000) Stress and health risks in repetitive work and supervisory monitoring work. In: R. Backs and W. Boucsein (Eds.), Engineering Psychophysiology: Issues and Applications. Lawrence Erlbaum, Hillsdale, NJ, pp. 339–359.

Lundberg, U., Granqvist, M., Hansson, T., Magnusson, M. and Wallin, L. (1989) Psychological and physiological stress responses during repetitive work at an assembly line. Work Stress, 3: 143–153.

Lundberg, U., Melin, B., Evans, G.W. and Holmberg, L. (1993) Physiological deactivation after two contrasting tasks at a video display terminal: learning vs repetitive data entry. Ergonomics, 36: 601–611.

Lundberg, U., Kadefors, R., Melin, B., Palmerud, G., Hassmén, P., Engström, M. and Elfsberg Dohns, I. (1994a) Psychophysiological stress and EMG activity of the trapezius muscle. Int. J. Behav. Med., 1: 354–370.

Lundberg, U., Mårdberg, B. and Frankenhaeuser, M. (1994b) The total workload of male and female white collar workers as related to age, occupational level, and number of children. Scand. J. Psychol., 35: 315–327.

Lundberg, U., Elfsberg Dohns, I., Melin, B., Sandsjö, L.,

Palmerud, G., Kadefors, R., Ekström, M. and Parr, D. (1999) Psychophysiological stress responses, muscle tension and neck and shoulder pain among supermarket cashiers. J. Occup. Health Psychol., 4(3): 1–11.

Lundberg, U., Forsman, M., Zachau, G., Eklöf, M., Palmerud, G., Melin, B. and Kadefors, R. (2002) Effects of experimentally induced mental and physical stress on trapezius motor unit recruitment. Work Stress, in press.

McEwen, B.S. (1998) Stress, adaptation and disease: Allostasis and allostatic load. N. Engl. J. Med., 338: 171–179.

Melin, B. (1993) Association between serum triglyceride levels and diastolic blood pressure during rest and exercise in healthy males and females. Scand. J. Behav. Ther., 22: 159–169.

Melin, B. (2001) Psychosocial stress, neck and shoulder disorders. In The 2nd PROCID Symposium — Prevention of Muscle Disorders in Computer Users: Scientific Basis and Recommendations, Göteborg, 8–10 March, 2001. National Institute for Working Life/West, Göteborg, pp. 67–70.

Melin, B. and Lundberg, U. (1997) A biopsychosocial approach to work-stress and musculoskeletal disorder. J. Psychophysiol., 11: 238–247.

Melin, B. and Sandqvist, D. (1994) Effects of thematically relevant visual stimuli in Raynaud's Disease. Scand. J. Behav. Ther., 23: 53–60.

Melin, B., Lundberg, U., Söderlund, J. and Granqvist, M. (1999) Psychophysiological stress reactions of male and female assembly workers: a comparison between two different forms of work organizations. J. Organ. Behav., 20: 47–61.

Melzack, R. and Wall, P.D. (1965) Pain mechanisms: a new theory. Science, 150: 971–979.

Melzack, R. and Wall, P.D. (1982) The Challenge of Pain. Basic Books, New York, NY.

Moon, S.D. and Sauter, S.L. (Eds.) (1996) Psychosocial Aspects of Musculoskeletal Disorders in Office Work. Taylor and Francis, London.

Odgen, J. (1997) Health Psychology: A Textbook. Open University Press, Philadelphia, PA.

Rissén, D., Melin, B., Sandsjö, L. and Lundberg, U. (2000) Surface EMG and psychophysiological stress reactions among female employees at supermarkets. Eur. J. Appl. Physiol., 83: 215–222.

Sandsjö, L., Melin, B., Rissén, D., Dohns, I. and Lundberg, U. (2000) Trapezius muscle activity, neck and shoulder pain, and subjective experiences during monotonous work in women. Eur. J. Appl. Physiol., 83: 235–238.

SBU — Statens Beredning för Medicinsk Utvärdering (2000) Ont i ryggen, ont i nacken. En evidensbaserad kunskapssammanställning. (Pain in the back, pain in the neck. An evidence-based review.) Vol. I och II, Rapport nr. 145/1 145/2 2000.

Schleifer, L.M. and Ley, R. (1994) End-tidal P_{CO_2} as an index of psychophysiological activity during VDT data-entry work and relaxation. Ergonomics, 37: 245–254.

Siegrist, J. (1996) Adverse health effects of high-effort/low-reward conditions. J. Occup. Health Psychol., 1: 27–41.

Sjøgaard, G., Lundberg, U. and Kadefors, R. (2000) The role of muscle activity and mental load in the development of pain and degenerative processes on the muscle cellular level during computer work. Eur. J. Appl. Physiol., 83: 99–105.

Statistics Sweden (2000). National Bureau of Statistics.

Svebak, S., Anjia, R. and Kårstad, S.I. (1993) Task-induced electromyographic activation in fibromyalgia subjects and controls. Scand. J. Rheumatol., 22: 124–130.

Theorell, T., Hasslehorn, H.-M. and Vingård, E. (2002) Endocrinological and immunological variables sensitive to psychological factors of possible relevance to computer work related musculoskeletal disorders. Work Stress, in press.

Timio, M. and Gentili, S. (1976) Adrenosympathetic overactivity under conditions of stress. Br. J. Prev. Soc. Med., 30: 262–265.

Timio, M., Gentili, S. and Pede, S. (1979) Free adrenaline and noradrenaline excretion related to occupational stress. Br. Heart J., 42: 471–474.

Veiersted, B. (1995) Stereotyped Light Manual Work, Individual Factors and Trapezius Myalgia. Doctoral dissertation, University of Oslo.

Veiersted, K.B., Westgaard, R.H. and Andersen, P. (1993) Electromyographic evaluation of muscular work pattern as a predictor of trapezius myalgia. Scand. J. Work Environ. Health, 19: 284–290.

Wellig, P. and Moschytz, G.S. (1999) Electromyogram decomposition using the single-linkage clustering algorithm and wavelets. In: Proceedings of the 6th IEEE International Conference on Electronics, Circuits, and Systems, Pafos, September 1999, Vol. 1, pp. 537–541.

Wik, G., Elbert, T., Fredrikson, M. and Hoke, M. (1996) Magnetic imaging in human classical conditioning. Neurorep. Int. J. Rapid Commun. Res. Neurosci., 7: 737–740.

Wærsted, M. (1997) Attention-Related Muscle Activity — A Contributor to Sustained Occupational Muscle Load. Doctoral dissertation, National Institute of Occupational Health, Oslo.

Wærsted, M., Bjørklund, R. and Westgaard, R. (1991) Shoulder muscle tension induced by two VDU-based tasks of different complexity. Ergonomics, 34: 137–150.

Section III

Early Identification and Preventive Interventions

Developing effective prevention strategies is a major challenge. How might the theoretical knowledge be transformed into practice? This section describes applications oriented towards early identification as well as towards intervention. Systematic application has produced some startling results.

Objectives are for the reader to:

• understand how early identification might be achieved
• gain knowledge about some early interventions and their effectiveness
• gain insights on how an effective early intervention might be derived from the existing body of knowledge

New Avenues for the Prevention of Chronic Musculoskeletal Pain and Disability
Pain Research and Clinical Management, Vol. 12
Edited by S.J. Linton

CHAPTER 12

Employing risk factors for screening of chronic pain disability

Carla B. Pulliam * and Robert J. Gatchel

Department of Psychiatry, University of Texas Southwestern Medical Center, 5323 Harry Hines Boulevard,
Dallas, TX 75235-8898, USA

Abstract: The development of chronic pain is a problem of staggering proportions. Yet factors associated with poor outcome following acute symptoms may provide insights into effective preventive measures. This chapter explores the possibility of employing risk factors for the early identification of patients who may develop persistent pain and disability. Factors such as the Minnesota Multiphasic Personality Inventory, coping strategies, psychopathology, compensation issues, and pain reports are reviewed to gain clarity about their role in poor outcome. The literature demonstrates that these variables all have predictive power. Considerable progress has been made in employing these risk factors in early identification, but also in targeting the intervention. Predictive models that help us to tailor interventions are in their infancy but show promise. Future research should utilize the large body of literature on risk factors in order to treat high-risk individuals preventively.

1. Introduction

Chronic musculoskeletal pain and the often concomitant disability have become issues of societal proportions. The costs are staggering in terms of financial outlay, as well as the emotional turmoil experienced by individuals afflicted with these disorders. Pain disorders account for approximately 80% of all physician visits, and the majority of the $70 billion in annual health-care expenditures (Gatchel and Epker, 1999). A recent survey found the 1-year prevalence of musculoskeletal pain among individuals aged 35–45 to be 66%. Twenty-five percent were deemed to have significant problems, including in-

tense pain episodes and significant functional impairment. These individuals averaged three health-care visits per person, per year, again making musculoskeletal pain one of the most frequently cited reasons for visits to health-care professionals today (Linton et al., 1998).

Of critical importance is the above use of the term 'chronic', as the majority of patients afflicted with musculoskeletal disorders will experience symptom resolution in the acute phase, without progressing towards chronic disability status. For example, approximately 70–80% of all individuals in industrialized countries will suffer from low back pain at some point during their lives (Deyo et al., 1991;

---
* Correspondence to: C.B. Pulliam, Department of Psychiatry, University of Texas Southwestern Medical Center, 5323 Harry Hines Boulevard, Dallas, TX 75235-8898, USA. E-mail: carla.pulliam@utsouthwestern.edu

Lanes et al., 1995). However, from the onset of symptoms, approximately 50% of patients with low back pain are no longer disabled within 2 weeks, 70% recover in 1 month, and approximately 90% recover within 3–4 months (Mayer and Gatchel, 1988). While others have found the prognosis to be more pessimistic, there nevertheless remains a significant portion of the population whose symptoms resolve relatively quickly. For example, in studies of populations in primary care, 27% of low back patients were completely better at a 3-month post-treatment assessment, 28% were improved, and 30% showed no change. Only 14% were worse or much worse at the 3-month post-treatment assessment (Croft et al., 1995; Jayson, 1997).

Mayer (1999) notes that the mean cost of low back pain care is more than ten times greater than the median cost. This suggests that the relatively small number of cases that become chronic account for the majority of expenditures in terms of direct (i.e., direct patient care) and indirect costs (i.e., loss of productivity, litigation, welfare expenditures). Some studies estimate that this approximate 10% will account for as much as 50–85% of the total cost (Spengler et al., 1986). Others have estimated that 15% of adults are totally and permanently disabled by chronic spinal disorders, and that $16 billion are subsequently spent on this small portion of the population. An approximate $27 billion is spent annually on all musculoskeletal patients (Gatchel et al., 1995b). Some have found that only 5% of musculoskeletal populations studied accounted for 50% of the health-care visits, with a correlation identified between health-care utilization and days of sick leave (Linton et al., 1998). This finding implies that this smaller portion of the population not only incurs additional costs through utilization of health-care services, but through lost productivity as well. In fact, it has been noted that health-care utilization, while costly, accounts for a small portion of the total expenditures associated with musculoskeletal pain and, in terms of point of intervention, may represent 'too little, too late' (Linton, 1999).

The above statistics highlight the importance of developing avenues for preventing the progression from acute to chronic musculoskeletal pain and disability. The literature in this area has historically focused on identifying risk factors, either intrinsic to the patient (i.e., psychological, social or functional difficulties) or external (i.e., factors specific to the work environment), with the goal of predicting which patients are at increased risk for progressing to chronic disability status following acute symptom presentation. Examination of these risk factors has traditionally been undertaken retrospectively, using baseline analyses as predictors of long-term outcome. The current authors are evaluating the benefits of using screening algorithms in the acute phase, in an effort to treat high-risk individuals prophylactically. The assumption underlying this approach is that early identification of patients allows for the application of targeted interventions geared towards preventing the emergence of more long-standing problems. In addition to preventing significant expenditures, early intervention could prevent the demoralizing effect that living with chronic pain has on the individual sufferer. In line with the above, more recent research has targeted the cost savings realized from intervening early in the illness progression. The current paper will examine research relative to predominant risk factors for progression from acute to chronic musculoskeletal pain, and will highlight issues relative to points of intervention (i.e., primary, secondary, or tertiary). Finally, the more recent studies examining the cost effectiveness of programs designed to prevent progression to chronic pain disability will be discussed.

Prior to embarking on a review of the risk factors that have received predominant attention in the literature, a brief perspective of the current *zeitgeist* for conceptualizing chronic musculoskeletal pain is in order. Historically, a unimodal, or biomedical, model has been used to approach the frequently problematic symptoms associated with this population. The traditional failure of physiological explanations to account for presenting symptomatology, however, has been widely reported with chronic pain. In fact, the associations between physical impairment and pain report and disability have been shown to be modest at best (Magora and Schwartz, 1980; Waddell and Main, 1984). Turk (1996) notes that chronic pain is more than a physical symptom, but rather a widespread problem resulting in significant and pervasive suffering. Typical symptoms include demoralization and affective disturbance, preoccupation with pain, limitation of personal, social, and work activities, and increased use of medications and health-care services.

The above factors led Turk and Rudy (1987) to develop the *biopsychosocial model of pain*, which currently predominates in the conceptualization of chronic pain. This model accounts for physiological, biological, cognitive, affective, behavioral, and social factors, and their interplay, in an effort to understand the individual patient's report of pain. For example, biologic conditions may initiate and perpetuate a psychological disturbance. Psychological factors may impact the patient's perception and assessment of physical stimuli, and social factors may impact the individual's behavior with respect to his or her pain experience. Turk (1996) notes that "no single factor in isolation — pathophysiological, psychological, or social — will adequately explain chronic pain status." As suffering increases, psychosocial factors are hypothesized to play an increasingly salient role in the perpetuation of pain and suffering. This model provides the foundation for the following discussion on risk factors associated with the progression from acute pain to chronic pain disability status. As the reader will note, a good portion of these factors are not pathophysiological in nature, but instead relate to aspects of the pain experience inherent in the patient's psychological make-up or surrounding environment.

2. Predictors of chronic pain

Given the existence of a somewhat distinct progression from acute to chronic pain (the course of which has been reviewed elsewhere; Gatchel, 1991), and the resulting financial and societal impact, it is not surprising that numerous researchers have attempted to predict which individuals with acute pain will have a propensity for developing more long-

standing, chronic problems. The ability to identify high-risk individuals early in the disease progression allows for the possibility of preventing the onset of chronic disability. In theory, the isolation of risk-related variables could potentially allow for the altering of these factors and subsequent alleviation of the risk (Linton, 1999).

As the upcoming review will elucidate, risk factors that have been associated with chronic musculoskeletal pain problems have included the Minnesota Multiphasic Personality Inventory (MMPI), coping strategies, psychopathology, compensation, and self-report of pain, together with some additional psychosocial variables. The above items have all demonstrated some predictive utility in identifying patients who are likely to develop chronic musculoskeletal pain following presentation with acute symptomatology.

2.1. The MMPI-2 as a predictor variable

The Minnesota Multiphasic Personality Inventory-2nd edition (MMPI-2) is a well-known psychological measure designed to assess acute areas of distress, as well as more stable personality traits. Clinicians have often used the MMPI in their efforts to identify psychosocial factors prominent in pain conditions. Hanvik (1951) conducted one of the earliest studies comparing psychological profiles and chronic pain disorders. This classic study resulted in the first identification of the 'Conversion V' pattern (elevated Hypochondriasis, Depression and Hysteria scales, with the Depression scale lower than the other two), which is frequently used to describe the psychological functioning of patients today. Although based on an overly simplistic model of pain, Hanvik's research was seminal in the application of the MMPI for use with chronic pain populations.

Overall scale elevations in different populations of musculoskeletal disorders have been identified as well. For example, Blanchard and Andrasik (1985) examined individuals with cluster headaches, migraine headaches, tension headaches and normal controls, and found that the first two groups did not differ significantly, while migraine sufferers exhibited significant elevations only on the Hysteria scale (Scale 3). However, individuals with tension headaches had elevated scores on the Hypochondriasis (Scale 1), Depression (Scale 2), Hysteria (Scale 3), Psychasthenia (Scale 7) and Schizophrenia (Scale 8) scales. Similar findings have been identified in a population of patients presenting with irritable bowel syndrome, with 20–30% of patients demonstrating significant elevations on various scales of the MMPI, versus 5–17% of non-treatment seeking patients and 0–4% of normal controls (Drossman et al., 1988).

Other studies have identified an elevated Hysteria scale in patients presenting with low back pain, leading this to be one of the most frequently investigated MMPI variables (Sternbach et al., 1973; Bigos et al., 1991; Fordyce et al., 1992; Gatchel et al., 1995a). An elevated Hysteria scale has been predictive of future development of low back pain in workers (Bigos et al., 1991), and has been more prevalent in a group of disabled men, relative to non-disabled controls (Frymoyer et al., 1985). The Hysteria scale is one component of the 'Neurotic Triad' [i.e., elevations on Hypochondriasis (Scale 1), Depression (Scale 2) and Hysteria (Scale 3)] which has been elevated in temporomandibular patients versus controls (Schumann et al., 1988; Etscheidt and Steiger, 1995). However, discriminant function analyses have not always resulted in patients and controls being correctly classified according to this distinction.

Regardless of the specific scale elevations, scores on the MMPI may increase as the duration of the disorder increases. However, Barnes et al. (1990) found that this trend can be reversed in low back pain patients following successful completion of a functional restoration program. These authors note that the scales are sensitive to situational stressors, and may be reflective of the injury and the ensuing life changes. Consistent with this argument, Bombardier et al. (1993) found that the MMPI profile appears more distressed as the patient experiences greater psychosocial problems.

Leavitt and Garron (1982) also found this to be true in their examination of the MMPI and low back pain. In this study, the MMPI differentiated three groups of patients: one group had no elevations; the second group exhibited the 'Conversion V' pattern; and a third group had a similar pattern but with more severe anguish and suffering reflected in higher profile elevations. These relative elevations in MMPI profiles correlated with self-reported measures of low back pain severity. Similarly, efforts to distinguish patient groups from MMPI profiles have been successful in the temporomandibular population. For example, McCreary et al. (1991) examined patients with myalgia, temporomandibular joint problems, and pain arising from muscle and joint problems. The first group evidenced profile elevations on Hypochondriasis (Scale 1), Depression (Scale 2), Hysteria (Scale 3), and Paranoia (Scale 6). These scores were additionally higher than the elevations on the same scales in the remaining two groups.

Despite the apparent consistencies in profiles of pain patients, attempts to categorize a typical pain profile with the MMPI have been unsuccessful, and the results have been inconsistent and strongly attacked (Main and Spanswick, 1995). Gatchel and Gardea (1999) note that one criticism concerns the overlap of test items and the symptomatology of given disorders. Pincus et al. (1987) demonstrated this problem in a population of patients with rheumatoid arthritis. These authors discovered five items on the MMPI that were indicative of both the presence and the severity of arthritis. Adjustments for positive responses demonstrated a four- to ten-point decrease in *T*-scores for the Hypochondriasis, Depression and Hysteria scales (Scales 1, 2 and 3).

In summary, it appears as though the Hysteria scale is beneficial in identifying patients at risk for developing chronic pain, and that the scale may be more elevated according to the degree of psychosocial disturbance experienced by the individual. Additionally, patterns of elevations, such as the Conversion V or Neurotic Triad, may also have some degree of clinical utility. However, efforts to identify characteristic 'pain' profiles have little predictive validity with respect to identifying subgroups of patients whose symptoms will resolve less rapidly following acute presentation.

2.2. Coping strategies as a predictor variable

Coping strategies have received much attention in the acute and chronic pain literatures as important variables to consider when assessing patients presenting with pain symptomatology. These studies have not consistently examined the predictive utility of investigating coping style variables and their relation to the progression from acute to chronic pain, but a clear relationship has emerged between chronic musculoskeletal pain and utilization of poor coping strategies. Among rheumatoid arthritis patients, for example, negative, exaggerated catastrophizing thoughts and/or feelings of loss of control were associated with increased pain perceptions (Keefe et al., 1989). Pre-treatment catastrophizing has also been found to predict changes in pain intensity after treatment in a group of patients suffering from chronic cervicobrachialgia (Samwel et al., 2000), and to lower self-efficacy for pain in patients presenting with osteoarthritis of the knees and persistent knee pain (Keefe et al., 1997). In this latter study, ignoring pain sensations and the use of coping self-statements were related to increased pain-related self-efficacy ratings (Keefe et al., 1997). Finally, self-efficacy ratings appear to be important in fibromyalgia patients as well, as pretreatment self-efficacy levels significantly predicted post-treatment outcome in this population (Buckelew et al., 1996).

Turk and Kerns (1983) and Kerns et al. (1985) suggest that a measure of a patient's coping strategies should be included in all pain assessments, as knowledge regarding patients' idiosyncratic appraisals of their pain and coping repertoires are critical for optimal treatment planning and for accurately evaluating treatment outcome. In part for this purpose, the above authors developed the West-Haven Yale Multidimensional Pain Inventory, or the Multidimensional Pain Inventory (MPI). The MPI is an empirically derived multidimensional instrument developed specifically for use with the chronic pain population. This instrument identifies clusters of coping abilities and styles (Dysfunctional, Interpersonally Distressed, or Adaptive Copers; Turk and Rudy, 1988) that have proven useful in classifying

and identifying appropriate interventions for patients presenting with chronic pain. *Dysfunctional* copers report that the severity of their pain and the extent to which it interferes with their lives is extreme. Patients with this coping style have demonstrated increased treatment failure, either conservative or surgical, and increased demand for radical therapy (Dahlstrom et al., 1997). Individuals with an *Interpersonally Distressed* coping style perceive a lack of support and understanding from their families and significant others. *Adaptive copers* report lower levels of pain severity, perceived interference from pain, and affective distress. They also report higher levels of daily activity and life control. In their 1988 study, Turk and Rudy found 43% of a heterogeneous group of pain patients to be Dysfunctional copers. Twenty-eight percent were identified as Interpersonally Distressed, and 29.5% described themselves as Adaptive copers. These findings were replicated with a second sample of patients.

Utilization of active and passive coping strategies also appears to affect pain experience, with active strategies generally decreasing pain and increasing functioning and social adjustment. Passive coping styles may increase dependence, feelings of helplessness, and experience of pain. For example, decreases in perception of pain helplessness have been linked to decreased pain severity (Burns et al., 1998). A notable caveat, however, is that coping styles may vary according to the degree of pain experienced. For example, 121 age-stratified patients with rheumatoid arthritis were found to use more active coping strategies while experiencing mild pain, but resorted to maladaptive strategies when the pain became severe. Additionally, older adults were more likely overall than younger patients to use maladaptive coping strategies when experiencing mild pain (Watkins et al., 1999). These findings highlight the importance of examining coping strategies in the context of overall pain experience, as the relationship between coping strategies and pain may not be consistently linear in nature.

Brown and Nicassio (1987) developed the *Vanderbilt Pain Management Inventory* to identify active and passive coping styles. They found active coping strategies such as staying busy, engaging in distraction techniques, and ignoring the pain to be associated with a reduction in pain perception. These active techniques may be related to the greater perceived life control and increased participation in daily activities characteristic of the Adaptive copers discussed above. Passive strategies, such as depending on others for pain relief, wishful thinking, and limiting activities, were associated with a perception of more severe pain, and are more consistent with items included in the Interpersonally Distressed and Dysfunctional coping categories.

Klapow et al. (1995) similarly examined passive versus active coping strategies, together with other variables, in an effort to discriminate groups of low back pain patients. These authors found that individuals presenting with a chronic pain syndrome had an increased reliance on passive/avoidant coping strategies, together with high levels of pain, disability, depression, life adversity, and less satisfaction with their social support structure. Kleinke (1994) found similar results in his investigation of the differences between acute and chronic pain individuals. He found that healthy emotional adjustment was related to employing active coping strategies, such as effective engagement in self-management strategies and utilization of social support. Poor emotional adjustment was related to passive strategies, which invoked feelings of helplessness and reliance on medical remedies. Similarly, Zautra and Manne (1992) identified a relationship between passive, avoidant, emotionally focused coping and lower self-esteem, poor adjustment and more negative affect, compared to counterparts utilizing more active strategies.

Numerous additional authors have identified the important role of coping strategies in the development and maintenance of chronic pain (Lazarus and Folkman, 1984; Fordyce et al., 1985; Turk and Flor, 1987; Boothby et al., 1999). It may be that active coping enables the individual to successfully manage the life-changing impact resulting from the onset of severe musculoskeletal pain, whereas passive coping results in an acceptance of a decrease in functioning. Regardless of the nature of the relationship, research has consistently supported the need to consider this variable in examination of the onset and maintenance of chronic pain.

2.3. Psychopathology as a predictor variable

A large body of evidence supports the idea that the presence of psychopathology is indicative of a poor prognosis in patients presenting with acute musculoskeletal pain. The presence of character pathology, in particular, has been associated with poor outcome in chronic pain patients (Peselow et al., 1992; Clark et al., 1994). As previously noted, however, physical illness and psychosocial distress play a reciprocal role in the development and maintenance of chronic pain. Consequently, significant research has focused on identifying which factor of the equation precedes the other.

Fishbain et al. (1997) conducted a review of 191 studies relating to the association between pain and depression. These authors concluded that depression is more common among chronic pain patients than controls because it is a consequence, not an antecedent, of the pain condition. In support of this conclusion, Timmermans and Sternbach (1976) demonstrated a nonsignificant trend showing that levels of reactive depression increased as subjective ratings of pain increased. The authors suggest that as the patient increasingly centers his or her life around the pain, it begins to have a greater impact on his or her daily functioning. Gatchel et al. (1995b) assessed 421 patients presenting with acute low back pain and followed them for 1 year. Their results likewise suggested that, if pre-injury psychopathology was present, it did not appear to predispose one to chronic pain disability.

Other authors have come to similar conclusions regarding the directional relationship between psychopathology and chronic pain. Dworkin et al. (1990) assessed multiple pain conditions and their association with affective disturbance, somatization, and psychological disturbance on 1016 enrollees of a large health maintenance organization. The authors asked respondents about the presence of five pain conditions, and then classified them based on pain severity, pain persistence, and pain-related disability days.

They found a highly significant association between number of pain conditions reported and elevated levels of somatization. Two or more pain conditions placed respondents at risk for an algorithm diagnosis of major depression, while individuals with one pain condition did not differ significantly from individuals with no pain condition. The authors concluded that patients with many physical complaints appear to be at greater risk for developing depression. Romano and Turner (1985) also found a relationship between pain and depression. However, it was unclear if the depression predisposed a person to develop chronic pain or if depression was a pathological sequela of it.

Research suggests that patients presenting with irritable bowel syndrome tend to be more psychologically disturbed than non-help seeking irritable bowel sufferers (Drossman et al., 1988), although it is unknown whether or not this relationship is causal (Blanchard, 1993). Similarly, individuals presenting with headaches tend to report depression as the most common co-disturbance (Adler et al., 1987), and depression appears to mediate treatment response in chronic pain patients presenting with temporomandibular disorders (Fricton and Olsen, 1996). However, as in other disorders, the interaction of biological, psychological, and social variables makes it difficult to ascertain whether the psychological disturbance preceded the emergence of pain or whether the inverse is true.

Evidence also exists to support the hypothesis that premorbid psychological conditions predispose the individual to develop chronic pain. For example, Blanchard et al. (1989) found that psychopathology may place an individual at greater risk for developing chronic headaches. Polatin et al. (1993) used the Structured Clinical Interview for the Diagnostic and Statistical Manual for Mental Disorders (SCID) in a sample of 200 chronic low back pain patients to examine the lifetime prevalence of psychopathology. These authors determined that 77% of their sample met criteria for lifetime prevalence of either a depressive, anxiety, or substance abuse disorder. Furthermore, many of these met criteria for a psychiatric disorder prior to the development of their pain condition (54% for depression, 94% for substance abuse, and 95% for

anxiety disorders), suggesting that psychopathology may have preceded, and thus influenced, the development of the chronic pain condition.

Gatchel (1996) further supported this hypothesis by observing that chronic low back pain patients have a considerably higher base rate of Axis I and Axis II diagnoses. In 1994, he and other authors examined a population of 152 chronic low back pain patients, and administered the SCID to ascertain the presence of psychopathology. These authors found that more than 90% of the patients met criteria for at least one Axis I disorder once treatment had been initiated. The most common diagnoses included somatoform pain disorder, substance abuse, and major depression. More than 50% of the patients examined met criteria for an Axis II diagnosis of character pathology. The most prevalent Axis II diagnosis was paranoid personality disorder (Gatchel et al., 1994). Fishbain et al. (1986) found similar results in their examination of 283 patients who had suffered from pain for more than 2 years. These authors found that more than 50% suffered from anxiety and/or depression, and 58.4% met criteria for an Axis II diagnosis. Men were more prone to exhibit paranoid and narcissistic personality traits, while women more frequently presented with traits characteristic of histrionic personality disorder.

The above-cited studies demonstrate the clear relationship between chronic pain and psychopathology. However, they also highlight the nebulous and complex nature of this relationship. Significant additional research will be required before the 'chicken or the egg' syndrome can be laid to rest once and for all. Regardless of the directional nature of the relationship, however, the significant co-morbidity between pain and psychological disturbance highlights the importance of considering these factors in predictive models geared towards identifying individuals at-risk for poorer prognosis when presenting with acute musculoskeletal pain.

2.4. Compensation as a predictor variable

Research suggests that receiving compensation following pain or injury serves as a powerful disincentive and barrier to recovery because of factors such as secondary gain (e.g., potential monetary gain; Gatchel and Gardea, 1999), and that compensation may therefore predispose individuals with acute pain to progress towards more chronic problems. Various outcome studies have supported this idea across a wide variety of presenting problems, including carpal tunnel syndrome, lumbar disc pathology, and inguinal hernias (Catts et al., 1994; Davis, 1994; Greenough et al., 1994; Roth et al., 1994).

'Compensation Neurosis' is a term used to describe "a conscious or unconscious tendency of some patients to amplify symptoms when there is a potential for financial gain. The essential feature of a compensation neurosis is that the claimant describes his or her capacity in terms of physical limitations and physical symptoms, but observers suspect that motivation factors underlie the complaints." (Robinson et al., 1997). The process of pursuing a disability claim is inherently adversarial, and it often encourages patients to escalate their presenting symptoms when reexamined or challenged. Even following resolution of the workers' compensation claim, patients retain ongoing disincentives to recover. For example, after presenting themselves as ill and disabled while advocating their claim, they may fear being perceived as malingerers should they recover, while at the same time continuing to fear a reexamination and withdrawal of benefits (Bellamy, 1997).

Beals (1984) demonstrated that active compensation has a significant effect on the continuance of disability. Similarly, Rohling et al. (1995) conducted a meta-analysis of all studies relating compensation to chronic pain. These authors found that receiving financial compensation is associated with increased experience of pain and decreased treatment efficacy. However, only 32 of the 157 reviewed studies utilized quantifiable data from treatment and control groups, suggesting that more rigorous research is needed.

Vaccaro et al. (1997) conducted a retrospective case series to identify factors influencing outcome in chronic back pain and low-grade spondylolisthesis. Twenty-four patients were evaluated for the influence of active litigation or workers' compensation claims,

as well as age, gender, radicular pain, concomitant laminectomy, fusion to L4 intervertebral disc bulge, and pseudoarthrosis. Poor treatment outcome was defined as continued similar pain level and functional limitation following surgery. Of the 24 patients, the 13 receiving workers' compensation or involved in pending litigation had fair or poor outcome, while 9 of 11 patients without secondary financial gain had good or excellent results.

Rainville et al. (1997) examined 192 patients referred for rehabilitation of chronic low back pain, and similar findings emerged. These authors divided patients into two groups based on whether or not they were receiving compensation (defined as workers' compensation, social security disability, private disability policy benefits, and/or plaintiffs in unsettled personal injury cases). Ninety-six of the 192 patients were involved with one or more forms of compensation. Groups were compared on pain and disability presentation, treatment recommendations and compliance with treatment. Comparisons took place at initial evaluation and at 3 and 12 months follow-ups. Overall, individuals in the compensation group reported a greater amount of pain, depression, and disability than the individuals in the noncompensation group. At 3 and 12 month follow-ups, both groups demonstrated improvement in depression and disability, although improvements in the compensation group were statistically and clinically less significant than the noncompensation group. At 12 months, the noncompensation group reported decreased pain, while the compensation group did not. Once again, this study highlights the important role that compensation plays in decreasing treatment efficacy, and the subsequent need to address this issue when the patient first presents with complaints of pain.

Sanderson et al. (1995) agree that work-related factors may influence disability, but they suggest that employment status may have more of an impact than compensation. These authors examined the relationship between compensation, work status and disability in 269 low back pain patients. The presence of unemployment and compensation resulted in increased disability. However, those who were employed and getting compensation reported less disability than the unemployed individuals who were receiving compensation for their injury. Therefore, even when compensation is present, additional mediating factors should continue to be explored. In particular, it may be important to investigate whether or not individuals have jobs to which they can return should they desire and become able to do so.

Other authors have suggested that the presence or absence of compensation may not fully account for the phenomenon of decreased treatment efficacy in chronic pain samples. For example, while compensation status may affect perceptions of pain intensity, financial remuneration does not necessarily affect the individual's decision to return to work. Tollison (1993) examined 43 patients involved in nonsurgical treatment of low back injury. At discharge, differences were identified between the two groups in subjective pain intensity and return-to-work status. At the 6-month follow-up, the differences in subjective pain intensity were still present. However, no differences in return-to-work status were identified between the two groups.

Absence from work in the acute phase of injury may affect return-to-work status as well, whether or not compensation issues are relevant. For example, the duration of preoperative sick leave has been linked to poor outcome following cervical discectomy (Bhandari et al., 1999) and surgery for lumbar disc herniation (Nygaard et al., 1994). Similarly, decreased length of unemployment, together with age, marital status, and education were predictive of return-to-work outcome in a sample of patients with chronic musculoskeletal pain (Tan et al., 1997).

Assuming that disability-related factors do, in fact, negatively impact return-to-work status, there is some evidence that effective interdisciplinary treatment can partially reverse this effect. Ambrosius et al. (1995) investigated a group of 35 patients with workers' compensation presenting for treatment in a highly structured functional restoration program, and compared them to 25 individuals in the same treatment program who were not receiving workers' compensation. Twenty-three of the workers' compensa-

tion patients were not working during treatment, compared to only one individual in the nonworkers' compensation group. At the end of treatment, however, 32 of the 35 workers' compensation patients had resumed their positions in the work force. All of the nonworkers' compensation patients had returned to work, resulting in return-to-work status for a full 91% of the treatment sample. These results suggest that effective treatment can overcome negative effects exerted by compensation status, and they provide promising avenues for future interventions with musculoskeletal patients.

The above studies underscore the importance of considering compensation status in efforts designed to identify high-risk, acute-pain patients. However, it is also evident from the current review that compensation status could potentially be mediated by other variables. Even when present, early identification and targeting of secondary gain issues can lead to significant mitigation of their effects. Education regarding the notoriously frustrating nature of the compensation system, and the emotional and financial costs inherent in adopting the sick role, can preemptively help individuals choose the path to recovery rather than passively progressing down the path towards disability.

2.5. Self-report of pain as a predictor variable

Reported pain level has also been identified as a factor predicting chronic disability. Self-report of pain is a subjective appraisal that involves social, cultural, and other factors that may play a role in confounding its validity as a measure. For example, Philips et al. (1991) investigated patients suffering from their first episode of back pain. Individuals reporting a severe amount of pain in the acute state were more likely to have pain at the 6-month follow-up. Von Korff et al. (1993) evaluated 1128 back patients 1 year after they had initially sought help. The most clinically significant measures that differentiated patients with poor outcome (defined as high disability with moderately or severely limiting back pain) from those with a good outcome were levels of pain intensity, pain-related disability, and pain persistence.

Number of days in pain, lower educational level, and female gender were also indicative of poor treatment response.

Similarly, Dworkin (1997a,b) has identified the severity of reported acute pain as a risk factor for three chronic pain syndromes: phantom pain, post-herpetic neuralgia and chronic back pain. The author cautions that future research should consider the distinction between sensory and affective components of pain, as well as specific pain qualities, when using severity of acute pain as a predictor.

2.6. Additional psychosocial factors as predictor variables

Variables as diverse as age (Lehto and Honkanen, 1995; Watkins et al., 1999), smoking (Lehto and Honkanen, 1995; Ohtsuka et al., 1995; Averns et al., 1996), family environment (Tota-Faucette et al., 1993) and gender (Gatchel et al., 1995b; Lehto and Honkanen, 1995) have also been noted to relate to chronic pain disability outcome. Family status, for example, has been identified in several studies as a factor worthy of attention. Lehmann et al. (1993) assessed 55 low back pain patients referred by occupational physicians. They found that married patients rejoined the work force more promptly than single patients. Volinn et al. (1991) found that age, wage, and family status affected risk of chronicity in patients suffering from back sprain. Patients who were widowed or divorced and had no children were twice as likely to develop chronic pain compared to single individuals with no children.

Barnes (1991) cites a variety of occupational factors that relate directly and indirectly to an individual's propensity to develop chronic low back pain. Physical job demands (e.g., lifting, twisting, bending, vibration, etc.) and work environment (e.g., noisy vs. quiet, quality of lighting, presence or absence of safety features) represent direct occupational factors that may lead to low back disability. Examples of indirect occupational factors include job satisfaction, supervisor ratings of job performance, and employee relationships with co-workers. Barnes additionally identified family response to injury/pain behaviors, attorney involvement in disability cases, and education level as social variables affecting the development of low back pain disability.

Bigos et al. (1991) also found that occupational factors relate to disability. In particular, they found that a predictive model, including work perceptions (i.e., how much subjects enjoyed their jobs), rendered subjects 3.3 times more likely to report a work-related back injury than a low risk group. Additional components of the model were high Scale 3 (Hysteria) on the MMPI and a history of back treatment. Frymoyer et al. (1983) also looked at work-related factors as predictors of disability. These authors evaluated 1221 men between the ages of 18 and 55. They found that severe low back pain was predicted by jobs requiring repetitive heavy lifting, use of jackhammers or machine tools, and operation of motor vehicles. Smoking also emerged as a risk factor for more severe pain.

In 1997, the National Advisory Committee on Health and Disability of New Zealand put out a document on psychosocial risk factors for the low back pain population (Kendall et al., 1998) that included a screening device (Linton and Halldén, 1989). These comprehensive guidelines included many of the risk factors reviewed above. They were designed as a tool to assist health-care professionals identify acute cases in danger of having a poor treatment response and developing a disabling low back pain condition. Identified risk factors included maladaptive attitudes and beliefs concerning back pain, frequent display of pain behaviors, reinforcement of pain behaviors by family members, heightened emotional reactivity, lack of social support, job dissatisfaction, and compensation issues. This screening device is indicative of a more recent move towards combining risk factors into comprehensive models. Examples of these are further discussed below.

3. Models predicting chronic pain disability

As the above review indicates, multiple variables have been identified as having some predictive utility in identifying high-risk acute patients who may develop chronic pain. While the research in this area has been helpful with regard to identifying the most robust predictive variables, investigators have only recently begun to combine these variables in an effort to develop predictive models. Block and Callewart (1999) used one such model in their clinical work with pre-surgical screenings. These authors evaluated numerous variables, including personality (MMPI scales), cognitive (coping ability), behavioral (spousal reinforcement, compensation, psychiatric history, marital distress, physical or sexual abuse, and substance abuse), and medical (chronicity, number of previous surgeries, surgical destruction, nonorganic signs of illness, previous health-care utilization, smoking, and obesity) factors. These factors are evaluated through a review of medical records, semi-structured interview, observation and psychological testing. Following the data gathering phase, the above factors are combined through an empirically derived procedure that allows the clinician to rate the patient in terms of good, fair, or poor candidates for surgical intervention. The authors report good results with this screening procedure (Bock, 1996).

Burton et al. (1997) examined 70 patients with a diagnosis of one or more chronic work-related upper-extremity disorders. Several factors emerged as contributors to a patient's ability to regain occupational functioning. Return to work at 1 year follow-up was predicted by the number of Axis I disorders, a past diagnosis of substance abuse, a past and/or current diagnosis of an anxiety disorder, a diagnosis of borderline personality disorder, a history of childhood abuse, self-report of depressed mood, and a moderate to high level of perceived disability. Additionally, age, race, length of disability, and prior surgical treatment predicted return-to-work rates.

In a sample of 1816 patients presenting for tertiary rehabilitation in a functional restoration program, Bendix et al. (1998) examined this same question. Age, days of sick leave, connection to the work force, and back pain intensity correlated to success at 1 year follow-up. Back muscle endurance, sports activity, performance on activities of daily living, and vibrations were additionally important for some

parameters predicting success following functional restoration treatment.

Finally, Maruta et al. (1979) examined a heterogeneous group of chronic pain patients who successfully completed a treatment program comprised of behavior modification, physical rehabilitation, medication management, education, group treatment, biofeedback/relaxation, family involvement, and supportive psychotherapy. At 1 year follow-up, those patients classified as 'successful' based on modification of attitude, reduction of pain-related medication, and improvement in physical function were distinguishable from those deemed 'failures' by duration of pain, lost work time, number of operations, subjective pain level, and drug dependency.

While the above models have combined predictive factors into comprehensive models, the included variables are often too numerous to have significant practical utility. In order for health-care providers to use models that identify patients presenting acutely who are at risk for developing chronic problems, it will be necessary to have parsimonious models with predictive algorithms that can be used quickly in the health-care setting. In this regard, Barnes et al. (1989) examined three groups of patients based on outcome and follow-up data 1 and 2 years after completion of a functional restoration program. These authors found that good outcome at follow-up was determined by certain MMPI and Millon Behavioral Health Inventory (MBHI) scale scores, prior surgical history, level of workers' compensation, and pain intensity ratings.

In 1995, Gatchel, Polatin, and Mayer further refined the above model. These authors systematically evaluated 421 patients presenting with acute low back pain in an effort to evaluate the predictive power of a comprehensive assessment of psychosocial and personality factors using a standard battery (Structured Clinical Interview for DSM-III-R Diagnosis, MMPI, and Millon Visual Pain Analog Scale). All patients had been symptomatic with lumbar pain for 6 weeks or less. Subjects were tracked every 3 months, culminating in a structured telephone interview conducted 1 year after initial evaluation to document return-to-work status. These authors found gender, self-reported pain and disability scores, scores on Scale 3 of the MMPI, and workers' compensation and personal injury insurance status correctly classified 90.7% of the cases. The authors note that the results suggest the presence of a robust 'psychosocial disability factor' that is associated with injured workers who are likely to progress from acute pain to a chronic pain state. Based on these data, Gatchel et al. (1995b) generated a statistical algorithm to identify those acute patients who will require early intervention to prevent development of chronic disability. This algorithm, which will be discussed further below, is currently being examined in terms of screening high-risk patient and offering prophylactic intervention to prevent the progression to chronic musculoskeletal pain and disability.

4. Points of intervention

The emerging ability to predict which patients are at-risk for progressing to chronic disability status raises the issue of identifying the appropriate point at which to intervene in order to accomplish effective prevention. Three intervention intervals are traditionally discussed: primary, secondary, or tertiary, and there is some literature to address efficacy at each of these periods in the course of illness. An exhaustive review of the outcome literature relevant to these efforts at prevention is beyond the scope of the current article. The reader is referred to Frank et al. (1996a,b) and Linton (1999) for impressive coverage of these topics. Nevertheless, salient issues involved in prevention are important to highlight, and are summarized in Table I. A brief discussion of these topics follows.

4.1. Primary prevention

Primary prevention of musculoskeletal pain is difficult to evaluate. Because musculoskeletal pain is not associated with well-defined medical findings, the traditional distinction between primary and secondary prevention can be nebulous at best. Despite the gargantuan effort that has been devoted to designing

TABLE I

Points of consideration with primary, secondary and tertiary treatment interventions

Primary prevention
- Cost
- Commitment to program change
- Identification of risk factors
- Previous intervention success
- Program compliance
- Program delivery
- Rigorous evaluation of outcomes
- Workstyle

Secondary prevention
- Health/behaviors, not medical pathology
- Open communication
- Patient self-management
- Prospective rather than retroactive
- Rigorous evaluation of outcomes
- Shift from "diagnose and cure" to active prevention
- Treatments based on empirical instead of theoretical factors
- Workstyle

Tertiary interventions
- Effective
- Too little, too late?

early prevention programs, few studies offer scientifically validated support that attest to their efficacy (Linton, 1999). In fact, some authors have concluded that there is a paucity of evidence to support the efficacy of primary prevention for back pain (Frank et al., 1996b), or for other musculoskeletal disorders at all, and that we know very little about primary prevention for these types of disorders (Spitzer, 1993).

There are several difficulties inherent in examining the efficacy of primary interventions (Frank et al., 1996b). In particular, effectiveness depends on many factors, such as previous success of the intervention, factors related to program delivery, and compliance and monitoring of implemented programs. In occupational settings, primary prevention occurs through two primary channels: (1) changing the workers, or teaching them appropriate techniques for lifting, etc.; or (2) changing the work, which implies a reduction of physical demands primarily through ergonomic techniques (Frank et al., 1996b).

Programs designed to change the workers, according to Frank and colleagues, often involve factors such as job training, behavior modification, and increasing trunk strength, with the assumption that increased conditioning and education of the worker will decrease the chances of experiencing injury. The authors report mixed results with these types of interventions. Of the above techniques, education appears to be the most common strategy, with the underlying assumption that individuals suffer more than necessary because they lack knowledge ranging from appropriate body mechanics to utilization of effective coping strategies (Linton, 1999). Educational interventions, which often take the form of back schools, present discussions regarding anatomy, biomechanics, lifting and postural changes related to work, as well as teaching appropriate exercises. Back schools involve educational principles, and they lend themselves particularly well to a group format, thereby increasing their popularity for primary prevention. Additionally, there is significant face validity and patients therefore appear to enjoy them. Despite these benefits, however, there is ongoing debate about their utility (Linton, 1999).

Linton (1999) additionally cites exercise as a commonly utilized primary prevention technique. While there is ample evidence for the benefits of exercise in chronic pain patients, the clinical utility of exercise programs for patients presenting acutely is more difficult to establish. Questions abound regarding appropriate type of exercise, whether there is improvement with exercise, whether exercise continues following completion of the program and whether or not exercise actually leads to reduced musculoskeletal pain (Linton, 1999). Nevertheless, there does appear to be a modest beneficial effect to using exercise as a preventative intervention (Gebhardt, 1994 cited in Linton, 1999).

Interventions designed to change the work environment have also proven difficult to evaluate, and very few interventions have demonstrated a clear reduction in the incidence of occupational low back pain with these strategies (Frank et al., 1996b). Factors that contribute to the challenging nature of demonstrating the efficacy of these programs include the high cost of redesigning the work place for preventative musculoskeletal difficulties, insufficient commitment to ergonomic interventions on behalf of workers or management, difficulty identifying the risk factors for injury (and consequently identifying which items require change), decisions regarding monitoring of outcomes, and weak study designs. Some authors note that there are no well-designed studies examining the effects of ergonomics (Karas and Conrad, 1996). Nevertheless, there is some evidence that ergonomic interventions result in direct reductions of occupational low back pain, providing promising paths for future research (Aaras, 1994 cited in Frank et al., 1996b).

In particular, the National Institute for Occupational Safety and Health undertook a comprehensive evaluation of the epidemiologic evidence for work-related musculoskeletal disorders (National Institute for Occupational Safety and Health, 1997). Each study was evaluated in terms of its methodological rigor and rated according to whether it provided 'strong evidence', 'evidence', 'insufficient evidence' or 'no evidence' for a causal relationship between physical work factors and musculoskeletal disorders. The review identified strong evidence for a causal relationship between postural factors and neck/shoulder difficulties. A combination of repetition, force, and postural factors were strongly linked to elbow difficulties, carpal tunnel syndrome, and tendonitis. Finally, vibration factors were linked to hand/arm vibration syndrome, and lifting/forceful movements and whole body vibrations were linked to back injuries. Moderate evidence was identified for 13 work-related factors and other musculoskeletal disorders. Overall, therefore, there does appear to be some evidence between physical work factors and the emergence of musculoskeletal pain, suggesting that this is a promising avenue of future research in the area of prevention.

More recently, proposed models have allowed for the interaction of work environment and worker factors in the development of work-related upper-extremity disorders. Several models have been noted to account for the precipitation of musculoskeletal injuries in the work place, the mechanisms of which are thought to interact in each individual to account for musculoskeletal difficulties (Kumar, 2001). In particular, the 'Multivariate Interaction Theory' describes the interplay between an individual's genetic endowment, morphological characteristics and psychosocial makeup, as well as with occupational biomechanical hazards. 'Differential Fatigue Theory' describes asymmetric occupational activities that result in differential fatigue of specific joints and muscles. Over time, the altered muscle kinetics may precipitate injury. 'Cumulative Load Theory' builds upon the idea that biological tissues have a finite capacity. Repeated load application can result in cumulative fatigue, and therefore alter the threshold at which tissues will fail. Finally, 'Overexertion Theory' describes the physical components of force, posture, motion, duration. These components and their complex interactions play a role in job-related injury (Kumar, 2001). The theories described above adopt the premise that occupational musculoskeletal injuries are biomechanical in nature. However, they hypothesize a complex interaction of factors between the individual and his or her environment to explain the precipitation of injury.

Other authors have also described the interaction of work place and worker when discussing the origin of work-related injuries. Feuerstein et al. (1999) have discussed the construct of workstyle, and its' contribution to upper-extremity disorders through direct and interactional effects. Workstyle is defined as "an individual pattern of cognitions, behaviors, and physiological reactivity that co-occur while performing job tasks" and that may be associated with alterations in physiological state. As the authors explain, once a physiological state has been repeatedly elicited, the development, exacerbation and/or maintenance of work-related musculoskeletal symptoms can be affected. Furthermore, an adverse workstyle, or style associated with an increased incidence of symptoms, can result from high work demands. Alternatively, self-imposed needs for achievement and/or acceptance can affect adverse workstyles. Fears of job loss, avoidance of negative consequence related to the job, and inadequate/improper training can also trigger adverse workstyles. The authors hypothesize that a sufficiently frequent, intense and enduring adverse workstyle can predispose an individual to develop upper-extremity disorders, particularly when exposed to suspected ergonomic risk factors. This model is attractive because it provides a context for considering both internal, or worker-related factors, and external, or job-related factors when considering the multidimensional construct of risk for chronic musculoskeletal disability. It is thereby more consistent with the predominant biopsychosocial model of conceptualizing individuals presenting with chronic pain.

4.2. Secondary interventions

As previously mentioned, a good portion of the literature focusing on forestalling progression from acute to chronic pain involves studying patients at points of secondary prevention, or when symptoms of pain have just begun. Often, researchers administer batteries of questionnaires when the patients first present, and then retrospectively examine which factors predict outcome. Few studies, however, have actually treated high-risk patients at this point in time with targeted interventions. In terms of cost effectiveness, this interval is potentially the most promising, as only individuals already afflicted with pain are targeted and, for high-risk patients, intervention can be administered before the astronomical expenditures associated with chronic disability status become entrenched.

A comprehensive review of factors relevant to the secondary prevention of chronic musculoskeletal pain in health-care settings has been reported elsewhere (Linton, 1999). Theoretical factors cited as particularly important include the timing of the intervention, with particular attention paid to reaching the patient before lifestyle changes have occurred. Secondly, a focus on health and behaviors, rather than on medical variables, is helpful as part of an overall emphasis on the active role the patient will play in the intervention. Including the patient as an active and engaged partner, rather than as a passive recipient of treatment, is beneficial. Finally, facilitating communication between all involved parties and following-up to effectively evaluate results are crucial components of effective preventative strategies (Linton, 1999).

With regard to occupational low back pain, Frank et al. (1996b) once again provide a cogent review of the relevant issues. They note that interventions can be based in the work place, such as providing modified duty in close proximity to injury onset, or encouraging employees to report injuries early on and obtain care at work. Conversely, interventions can be based in the health-care system, including the use of standardized treatment guidelines, which raise particular issues with regard to physician compliance and successful implementation of established guidelines.

In the health-care systems, Linton et al. (1993) found that an early intervention comprised of information regarding results of the doctor examination, prognosis, treatment, and advice about how to improve and what activities to engage in, resulted in fewer sick days for patients with acute musculoskeletal pain. Similarly, an intervention in a primary care setting in the Netherlands compared a standard general practitioner intervention to this same intervention plus exercise, massage, and physical therapy, and found the more extensive treatment group to have a greater overall perceived treatment effect at 6 and 12 month follow-ups. A manipulative therapy group achieved similarly positive long-term outcomes (Koes et al., 1993).

Others have suggested that patient self-management is an important component in managing both recurrent and chronic pain, and that collaboration between patients and health-care providers is critical for effective and cost containing intervention (Von Korff et al., 1997). Ongoing monitoring on behalf of the patient, combined with effective communication with physicians, could result in appropriate care being administered in the acute phase, before the illness becomes more entrenched. Furthermore, this approach to patient care is consistent with the outlooks of both patients and physicians. When primary care back pain patients and their physicians were asked who should have primary responsibility for directing patient back pain care, both patients and physicians responded that the two should either share

the responsibility, or that care should be primarily directed by the patient (Turner et al., 1998). This increased responsibility on behalf of the patient could potentially play a critical role in secondary prevention, in terms of seeking out appropriate management early enough in the illness presentation to prevent the progression to more longstanding difficulties.

While a good deal has been done to screen patients presenting acutely to identify those who are at higher risk for chronic pain progression, many interventions to date have been based solely on theory, rather than on known causal factors. This has occurred primarily as a result of our lack of understanding regarding the etiology of many musculoskeletal difficulties (Linton, 1999). As previously mentioned, the current authors are undertaking a systematic examination of risk factors identified through earlier research (Gatchel et al., 1995b) to identify high-risk patients. These individuals are then treated prophylactically with an interdisciplinary intervention (discussed below) in an effort to return them to work and forestall progression to chronic pain disability status. Should this intervention prove effective, numerous practical implications could potentially be realized, such as decreased costs of long-term patient care, reduced loss of productivity, and alleviated pain and suffering on behalf of the patient. In fact, Linton (1999) notes that the point of first contact with health-care personnel may provide an excellent opportunity for early, preventative interventions. This shift from the traditional model of 'diagnosing and curing' patients towards a more active stance involving patient involvement and preventative care might affect patient attitudes as well as help them to engage in important behavioral changes (Linton, 1999). Research demonstrating the efficacy of active, preventative strategies such as these could ultimately revolutionize our current approach to patient care.

4.3. Tertiary interventions

Numerous studies attest to the efficacy of tertiary interventions, particularly as they relate to interdisciplinary interventions. Interdisciplinary treatment frequently takes place in pain clinics, or pain centers, and it is often recommended for a number of chronic pain conditions. Geisser and Colwell (1999) note that, while the specific components of interdisciplinary, or multidisciplinary treatment vary, they generally include ongoing medical care, exercise or physical therapy interventions, psychosocial interventions, and occupational/vocational rehabilitation. Interdisciplinary, versus multidisciplinary, treatment centers, represent the gold standard, and are to be differentiated from the latter based on the quality of the communication between the providers (Gatchel and Turk, 1999).

Okifuji et al. (1999) reviewed the available literature and concluded that multidisciplinary pain centers are effective in pain reduction, decreased opioid use, return to work, decreased health-care utilization, and closure of disability claims. Similarly, Linton et al. (1989) found interdisciplinary treatment to be effective in decreasing pain intensity, anxiety, fatigue ratings, observed pain behaviors, and feelings of helplessness. The treatment was additionally effective in increasing sleep quality, activities, and mood.

A subtype of interdisciplinary treatment is the functional restoration approach developed by Mayer and Gatchel (1988). This approach involves intensive interdisciplinary care for patients with low back injury, as well as other musculoskeletal disabilities, and involves an extensive functional capacity evaluation involving objectively quantified measures of physical and psychological functioning. Patients participate in intensive programs involving numerous disciplines, and treatment is guided by repeat testing with emphasis on feeding progress data back to the patient to enhance spinal mobility and strength. Psychological intervention involves multimodal disability management focusing on four major areas: behavioral stress management, cognitive-behavioral skills training, individual and group counseling from a crisis intervention model, and family counseling (Mayer et al., 1987). The functional restoration approach has been tremendously successful in rehabilitating patients with low back injury (e.g., Mayer et al., 1985, 1987; Mayer and Gatchel, 1988).

As demonstrated above, the efficacy of interdisciplinary/multidisciplinary interventions for tertiary rehabilitation of chronic musculoskeletal disorders is indisputable, and is extensively reviewed elsewhere (Flor et al., 1992; Okifuji et al., 1999). However, optimal savings might be best realized by intervening prior to the onset of chronic pain disability. Increasingly, researchers are evaluating the cost effectiveness of interventions occurring early in the disease course, and the literature is growing with respect to the staggering savings realized by these preventative measures.

5. Cost effectiveness of preventative interventions

While cost reduction is frequently cited as a justification for using preventative interventions with chronic musculoskeletal pain, few adequate analyses have been reported (Linton and Bradley, 1996). As mentioned, however, the few high-quality studies that have attempted to quantify cost savings have identified promising figures in terms of justifying interventions of this sort. For example, focusing solely on decreased health-care utilization has been found to save $78,960 over 1 year in a sample of 61 heterogeneous chronic pain patients treated in a military setting (Peters et al., 2000).

When authors expand their cost savings analyses to include indirect measures, the figures become even more staggering. Linton et al. (1989) examined the effects of a secondary prevention program on sick-listing and associated costs among nurses with subacute back pain. In this study, sources for absenteeism estimates were derived from The National Health Insurance Authority in Sweden, which reportedly records all lost work days for employees. At 6 month follow-up, participants in the program had significantly fewer days off than waiting-list controls. An 18-month follow-up evaluation indicated that the mean reduction in sick days relative to pretreatment trends was 76.5 days per person, resulting in a savings of nearly $10,000 per person, or approximately twice the cost of the intervention.

One group of authors examined costs of a health-care model emphasizing early intervention through a managed care program (Matheson et al., 1995).

The treatment model adopted an occupational rehabilitation orientation, with the primary focus being return to work. Patients were triaged by a diagnostic team comprised of a physician case manager, physical therapist, and clinical case manager. Treatment was described as intense and 'front-end loaded' with more activity in the early stages. At-home rest, specialty referrals, and expensive diagnostic procedures or surgeries were limited. Data were analyzed for the 294 cases on which complete medical charges were obtained. The average cost was $2330 per case, although a small proportion was responsible for an inordinate proportion of the costs. The 30 most costly cases accounted for 53% of the total medical costs, while the 60 most costly cases accounted for 73% of the medical expenditures. Two hundred and twenty-five subjects missed no days of work following injury, and an additional 32 returned to work within 2 days or less. Medical costs were 296% higher for those 70 injured workers who lost at least 1 day of work. Mean case costs were $4701 for this group, compared to $1588 for the 224 patients who returned to work immediately. While the above study did not provide a control group, the authors compared their results to published data and calculated a savings of $151 per case overall and $244 per back pain case.

Analysis of costs savings based on the previously mentioned review article published by Flor et al. (1992) resulted in estimates of savings as much as $18 million in medical treatment for a sample of 2318 patients in the first year following treatment. The authors note that these figures do not consider savings that might accrue from indirect costs such as reduced disability payments, gains in productivity and gains in revenue from taxes paid by successfully treated patients (Turk and Okifuji, 1998a).

Okifuji et al. (1999) used published figures to estimate treatment costs for different procedures based on a hypothetical annual cohort of 17,600 patients. The authors note that the cohort figure was derived from the assumption that each multidisciplinary pain center treats at least 50 patients annually. Based on figures from the American Pain Society, the authors suggest that multidisciplinary treated patients would spend a total of $280 million less in medical costs and additional surgery in the year following treatment than would these same patients treated with the conventional approach. Compared to patients originally treated with surgery, these authors estimated that multidisciplinary pain treated patients would spend $63 million less for possible future surgeries required due to pain. They go on to examine differences in terms of disability payments and return-to-work status, and they calculated a total cost difference between the annual cohort of multidisciplinary treated versus conventionally treated patients to be $2,200,352,400 versus $5,186,000, respectively.

As the cost effectiveness of preventative interventions is just emerging as an area of study, the issues relevant to this type of research are only now becoming evident. For example, two groups of authors have noted the importance of examining outcome of chronic pain patients from multiple perspectives due to the multifactorial nature of chronic pain. They, therefore, suggest that cost savings be addressed from several vantage points. Additionally, they point out the numerous assumptions inherent in this type of analysis, particularly with regard to cost of disability, treatment costs, general inflation, and inflation in medical expenses (Turk and Okifuji, 1998b).

The above studies make evident the tremendous potential savings of preventative intervention in the acute stage of musculoskeletal pain. More studies with greater attention to issues such as prospective designs, standardization of treatment, randomization of samples, and reliability with regard to data collection (i.e., using administrative databases or other objective sources to quantify utilization) would be helpful in further elucidating the issues under discussion. The literature already demonstrates a trend in this direction. For example, Linton et al. (1989) cite the source of their data for absenteeism as a published administrative database, and Okifuji et al. (1999) provide detailed explanations regarding the sources of their financial data and the assumptions underlying their analyses. The preliminary research cited above suggests that early intervention with musculoskeletal patients represents a promising means for breaking the cycle of progression from acute to chronic pain, thus providing an opportunity to decrease the significant financial expenditures and personal suffering resulting from this health-care dilemma.

6. Summary and conclusions

Great strides have been made regarding preventative strategies for chronic musculoskeletal pain and disability. These strides have evolved primarily through the identification of risk factors associated with negative treatment outcome following acute symptom presentation. Risk factors have traditionally reflected the biopsychosocial model of chronic musculoskeletal pain that predominates today, and have included variables such as pathophysiology, psychopathology, coping strategies, secondary gain issues and work and family variables.

Similarly, effective interdisciplinary interventions involving on-site treatment coordination, with open channels of communication between health-care providers dedicated to the functional restoration of patients, have demonstrated efficacy with heterogeneous groups of chronic pain patients. However, these interventions have frequently been implemented in the tertiary rehabilitation stage of illness progression, after significant financial and emotional expenditures have accrued on behalf of society and the individual patient.

Parsimonious predictive models that enable targeted interventions to be offered to high-risk patients in the acute phase are only recently being developed. Future avenues of research should increasingly capitalize on the substantial body of knowledge regarding risk factors, in order to treat high-risk individuals prospectively, as opposed to retrospectively. Interventions of this sort could have a tremendous impact on the substantial financial and treatment issues that become increasingly salient as chronic disability status becomes entrenched, and could revolutionize our approach to patient care with this often recalcitrant population.

Acknowledgements

Supported in part by Grant Nos. 2R01-MH46452, 2KO2-MH01107, and 2RO1-DE10713 from the National Institutes of Health.

References

Aaras, A. (1994) The impact of ergonomic intervention on individual health and corporate prosperity in a telecommunications environment. Ergonomics, 37: 1679–1696.

Adler, C.S., Adler, S.M. and Packard, R.C. (1987) Psychiatric Aspects of Headache. Williams and Wilkins, Baltimore, MD.

Ambrosius, F.M., Kremer, A.M., Herkner, P.B., DeKraker, M. and Bartz, S. (1995) Outcome comparison of workers' compensation and noncompensation low back pain in a highly structured functional restoration program. J. Orthop. Sports Phys. Ther., 21: 7–12.

Averns, H.L., Oxtoby, J., Taylor, H.G., Jones, P.W., Dziedzic, K. and Dawes, P.T. (1996) Smoking and outcome in ankylosing spondylitis. Scand. J. Rheumatol., 25(3): 138–142.

Barnes, D. (1991) Social factors affecting pain. In: T.G. Mayer, V. Mooney and R.J. Gatchel (Eds.), Contemporary Conservative Care for Painful Spinal Disorders. Lea and Febiger, Philadelphia, PA, 143–148.

Barnes, D., Smith, D., Gatchel, R.J. and Mayer, T.G. (1989) Psychosocioeconomic predictors of treatment success/failure in chronic low-back pain patients. Spine, 14(4): 427–430.

Barnes, D., Gatchel, R.J., Mayer, T.G. and Barnett, J. (1990) Changes in MMPI profiles of chronic low back pain patients following successful treatment. J. Spinal Disord., 3: 353–355.

Beals, R. (1984) Compensation and recovery from injury. West. J. Med., 140: 233–237.

Bellamy, R. (1997) Compensation neurosis. Financial reward for illness as nocebo. Clin. Orthop., 336: 94–106.

Bendix, A.F., Bendix, T. and Haestrup, C. (1998) Can it be predicted which patients with chronic low back pain should be offered tertiary rehabilitation in a functional restoration program? A search for demographic, socioeconomic and physical predictors. Spine, 23: 1775–1784.

Bhandari, M., Louw, D. and Reddy, K. (1999) Predictors of return to work after anterior cervical discectomy. J. Spinal Disord., 12(2): 94–98.

Bigos, S.J., Battie, M.C., Spengler, D.M., Fisher, L.D., Fordyce, W.E., Hansson, T.H., Nachemson, A.L. and Wortley, M.D. (1991) A prospective study of work perceptions and psychosocial factors affecting the report of back injury. Spine, 16(1): 1–6.

Blanchard, E.B. (1993) Irritable Bowel Syndrome. In: R.J. Gatchel and E.B. Blanchard (Eds.), Psychophysiological Disorders. American Psychological Association, Washington, WA, pp. 23–62.

Blanchard, E.B. and Andrasik, F. (1985) Management of Chronic

Headache: A Psychological Approach. Pergamon Press, Elmsford, NY.

Blanchard, E.B., Kirsch, C.A., Applebaum, K.A. and Jaccard, J. (1989) Role of psychopathology in chronic headache: Cause or effect. Headache, 29: 295–301.

Block, A.R. and Callewart, C.N.Y.G.P., Inc. (1999) Surgery for chronic spine pain: Procedures for patient selection and outcome enhancement. In: R.J. Gatchel and D.C. Turk (Eds.), Psychological Approaches to Pain Management: A Practitioner's Handbook. Guilford Publications, New York, NY, pp. 33–52.

Bock, A.R. (1996) Presurgical Psychological Screening in Chronic Pain Syndromes: A Guide for the Behavioral Health Practitioner. Lawrence Erlbaum, Mahwah, NJ.

Bombardier, C.H., Divine, G.W., Jordan, J.S., Brooks, W.B. and Neelon, F.A. (1993) Minnesota Multiphasic Personality Inventory (MMPI) cluster groups among chronically ill patients: Relationship to illness adjustment and treatment outcome. J. Behav. Med., 16: 467–484.

Boothby, J.L., Thorn, B.E., Stroud, M.W. and Jensen, M.P. (1999) Coping with pain. In: R.J. Gatchel and D.A. Turk (Eds.), Psychosocial Factors in Pain: Critical Perspectives. Guilford Press, New York, NY, pp. 343–359.

Brown, G.K. and Nicassio, P.M. (1987) Development of questionnaire for the assessment of active and passive coping strategies in chronic pain patients. Pain, 31: 53–64.

Buckelew, S.P., Huyser, B., Hewett, J.E., Parker, J.C., Johnson, J.C., Conway, R. and Kay, D.R. (1996) Self-efficacy predicting outcome among fibromyalgia subjects. Arthritis Care Res., 9(2): 97–104.

Burns, J.W., Johnson, B.J., Mahoney, N., Devine, J. and Pawl, R. (1998) Cognitive and physical capacity process variables predict long-term outcome after treatment of chronic pain. J. Consult. Clin. Psychol., 66(2): 434–439.

Burton, K., Polatin, P.B. and Gatchel, R.J. (1997) Psychosocial factors and the rehabilitation of patients with chronic work-related upper extremity disorders. J. Occup. Rehabil., 7: 139–153.

Catts, P.F., Aroney, M. and Indyk, J.S. (1994) Laparoscopic repair of inguinal hernia. Med. J. Aust., 161: 243–248.

Clark, L.A., Watson, D. and Mineka, S. (1994) Temperament, personality and the mood and anxiety disorders. J. Abnorm. Psychol., 103: 103–116.

Croft, P.R., Papageorgiou, A.C., Ferry, S., Thomas, E., Jayson, M.I.V. and Silman, A.J. (1995) Psychological distress and low back pain. Evidence from a prospective study in the general population. Spine, 20: 2731–2737.

Dahlstrom, L., Widmark, G. and Carlsson, S.G. (1997) Cognitive-behavioral profiles among different categories of orofacial pain patients: diagnostic and treatment. Eur. J. Oral Sci., 105(5 PT 1): 377–383.

Davis, R.A. (1994) A long-term outcome analysis of 984 surgically treated herniated lumbar discs. J. Neurosurg., 80: 415–421.

Deyo, R.A., Cherkin, D., Conrad, D. and Volinn, E. (1991) Cost, controversy, crisis: Low back pain and the health of the public. Annu. Rev. Public Health, 12: 141–156.

Drossman, D.A., McKee, D.C., Sandler, R.S., Mitchell, C.M., Cramer, E.M., Lowman, B.C. and Burger, A.L. (1988) Psychosocial factors in the irritable bowel syndrome: A multivariate study of patients and nonpatients with irritable bowel syndrome. Gastroenterology, 95: 701–708.

Dworkin, R.H. (1997a) Toward a clearer specification of acute pain risk factors and chronic pain outcomes. Pain Forum, 6: 148–150.

Dworkin, R.H. (1997b) Which individuals with acute pain are most likely to develop a chronic pain syndrome. Pain Forum, 6: 127–136.

Dworkin, S.F., Von Korff, M.R. and LeResche, L. (1990) Multiple pains and psychiatric disturbance: An epidemiologic investigation. Arch. Gen. Psychiatry, 47: 239–244.

Etscheidt, M.A. and Steiger, H.G. (1995) Multidimensional Pain Inventory profile classification and psychopathology. J. Consult. Clin. Psychol., 51(1): 29–36.

Feuerstein, M., Huang, G.D. and Pransky, G. (1999) Workstyle and work-related upper extremity disorders. In: R.J. Gatchel and D.A. Turk (Eds.), Psychosocial Factors in Pain: Critical Perspectives. Guilford Press, New York, NY, pp. 175–192.

Fishbain, D.A., Goldberg, M., Meagher, B.R., Steele, R. and Rosomoff, H. (1986) Male and female chronic pain patients categorized by DSM-III psychiatric diagnostic criteria. Pain, 26: 181–197.

Fishbain, D.A., Cutler, R., Rosomoff, H.L. and Rosomoff, R.S. (1997) Chronic pain-associated depression: Antecedent or consequence of chronic pain? A review. Clin. J. Pain, 13: 116–137.

Flor, H., Fydrich, T. and Turk, D. (1992) Efficacy of multidisciplinary pain treatment centers: A meta-analytic flow. Pain, 49: 221–230.

Fordyce, W.E., Roberts, A.H. and Sternbach, R.A. (1985) The behavioral management of chronic pain: A response to critics. Pain, 22: 112–125.

Fordyce, W., Bigos, S., Battie, M. and Fisher, L. (1992) MMPI scale 3 as a predictor of back injury report: What does it tell us. Clin. J. Pain, 8: 222–226.

Frank, J.W., Brooker, A., DeMaio, S.E., Kerr, M.S., Maetzel, A., Shannon, H.S., Sullivan, T.J., Norman, R.W. and Wells, R.P. (1996a) Disability resulting from occupational low back pain. Part II: What do we know about secondary prevention? A review of the scientific evidence on prevention after disability begins. Spine, 21: 2918–2929.

Frank, J.W., Kerr, M.S., Brooker, A., DeMaio, S.E., Maetzel, A., Shannon, H.S., Sullivan, T.J., Norman, R.W. and Wells, R.P. (1996b) Disability resulting from occupational low back pain. Part I. What do we know about primary prevention? A review of the scientific evidence on prevention before disability begins. Spine, 21(24): 2908–2917.

Fricton, J.R. and Olsen, T. (1996) Predictors of outcome for treatment of temporomandibular disorders. J. Orofacial Pain, 10(1): 54–65.

Frymoyer, J.S., Pope, M.H., Clements, J.H., Wilder, D.G., MacPherson, B. and Ashikaga, K. (1983) Risk factors in low back pain: An epidemiological survey. J. Bone Joint Surg., 65: 213–218.

Frymoyer, J., Rosen, J., Clements, J. and Pope, M. (1985) Psychological factors in low back pain disability. J. Clin. Orthop., 195: 178–184.

Gatchel, R.J. (1991) Early development of physical and mental deconditioning in painful spinal disorders. In: T.G. Mayer, V. Mooney and R.J. Gatchel (Eds.), Contemporary Conservative Care for Painful Spinal Disorders. Lea and Febiger, Philadelphia, PA, pp. 278–289.

Gatchel, R.J. (1996) Psychological disorders and chronic pain: Cause and effect relationships. In: R.J. Gatchel and D.C. Turk (Eds.), Psychological Approaches to Pain Management: A Practitioner's Handbook. Guilford Publications, New York, NY, pp. 33–52.

Gatchel, R.J. and Epker, J.T. (1999) Psychosocial predictors of chronic pain and response to treatment. In: R.J. Gatchel and D.C. Turk (Eds.), Psychosocial Factors in Pain: Critical Perspectives. Guilford Publications, New York, NY, pp. 412–434.

Gatchel, R.J. and Gardea, M.A. (1999) Psychosocial issues: their importance in predicting disability, response to treatment, and search for compensation. Neurol. Clin., 17(1): 149–166.

Gatchel, R.J. and Turk, D.C. (1999) Interdisciplinary treatment of chronic pain patients. In: R.J. Gatchel and D.C. Turk (Eds.), Psychosocial Factors in Pain: Critical Perspectives. Guilford Press, New York, NY, pp. 435–444.

Gatchel, R.J., Polatin, P.B., Mayer, T.G. and Garcy, P.D. (1994) Psychopathology and the rehabilitation of patients with chronic low back pain disability. Arch. Phys. Med. Rehabil., 75(6): 666–670.

Gatchel, R.J., Polatin, P.B. and Kinney, R.K. (1995a) Predicting outcome of chronic back pain using clinical predictors of psychopathology: a prospective analysis. Health Psychol., 14(5): 415–420.

Gatchel, R.J., Polatin, P.B. and Mayer, T.G. (1995b) The dominant role of psychosocial risk factors in the development of chronic low back pain disability. Spine, 20(24): 2702–2709.

Gebhardt, W.A. (1994) Effectiveness of training to prevent job-related back pain: A meta-analysis. Br. J. Clin. Psychol., 33: 571–574.

Geisser, M.E. and Colwell, M.O. (1999) Chronic back pain: Conservative approaches. In: A.R. Block, E.F. Kremer and E. Fernandez (Eds.), Handbook of Pain Syndromes: Biopsychosocial Perspectives. Lawrence Erlbaum, NJ, pp. 169–190.

Greenough, C.G., Taylor, L.J. and Fraser, R.D. (1994) Anterior lumbar fusion: A comparison of noncompensation patients with compensation patients. Clin. Orthop., 300: 30–37.

Hanvik, L.J. (1951) MMPI profiles in patients with low back pain. J. Consult. Psychol., 15: 350–353.

Jayson, M.I.V. (1997) Presidential address: Why does acute back pain become chronic. Spine, 22: 1053–1056.

Karas, B.E. and Conrad, K.M. (1996) Back injury prevention interventions in the workplace: An integrative review. Am. Assoc. Occup. Health Nurse J., 44(4): 189–196.

Keefe, F.J., Brown, G.K., Wallston, K.A. and Caldwell, D.S. (1989) Coping with rheumatoid arthritis pain: Catastrophizing as a maladaptive strategy. Pain, 37: 51–56.

Keefe, F.J., Kashikar-Zuck, S., Robinson, E., Salley, A., Beaupre, P., Caldwell, D., Baucom, D. and Haythornwhite, J. (1997) Pain coping strategies that predict patients' and spouses' ratings of patients' self-efficacy. Pain, 73(2): 191–199.

Kendall, N.A.S., Linton, S.J. and Main, C. (1998) Psychosocial yellow flags for acute low back pain: 'Yellow Flags' as an analogue to 'Red Flags'. Eur. J. Pain, 2: 87–89.

Kerns, R., Turk, D. and Rudy, T. (1985) The West Haven-Yale Multidimensional Pain Inventory. Pain, 23: 345–356.

Klapow, J.C., Slater, M.A., Patterson, T.L., Atkinson, J.H., Weickgenant, A.L., Grant, I. and Garfin, S.R. (1995) Psychosocial factors discriminate multidimensional clinical groups of chronic low back pain patients. Pain, 62: 349–355.

Kleinke, C.L. (1994) MMPI scales as predictors of pain-coping strategies preferred by patients with chronic pain. Rehabil. Psychol., 39: 123–128.

Koes, B.W., Bouter, L.M., van Mameren, H., Essers, A.H., Verstegen, G.M., Hofhuizen, D.M., Houben, J.P. and Knipschild, P.G. (1993) A randomized clinical trial of manual therapy and physiotherapy for persistent back and neck complaints: subgroup analysis and relationship between outcome measures. J. Manipulative Physiol. Ther., 16: 211–219.

Kumar, S. (2001) Theories of musculoskeletal injury causation. Ergonomics, 44(1): 17–47.

Lanes, T.C., Gauron, E.F., Spratt, K.F., Wernimott, T.J., Found, E.M. and Weinstein, J.N. (1995) Long-term follow-up of patients with chronic back pain treated in a multidisciplinary rehabilitation program. Spine, 18: 1103–1112.

Lazarus, R. and Folkman, J. (1984) Stress, Appraisal, and Coping. Springer, New York, NY.

Leavitt, F. and Garron, D.C. (1982) Patterns of psychological distress and pain report in patients with low back pain. J. Psychosom. Res., 26: 301–307.

Lehmann, T.R., Spratt, K.F. and Lehmann, K.K. (1993) Predicting long-term disability in low back injured workers presenting to a spine consultant. Spine, 18: 1103–1112.

Lehto, M.U. and Honkanen, P. (1995) Factors influencing the outcome of operative treatment for lumbar spinal stenosis. Acta Neurochir., 137(1–2): 25–28.

Linton, S.J. (1999) Prevention with special reference to chronic musculoskeletal disorders. In: R.J. Gatche and D.A. Turk (Eds.), Psychosocial Factors in Pain: Critical Perspectives. Guilford Press, New York, NY, pp. 374–389.

Linton, S.J. and Bradley, L.A. (1996) Strategies for the prevention of chronic pain. In: R.J. Gatchel and D.C. Turk (Eds.), Psychological Approaches to Pain Management: A Practitioner's Handbook. Guilford Publications, New York, NY, pp. 438–457.

Linton, S.J. and Halldén, K. (1989) Can we screen for problematic back pain? A screening questionnaire for predicting outcome in acute and subacute back pain. Clin. J. Pain, 14: 209–215.

Linton, S.J., Bradley, L.A., Jensen, I., Spangfort, E. and Sundell, L. (1989) The secondary prevention of low back pain: a controlled study with follow-up. Pain, 36: 197–207.

Linton, S.J., Hellsing, A.L. and Andersson, D. (1993) A controlled study of the effects of an early intervention on acute musculoskeletal pain problems. Pain, 54: 353–359.

Linton, S.J., Hellsing, A.L. and Halldén, K. (1998) A population based study of spinal pain among 35- to 45-year-olds: Prevalence, sick leave, and health-care utilization. Spine, 23: 1457–1463.

Magora, A. and Schwartz, A. (1980) Relation between the low back pain syndrome and X-ray findings. Scand. J. Rehabil. Med., 12: 9–15.

Main, C.J. and Spanswick, C.C. (1995) Personality assessment and the Minnesota Multiphasic Personality Inventory: 50 years on: Do we still need our security blanket. Pain Forum, 4: 90–96.

Maruta, T., Swanson, D.W. and Swenson, W.M. (1979) Chronic pain: Which patient may a pain management program help. Pain, 7: 321–329.

Matheson, L.N., Brophy, R.G., Vaughan, K.D., Nunez, C. and Saccoman, K.A. (1995) Workers' compensation managed care: Preliminary findings. J. Occup. Rehabil., 5: 27–36.

Mayer, T.G. (1999) Rehabilitation. What do we do with the chronic patient. Neurol. Clin. North Am., 17: 131–147.

Mayer, T.G. and Gatchel, R.J. (1988) Functional Restoration for Spinal Disorders: The Sports Medicine Approach. Lea and Febiger, Philadelphia, PA.

Mayer, T.G., Gatchel, R.J., Kishino, N., Keeley, J., Capra, P., Mayer, H., Barnett, J. and Mooney, V. (1985) Objective assessment of spine function following industrial injury. A prospective study with comparison group and one-year follow-up. Spine, 10(6): 482–493.

Mayer, T.G., Gatchel, R.J., Mayer, H., Kishino, N.D., Keeley, J. and Mooney, V. (1987) A prospective two-year study of functional restoration in industrial low back injury. An objective assessment procedure [published erratum appears in JAMA 1988 Jan 8;259(2):220]. JAMA, 258(13): 1763–1767.

McCreary, C.P., Clark, G.T., Merril, R.L., Flack, V. and Oakley, M.E. (1991) Psychological distress and diagnostic subgroups of temporomandibular disorder patients. Pain, 44: 29–34.

National Institute for Occupational Safety and Health (1997) Musculoskeletal disorders and workplace factors: A critical review of epidemiologic evidence for work-related musculoskeletal disorders of the neck, upper extremity, and low back (pp. x–xv). Cincinnati, OH.

Nygaard, O.P., Romner, B. and Trumpy, J.H. (1994) Duration of symptoms as a predictor of outcome after lumbar disc surgery. Acta Neurochir., 128(1–4): 53–56.

Ohtsuka, Y., Munakata, M., Tanimura, K., Ukita, H., Kusaka, H., Masaki, Y., Doi, I., Ohe, M., Amishima, M. and Homma, Y. (1995) Smoking promotes insidious and chronic farmer's lung disease, and deteriorates the clinical outcome. Intern. Med., 34(10): 966–971.

Okifuji, A., Turk, D.A. and Kalauokalani, D. (1999) Clinical outcomes and economic evaluation of multidisciplinary pain centers. In: A.R. Block, E.F. Kremer and E. Fernandez (Eds.), Handbook of Pain Syndromes. Lawrence Erlbaum, Mahwah, NJ, pp. 169–191.

Peselow, E.D., Fieve, R.R. and DiFiglia, C. (1992) Personality traits and response to desipramine. J. Affect. Disord., 24: 209–216.

Peters, L., Simon, E.P., Folen, R.A., Umphress, V. and Lagana,

L. (2000) The COPE Program: Treatment efficacy and medical utilization outcome of a chronic pain management based at a major military hospital. Mil. Med., 165: 954–960.

Philips, H.C., Grant, L. and Berkowitz, J. (1991) The prevention of chronic pain and disability: A preliminary investigation. Behav. Res. Ther., 29: 443–450.

Pincus, T., Callahan, L.F., Bradley, L.A., Vaughn, W.K. and Wolfe, F. (1987) Elevated MMPI scores for hypochondriasis, depression and hysteria in patients with rheumatoid arthritis reflect disease rather than psychological status. Arthritis Rheum., 29: 1456–1466.

Polatin, P.B., Kinney, R.K., Gatchel, R.J., Lillo, E. and Mayer, T.G. (1993) Psychiatric illness and chronic low-back pain. The mind and the spine — which goes first. Spine, 18(1): 66–71.

Rainville, J., Sobel, J., Hartigan, C. and Wright, A. (1997) The effect of compensation involvement of the reporting of pain and disability by patients referred for rehabilitation of chronic low back pain. Spine, 22(17): 2016–2024.

Robinson, J.P., Rondinelli, R.D., Scheer, S.J. and Weinstein, S.M. (1997) Industrial rehabilitation medicine. 1. Why is industrial rehabilitation medicine unique. Arch. Phys. Med. Rehabil., 78(Suppl.): S3–S9.

Rohling, M.L., Binder, L.M. and Langhinrichsen-Rohling, J. (1995) Money matters: A meta-analytic review of the association between financial compensation and the experience of treatment of chronic pain. Health Psychol., 14: 537–547.

Romano, J.M. and Turner, J.A. (1985) Chronic pain and depression: Does the evidence support a relationship. Psychol. Bull., 97: 18–34.

Roth, J.H., Richards, R.S. and Macleod, M.D. (1994) Endoscopic carpal tunnel release. Can. J. Surg., 37: 189–193.

Samwel, H., Slappendel, R., Crul, B.J. and Voerman, V.F. (2000) Psychological predictors of the effectiveness of radiofrequency lesioning of the cervical spinal dorsal ganglion (RF-DRG). Eur. J. Pain, 4(2): 149–155.

Sanderson, P.L., Todd, B., Holt, G.R. and Getty, C.J.M. (1995) Compensation, work status, and disability in low back pain patients. Spine, 20: 554–556.

Schumann, N., Zweiner, U. and Nebrick, A. (1988) Personality and quantified neuromuscular activity of the masticatory system in patients with temporomandibular joint dysfunction. J. Oral Rehabil., 15: 35–47.

Spengler, D., Bigos, S.J., Martin, N.Z., Zeh, J., Fisher, L. and Nachemson, A. (1986) Back injuries in industry: A retrospective study, I. Overview and cost analysis. Spine, 11: 241–245.

Spitzer, W.O. (1993) Low back pain in the workplace: Attainable benefits not attained. Br. J. Ind. Med., 50(5): 245–250.

Sternbach, R.A., Wolf, S.R., Murphy, R.W. and Akeson, W.H. (1973) Traits of pain patients: The low-back 'loser'. Psychosomatics, 14: 226–229.

Tan, V., Cheatle, M.D., Mackin, S., Moberg, P.J. and Esterhai, J.L.J. (1997) Goal setting as a predictor of return to work in a population of chronic musculoskeletal pain patients. Int. J. Neurosci., 92(3–4): 161–170.

Timmermans, G. and Sternbach, R.A. (1976) Human chronic

pain and personality: A canonical correlation analysis. Adv. Pain Res. Ther., 1: 307–310.

Tollison, C.D. (1993) Compensation status as a predictor of outcome in nonsurgically treated low back injury. South. Med. J., 86: 1206–1234.

Tota-Faucette, M.E., Gil, K.M., Williams, D.A., Keefe, F.J. and Goli, V. (1993) Predictors of response to pain management treatment. The role of family environment and changes in cognitive processes. Clin. J. Pain, 9(2): 115–123.

Turk, D.C. (1996) Biopsychosocial perspective on chronic pain. In: R.J. Gatchel and D.C. Turk (Eds.), Psychological Approaches to Pain Management: A Practitioner's Handbook. Guilford Publications, New York, NY, pp. 3–32.

Turk, D.C. and Flor, H. (1987) Pain greater than pain behaviors. The utility of the pain behavior construct. Pain, 31: 277–295.

Turk, D.C. and Kerns, R.D. (1983) Conceptual issues in the assessment of clinic pain. Int. J. Psychiatr. Med., 13: 15–26.

Turk, D. and Okifuji, A. (1998a) Directions in prescriptive chronic pain management based on diagnostic characteristics of the patient. APS Bull., 8: 5–11.

Turk, D.C. and Okifuji, A. (1998b) Treatment of chronic pain patients: Clinical outcomes, cost-effectiveness, and cost–benefits of multidisciplinary pain centers. Crit. Rev. Phys. Rehabil. Med., 10: 181–208.

Turk, D.C. and Rudy, T.E. (1987) Towards a comprehensive assessment of chronic pain patients. Behav. Res. Ther., 25: 237–249.

Turk, D.C. and Rudy, T.E. (1988) Toward an empirically derived taxonomy of chronic pain patients: Integration of psychological assessment data. J. Consult. Clin. Psychol., 56: 233–238.

Turner, J.A., LeResche, L., Von Korff, M. and Ehrlich, K. (1998) Back pain in primary care. Patient characteristics, content of initial visit, and short-term outcomes. Spine, 23(4): 463–469.

Vaccaro, A.R., Ring, D., Scuderi, G., Cohen, D.S. and Garfin, S.R. (1997) Predictors of outcome in patients with chronic back pain and low-grade spondylolisthesis. Spine, 22: 2030–2035.

Volinn, E., Van Koevering, D. and Loeser, J. (1991) Back sprain in industry: The role of socioeconomic factors in chronicity. Spine, 16(5): 542–548.

Von Korff, M., Deyo, R., Cherkin, D. and Barlow, W. (1993) Back pain in primary care: Outcomes of 1 year. Spine, 18: 855–862.

Von Korff, M., Gruman, J., Schaefer, J., Curry, S.J. and Wagner, E.H. (1997) Collaborative management of chronic illness. Ann. Intern. Med., 127: 1097–1102.

Waddell, G. and Main, C.J. (1984) Assessment of severity in low back disorders. Spine, 9: 204–208.

Watkins, K.W., Shifren, K., Park, D.C. and Morrell, R.W. (1999) Age, pain, and coping with rheumatoid arthritis. Pain, 82(3): 217–228.

Zautra, A.J. and Manne, S.L. (1992) Coping with rheumatoid arthritis: A review of a decade of research. Ann. Behav. Med., 14: 31–39.

New Avenues for the Prevention of Chronic Musculoskeletal Pain and Disability
Pain Research and Clinical Management, Vol. 12
Edited by S.J. Linton

Early assessment of psychological factors: the Örebro Screening Questionnaire for Pain

Katja Boersma * and Steven J. Linton

Department of Occupational and Environmental Medicine, Örebro University Hospital, S-701 85 Örebro, Sweden

Abstract: This chapter focuses on the use of a screening procedure to identify patients at risk for developing long-term musculoskeletal pain disability. It presents a description of the Örebro Screening Questionnaire for Pain. This self-administered instrument is targeted to be a tool for health-care professionals in making a judgment about the risk an individual with acute or sub-acute pain has for developing a chronic pain problem. In addition, it may be of value in identifying problem areas, discussing the problem with patients, and planning intervention strategies. The questionnaire focuses on yellow flags, i.e., the psychological risk factors identified. After a description of the instrument, some of the reported results are presented as well as an outline for how the questionnaire may be utilized clinically. The results of the reported studies demonstrate that the questionnaire is a clinically reliable and valid instrument that may have utility in the early identification of patients at risk for developing persistent pain problems. The instrument appears to be most helpful in predicting future functional problems as well as sick absenteeism. However, the predictive validity of the instrument for pain is low relative to the predictive validity for function or sick absenteeism. Taken together, the results suggest that the instrument could be of value in isolating patients in need of early interventions and in promoting the use of appropriate interventions for patients with psychological risk factors.

1. Introduction

The prevention of the development of persistent musculoskeletal pain would be greatly enhanced if only we could identify patients most in need at a very early point in time. This would allow us to concentrate vital, but restricted resources on those cases that might best benefit from the intervention. Moreover, it might help clinicians and researchers to target better the content of the intervention to the actual problems fueling the development. Preventive programs presuppose a crisp screening procedure to identify patients at risk of developing the problem.

As musculoskeletal pain is a frequent problem, often recurrent in nature, screening may be essential for the elaboration of a successful prevention program. Most people will suffer from spinal pain at some point and have recurrences (Crombie et al., 1999). However, only a small percentage (3–10%) are estimated to develop a long-term work absence after an acute bout of back pain (Reid et al., 1997). Moreover, these few patients consume enor-

* Correspondence to: K. Boersma, Department of Occupational and Environmental Medicine, Örebro University Hospital, S-701 85 Örebro, Sweden. E-mail: katja.boersma@orebroll.se

mous amounts of resources (Waddell, 1996, 1998; Nachemson and Jonsson, 2000). As a result, providing every patient with acute pain with a preventive intervention would be costly and raise logistic concerns. On the other hand, being able to effectively intervene for those patients who truly risk developing a persistent disability would offer a great opportunity for reducing suffering and costs. An important question is how screening might be achieved.

Research during the past decade has established a firm link between psychological factors and the development of a chronic pain problem (Turk, 1996, 1997; Waddell, 1998; Turk and Flor, 1999; Linton, 2000; Main and Spanswick, 2000; Vlaeyen and Linton, 2000). It seems, in fact, that psychosocial risk factors play a major role in the transition from acute pain to a chronic pain problem (Burton et al., 1995; Turk, 1997). These psychological factors have also been conceptualized as 'yellow flags', meaning that these factors may impede recovery (Kendall et al., 1997). In this view 'red flags' represent the rare but important biological risks factors that need immediate attention such as fractures, infections and tumors, while yellow flags represent psychosocial factors that may be barriers to recovery. Psychosocial factors then might represent key factors that could be utilized in screening (Gatchel et al., 1995; Linton, 2000).

Screening might be useful in several other respects. As stated above, screening may be beneficial in directing preventive interventions specifically to those individuals who need it the most. In addition, early screening might elucidate and direct attention to those psychosocial factors that are most pertinent. Finally, screening might complement primary care facilities that often are simply not equipped in or lack the time and resources for assessing psychosocial factors. Assessing the large number of identified psychosocial risk factors through an interview would, for instance, be time-consuming, especially considering the large number of individuals seeking care for musculoskeletal pain. Some health-care professionals may find it difficult to address delicate psychosocial issues such as depression or anxiety and lack skills in how these issues should be handled.

So, although there exists a large body of research on risk factors for development of chronic musculoskeletal pain, it is still a huge challenge for the health-care professional to put this knowledge into practice with respect to how to asses risk, to communicate and consequently treat.

In order to aid in the assessment of psychosocial factors as well as to communicate with patients and implement early intervention, the Örebro Musculoskeletal Pain Screening Questionnaire was developed and tested (Linton and Halldén, 1997, 1998). This questionnaire is a self-administered screening instrument for individuals with acute or sub-acute musculoskeletal pain, containing 25 questions and meant to be used by health-care professionals. The questionnaire is targeted to be a tool for the health-care professional in making a judgment of the risk an individual with acute or sub-acute pain has, in developing a chronic pain problem. In addition, it may be of value in identifying problem areas, discussing the problem with patients, and planning intervention strategies.

The aim of this chapter is to describe the use of the Örebro Screening Questionnaire in the early identification of patients at risk of developing a persistent pain problem. The questionnaire is currently being used in various settings and the results from some of the first studies are now available (Kendall, 1999; Hurley et al., 2000, 2001). We will describe the development of the questionnaire, present some of the reported results, as well as outline how the questionnaire may be utilized clinically.

2. Örebro Musculoskeletal Pain Screening Questionnaire

2.1. Constructing the questionnaire

The Örebro Screening Questionnaire was constructed with a number of criteria in mind. In order to be useful a screening questionnaire should utilize the most potent psychosocial risk factors. Second it should be a reliable and valid measure of the constructs employed. It should moreover have good predictive validity, that is, actually identify those who develop disability. Finally, the instrument should be practical to use in clinical settings. Thus, administration, scoring and interpretation should be relatively easy and fast.

After a review of the literature on psychological risk factors, a list of 98 possible variables was assembled. Of these, 67 were omitted because of a clear overlap. For the remaining 31 variables questions were located in other psychometrically sound instruments. Employing such items is believed to enhance reliability and validity.

The items included in the questionnaire are shown in Table I. After item analyses in pilot work, the number of items was reduced from 31 to 25. Six questions deal with background factors and 19 items deal with a variety of psychological factors. In order to give all items equal weight and to enhance clarity for patients, all items have a range from 0 to 10 points. For scoring purposes some items are inverted so that higher scores indicate higher levels of risk. Then the scores from the individual items are summed to form a total score. Since the background items (1 to 4) were not found to contribute statistically, they are not included in the calculation of the total score.

The properties of the Örebro Screening Questionnaire were subsequently tested.

2.2. Utility

In this section we will briefly summarize the results of some of the studies reporting results on the utility of the Örebro Screening Questionnaire. In the first study conducted with the instrument, the screening instrument was found to have satisfactory test–retest reliability (0.83) and validity in a study of 142 patients where outcome was sick absenteeism (Linton and Halldén, 1997, 1998). When using a cut-off score of 105 (the maximum score is 210), the specificity was found to be 0.75 and the sensitivity 0.88. This means that the chance of correctly classifying a person as 'healthy' with regard to no sick leave in the next 6 months was 75%. At that same cut-off point the chance of accurately classifying someone as at risk for future sick leave would be 88%. Kendall

(1999) tested the instrument on a population of more than a hundred acute-pain patients in New Zealand and found that a cut-off score of 105 was related to future disability. Hurley et al. (2000) investigated the instruments predictive ability with regard to return-to-work after physical therapy. They reported that a cut-off point of 112 correctly identified 80% of patients failing to return to work at the end of treatment (sensitivity), while at the same time 59% of those returning to work were identified (specificity).

Currently we are conducting a replication study that has included 107 patients seeking health care for acute or sub-acute spinal pain. The participants were recruited through primary health-care clinics and physiotherapy clinics in middle Sweden. Volunteers were first asked to complete the questionnaire at the first visit. Responses were mailed to the research team and were consequently blind to the clinicians. Outcome was assessed 6 months later via a postal questionnaire pertaining accumulated sick absenteeism, level of functioning, and pain.

The average age of the participants was 41 years (range 22–66), 48% were female and 93% were born in Sweden. The participants reported multiple pain sites (53% had lower back pain, 44% shoulder pain, and 44% neck pain). The average scores and standard deviations for the individual items are shown in Table II.

Univariate analyses showed good test–retest (0.80) and most questions in the screening questionnaire had a significant relation with sick leave, level of function, and pain intensity.

Multivariate analyses showed that, after a two-step discriminant analysis, three items correctly classified 68.3% of the people in three classes of sick absenteeism (0 days, 1–30 days and <30 days). The three significant items were (1) gender, (2) sick leave, and (3) difficulties in doing shopping. Table III shows that the specificity (classifying a healthy person as healthy) was 71%, whereas the sensitivity (the correct classification of those who will be sick listed from work) was 58% for the 1–30-days group and 72% for the <30-days group.

Since functional disability is a key variable in the development of a persistent pain problem as well,

TABLE I

Screening questionnaire for problematic back pain

Question			Variable name
1.	What year were you born?	Fill in blank	Age
2.	Are you	Male/Female	Gender
3.	What is your current employment status?	Categories	Employed
4.	Are you born in Sweden?	Yes/No	Nationality
5.	Where do you have pain?	Categories	Pain site
6.	How many days of work have you missed (sick leave) because of pain during the past 12 months?	Categories	Sick leave
7.	How many weeks have you suffered from your current pain problem?	Categories	Duration
8.	Is your work heavy or monotonous?	0–10	Heavy work
9.	How would you rate the pain you have had during the past week?	0–10	Current pain
10.	In the past 3 months, on average, how intense was your pain?	0–10	Average pain
11.	How often would you say that you have experienced pain episodes, on average, during the past 3 months?	0–10	Frequency
12.	Based on all things you do to cope or deal with your pain, on an average day, how much are you able to decrease it?	0–10	Coping
13.	How tense or anxious have you felt in the past week?	0–10	Stress
14.	How much have you been bothered by feeling depressed in the past week?	0–10	Depression
15.	In your view, how large is the risk that your current pain may become persistent (may not go away)?	0–10	Risk chronic
16.	In your estimation, what are the chances that you will be working in 6 months?	0–10	Chance working
17.	If you take into consideration your work routines, management, salary, promotion possibilities, and work mates, how satisfied are you with your job?	0–10	Job satisfaction
18.	Physical activity makes my pain worse.	0–10	Belief: increase
19.	An increase in pain is an indication that I should stop what I am doing until the pain decreases.	0–10	Belief: stop
20.	I should not do my normal work with my present pain.	0–10	Belief: not work
21.	I can do light work for an hour.	0–10	Light work
22.	I can walk for an hour.	0–10	Walk
23.	I can do ordinary household chores.	0–10	Household work
24.	I can do the weekly shopping.	0–10	Shopping
25.	I can sleep at night.	0–10	Sleep

the predictive power of the questionnaire was also determined with regard to two classes of functioning: 'functional recovery' versus 'functional disability'. Multivariate analyses isolated four significant items: (1) sleep, (2) sick leave, (3) pain site, and (4) chance working. This solution correctly classified 81% of the patients (sensitivity = 79%; specificity = 83%), which is, given an even distribution, higher than the random level of 50%.

To increase validity and utility of the Örebro Screening Questionnaire, employing a total score solution for determining risk and cut-off scores has been suggested. Therefore, a total score analysis was conducted for the three categories of sick leave (0 days, 1–30 days, >30 days of sick leave). Total score distributions were then generated for each group, to compare and evaluate the overall differences, and possible cut-off points.

For the whole sample, the mean total score was 95, the range 32–166, and the standard deviation 28. The three groups differed significantly in their total score ($p < 0.001$). Post hoc tests indicated that the total score for the group with no sick leave (0 days, mean score 84) was significantly different from both the 1–30-days group (mean score 105) and the >30-days group (mean score 116).

TABLE II

Average scores and standard deviations for each item

Question		Mean [a]	S.D.
1.	What year were you born?	41.1	range 22–66
2.	Are you	48% F	
3.	What is your current employment status?	84% working	
4.	Are you born in Sweden?	93% born in Sweden	
5.	Where do you have pain?	56% lower back, 44% neck, 44% shoulder	
6.	How many days of work have you missed (sick leave) because of pain during the past 12 months?	49% 0 days	
7.	How many weeks have you suffered from your current pain problem?	43% > 24 weeks	
8.	Is your work heavy or monotonous?	5.1	3.0
9.	How would you rate the pain you have had during the past week?	6.2	2.1
10.	In the past 3 months, on average, how intense was your pain?	5.1	2.2
11.	How often would you say that you have experienced pain episodes, on average, during the past 3 months?	6.1	2.9
12.	Based on all things you do to cope or deal with your pain, on an average day, how much are you able to decrease it?	5.0	2.3
13.	How tense or anxious have you felt in the past week?	5.0	3.0
14.	How much have you been bothered by feeling depressed in the past week?	3.4	3.0
15.	In your view, how large is the risk that your current pain may become persistent (may not go away)?	6.3	2.9
16.	In your estimation, what are the chances that you will be working in 6 months?	0.9	1.6
17.	If you take into consideration your work routines, management, salary, promotion possibilities, and work mates, how satisfied are you with your job?	2.9	2.6
18.	Physical activity makes my pain worse.	6.1	3.4
19.	An increase in pain is an indication that I should stop what I am doing until the pain decreases.	6.9	2.9
20.	I should not do my normal work with my present pain.	5.1	3.4
21.	I can do light work for an hour.	3.3	2.9
22.	I can walk for an hour.	3.2	3.3
23.	I can do ordinary household chores.	3.5	2.9
24.	I can do the weekly shopping.	3.6	3.4
25.	I can sleep at night.	4.0	2.9

[a] High scores indicate increased risk. S.D. = standard deviation.

Table IV shows the results of different cut-off points for the accuracy to predict sick leave. It provides information concerning the numbers of 'hits' and 'misses' different cut-off points would entail. A cut-off point of 100 for example, correctly identifies (hits) 76% of those persons sick listed for more than 30 days. It would incorrectly identify (miss) 24% as a false positive (those persons identified as at risk when in fact they did not develop a problem). On the other hand, a cut-off point of 100 correctly identifies 74% of those persons who do not go on sick leave, meaning that 26% would be false negatives (those persons identified as not at risk when in fact they did develop sick leave).

To be able to compare the questionnaire's potential as a screening instrument over more than one main outcome, a total score analysis of functional ability was conducted as well. Participants were divided into 'recovered' and 'not recovered' classes. Total score distributions were generated for each group, to compare and evaluate the overall differences, and possible cut-off points.

TABLE III

Discriminant analyses of sick leave (% correctly classified)

Sick leave	Recovered	1–30 days	>30 days
Recovered	**71%**	19%	10%
1–30 days	17%	**58%**	25%
>30 days	17%	11%	**72%**

Correctly classified = 68.3%; the three significant items were (1) gender, (2) sick leave, and (3) difficulties in doing shopping.

TABLE IV

Examples of the effect of different cut-off scores on the prediction of sick listing

Cut-off score	0 days (specificity)	1–30 days (sensitivity)	>30 days
90	65%	67%	89%
100	74%	45%	76%
105	81%	40%	67%
110	86%	38%	63%
120	94%	28%	36%

TABLE V

Examples of the effect of different cut-off scores on the prediction of functional ability

Cut-off score	Recovered (specificity)	Not recovered (sensitivity)
80	63%	88%
90	79%	74%
100	87%	54%
105	95%	49%
110	97%	48%

With regard to functional ability, the two groups differed significantly in their total score (mean score 'recovered' group = 74, mean score 'not recovered' group = 107; $p < 0.001$). Table V shows the results of different cut-off points.

A cut-off point of, for example, 90, correctly identifies (hits) 74% of those persons who do not recover. It would incorrectly identify (miss) 26% as false positives. At the same time, a cut-off point of 90 correctly identifies 79% of those persons who do recover, meaning that 21% would be false negatives.

A cut-off score of 100 would increase the correct classification of those who recover to 87%. The percentage of 'hits' for those persons who do not recover though, would decrease to 54%.

As the tables with the cut-off scores for sick leave and functional disability show, the lower the cut-off score, the higher the percentages of those 'sick listed' or 'not recovered' that are classified correctly. At the same time, the percentage 'recovered' that is classified correctly decreases. Higher cut-off points increase the percentage of correctly identified people with a good prognosis, but at the same time decreases the percentage identified with a poorer prognosis. Depending on the objectives of the user of the instrument, the one or the other may be of more importance.

2.3. Conclusions

The results show that the total score of the screening questionnaire is related to future sick leave and functional ability; the higher the score, the higher the risk for long-term sick leave and the development of a chronic functional problem. The cut-off scores are slightly lower than in former studies but the questionnaire still predicts well between those recovering and those not recovering.

The cut-off scores for a 'best prediction' of chronic problems vary slightly between the different studies conducted with the questionnaire. In the former study (Linton and Halldén, 1998) as well as in the study done by Kendall (1999) a cut-off score of 105 was found to give the best prediction. In the study of Hurley et al. (2000), a cut-off score of 112 correctly classified 80% of those off-work after treatment. A cut-off score of 105 worked nearly as well (80% correctly classified as off-work) but had a somewhat lower specificity (52% correctly classified as returning to work). In the present study the cut-off score ranges from 90 to 105 depending on the outcome criteria that were used and the objective of the researcher. If, for example, the objective is to isolate only those patients who are extremely likely to have a poor prognosis, the cut-off point goes up, while if the objective is not to miss anyone likely to develop problems, the cut-off point is lowered. In other words, the cut-off point in part depends on the need of the health-care professional.

Therefore, caution is warranted in applying the cut-off points strictly and without regard to population, setting and purpose. The variations in cut-off scores also underline the importance examining not only the total score but the individual items as well. The screening instrument can be a useful diagnostic aid that adds information and provides a guideline for risk assessment, as well as it can be a tool for communication with the patient. Using the questionnaire as a golden standard with regard to cut-off scores would be unwise since, although the prediction is far better than chance, it is also far from being perfect.

3. Practical use with patients

A number of important issues arise concerning the implementation of the screening questionnaire in clinical practice. In this section we address some of the most common practical aspects of employing this instrument.

3.1. Who, when, and where

The screening questionnaire is targeted to individuals seeking care with acute, sub-acute or recurrent musculoskeletal pain. It can be used in, for example, primary health-care settings and physiotherapy clinics.

3.2. Time investment

The questionnaire is designed to be a self-administered instrument and requires basic language skills. Filling out the instrument should normally take between 5 and 10 min, and could for example take place while waiting to see the health-care professional. There are 21 items to be scored which takes 2–3 min for the trained observer. With training the feedback session can take as little as 5 min for patients with 'at risk' scores, and less for those with low risk scores.

3.3. Targeting problems by using the total score

3.3.1. Adjusting the cut-off score to the goal of the health-care professional

The optimal cut-off score is dependent on the population under study and the goal of the health-care professional. Further, employing a cut-off score always entails so-called 'false positives' and 'false negatives'. Increasing the cut-off level, for example, reduces one's chance of incorrectly identifying persons as 'at risk' ('false positives'), while at the same time increasing the percentage of people 'at risk' that is missed ('false negatives'). So, is the goal not to miss anyone who is 'at risk', the cut-off score should be lowered. The cut-off score should be heightened when, for example, interventions are very expensive and one does not want to include anyone who is not truly 'at risk'.

3.3.2. Adjusting the cut-off score to the population

With the slightly different cut-off scores in the different studies in mind (with intermediate cut-off scores ranging from 90 to 112 when investigating the prediction of sick leave in the different studies), one should consider the sort of population when determining relevant cut-off scores, especially with scores falling within this range. Scores over and under this range indicate respectively a high and a low risk of future sick listing.

3.4. Targeting problems by evaluating individual items

When the questionnaire is examined on an item basis, one can isolate areas of special importance for risk judgment, as well as topics that can be taken up in an interview. In this way, the questionnaire can aid as a tool of communication between patient and professional. Areas of concern such as a high score on the fear–avoidance items or a high score on the depression item can be identified. They can be followed up with appropriate action such as further assessment in the case of a suspected depression, or education and the promotion of active self-care skills in the case of fear avoidance. This can even take place when the low total score indicates a low risk. The patient can have one or two items with a 'high risk' rating such as on job satisfaction and on heavy or monotonous work. Although the overall risk is low, one might want to discuss these items, as they could be relevant for further problems.

3.5. Providing feedback and planning intervention

Probably one of the most important aspects of screening is providing the patient with appropriate feedback. Most people are very curious as to what the result of their effort is, when asked to fill out a questionnaire. Thereby, it is likely that people are somewhat anxious, particularly when they are insecure about the extent of their pain problem. A clear explanation and careful wording can counteract this insecurity and can motivate the patients in an active participation in handling their pain problem.

When communicating the concept 'risk' careful choice of wording is especially important. The word 'risk' in itself is often too difficult to grasp and has a dichotomous connotation as in 'no risk, risk', 'normal, abnormal', or 'positive, negative'. Having a higher risk means no more than having a similar score as previous people who have developed a problem. The total score and scrutiny of the individual items should serve as a starting point for further assessment or further treatment planning. Not in the least can it function as an educational tool to promote active self-help and a broad view on the problem.

3.6. Recapitulation

The Örebro Screening Questionnaire can serve as an aid in screening patients so that resources may be utilized effectively. The questionnaire is a complement to usual medical examinations that may help clinicians delve into psychosocial aspects in an effective manner. It introduces the topic, shows a holistic approach, may be educative, and may be used to enhance commitment and active self-help. It can help to identify and communicate important and sensitive issues.

References

Burton, A.K., Tillotson, K.M., Main, C.J. and Hollis, S. (1995) Psychosocial predictors of outcome in acute and subchronic low back trouble. Spine, 20(6): 722–728.

Crombie, I.K., Croft, P.R., Linton, S.J., LeResche, L. and Von Korff, M. (1999) Epidemiology of Pain. IASP Press, Seattle, WA.

Gatchel, R.J., Polatin, P.B. and Kinney, R.K. (1995) Predicting outcome of chronic back pain using clinical predictors of psychopathology: a prospective analysis. Health Psychol., 14(5): 415–420.

Hurley, D., Dusoir, T., McDonough, S., Moore, A., Linton, S.J. and Baxter, G. (2000) Biopsychosocial screening questionnaire for patients with low back pain: preliminary report of utility in physiotherapy practice in Northern Ireland. Clin. J. Pain, 16(3): 214–228.

Hurley, D.A., Dusoir, T.E., McDonough, S.M., Moore, A.P. and Baxter, G.D. (2001) How effective is the Acute Low Back Pain Screening Questionnaire for predicting 1-year follow-up in patients with low back pain? Clin. J. Pain, 17: 256–263.

Kendall, N. (1999) Screening and early interventions: the New Zealand experience. Paper presented at the International Association for the Study of Pain, Vienna.

Kendall, N.A.S., Linton, S.J. and Main, C.J. (1997) Guide to assessing psychosocial yellow flags in acute low back pain: risk factors for long-term disability and work loss. Accident Rehabilitation and Compensation Insurance Corporation of New Zealand and the National Health Committee, Wellington.

Linton, S.J. (2000) A review of psychological risk factors in back and neck pain. Spine, 25(9): 1148–1156.

Linton, S.J. and Halldén, K. (1997) Risk factors and the natural course of acute and recurrent musculoskeletal pain: developing a screening instrument. In: T.S. Jensen, J.A. Turner and Z. Wiesenfeld-Hallin (Eds.), Proceedings of the 8th World Congress on Pain: Progress in Pain Research and Management. IASP Press, Seattle, WA, pp. 527–536.

Linton, S.J. and Halldén, K. (1998) Can we screen for problematic back pain? A screening questionnaire for predicting outcome in acute and subacute back pain. Clin. J. Pain, 14(3): 209–215.

Main, C.J. and Spanswick, C.C. (2000) Pain Management: An Interdisciplinary Approach. Churchill Livingstone, Edinburgh.

Nachemson, A. and Jonsson, E. (Eds.) (2000) Neck and Back Pain: The Scientific Evidence of Causes, Diagnosis, and Treatment. Lippincott Williams and Wilkins, Philadelphia, PA.

Reid, S., Haugh, L.D., Hazard, R.G. and Tripathi, M. (1997) Occupational low back pain: recovery curves and factors associated with disability. J. Occup. Rehabil., 7(1): 1–14.

Turk, D.C. (1996) Biopsychosocial perspective on chronic pain. In: R.J. Gatchel and D.C. Turk (Eds.), Psychological Approaches to Pain Management: A Practitioner's Handbook. Guilford Press, New York, NY, 1st ed., pp. 3–32.

Turk, D.C. (1997) The role of demographic and psychosocial factors in transition from acute to chronic pain. In: T.S. Jensen, J.A. Turner and Z. Wiesenfeld-Hallin (Eds.), Proceedings of the 8th World Congress on Pain, Progress in Pain Research and Management. IASP Press, Seattle, WA, pp. 185–213.

Turk, D.C. and Flor, H. (1999) Chronic pain: a biobehavioral perspective. In: R.J. Gatchel and D.C. Turk (Eds.), Psychosocial Factors in Pain: Critical Perspectives. Guilford Press, New York, NY, pp. 18–34.

Vlaeyen, J.W.S. and Linton, S.J. (2000) Fear-avoidance and its consequences in chronic musculoskeletal pain: a state of the art. Pain, 85: 317–332.

Waddell, G. (1996) Low back pain: A twentieth century health care enigma. Spine, 21(24): 2820–2825.

Waddell, G. (1998) The Back Pain Revolution. Churchill Livingstone, Edinburgh.

New Avenues for the Prevention of Chronic Musculoskeletal Pain and Disability
Pain Research and Clinical Management, Vol. 12
Edited by S.J. Linton

CHAPTER 14

Secondary prevention and the workplace [1]

William S. Shaw [1,*], Michael Feuerstein [2,3] and Grant D. Huang [2]

[1] *Liberty Mutual Center for Disability Research, 71 Frankland Road, Hopkinton, MA 01748, USA*
[2] *Department of Medical and Clinical Psychology and Department of Preventive Medicine and Biometrics, Uniformed Services University of the Health Sciences, 4301 Jones Bridge Road, Bethesda, MD 20814, USA*
[3] *Georgetown University Medical Center, Washington, DC 20057, USA*

Abstract: Secondary preventive interventions in the workplace have been suggested to reduce the impact of work-related musculoskeletal disorders. The purpose of this chapter is to review evidence concerning such programs and recommend future directions for program development and research. Secondary prevention programs may entail two distinct aspects. First, such programs may focus on the early detection and treatment of mild to moderate symptoms. Second, accommodating temporary functional limitations may aid recovery and reduce the likelihood of recurrence. From this framework, risk factors are reviewed that might direct intervention goals. Several interventions are examined that attempt to prevent musculoskeletal pain at the workplace such as those aimed at the physical work environment, modified duty, educational and exercise approaches, case management, and programs for supervisors. As a whole the evidence shows that there is considerable potential for these approaches to reduce the disability and recurrence associated with work-related musculoskeletal pain. Efforts to reduce ergonomic risk factors, to enhance education or fitness as well as to influence case managers and supervisors provide opportunities for effective secondary prevention. The themes of integrating care and facilitating communication among workers, health-care providers and the workplace emerge as particularly salient. Future research will need to identify the most efficient methods in controlled outcome studies.

1. Introduction

High medical costs and prolonged disability for a subset of workers with musculoskeletal disorders have led employers and health-care providers to seek innovative methods for identifying and modifying factors that contribute to musculoskeletal pain and disability. A growing body of evidence linking physical work to rates of musculoskeletal injuries (National Research Council, 1998; National Research Council and Institute of Medicine, 2001) has supported the need to address ergonomic stressors to reduce workplace disability. Slow, steady progress has been made by many industries to reduce workplace ergonomic risk factors. However, these primary prevention efforts have not substantially curbed the problem. Sprains, strains, muscle tears, carpal tunnel syndrome, and tendonitis continue to account

---

[1] The opinions or assertions contained herein are the private ones of the authors and are not to be construed as official views of the Department of Defense or the Uniformed Services University of the Health Sciences.
* Correspondence to: W.S. Shaw, Liberty Mutual Center for Disability Research, 71 Frankland Road, Hopkinton, MA 01748, USA. E-mail: william.shaw@libertymutual.com

for half of all lost-time non-fatal work injuries (Bureau of Labor Statistics, 2001). *Secondary prevention*, that strives to reduce the chronicity, duration, or recurrence of pain and onset of disability represents a feasible adjunct to primary prevention efforts for reducing this leading source of disability. Secondary prevention can be offered to fewer individuals and potentially with greater effect, thus providing a higher cost-to-benefit ratio. In this chapter, the authors review epidemiological evidence and describe workplace interventions in support of a secondary prevention approach to work-related musculoskeletal disorders.

2. Defining secondary prevention for musculoskeletal disorders

Secondary prevention can include any effort designed to reduce the likelihood that a given disorder will develop or advance once early signs or symptoms are detected. These efforts contrast with those of *primary prevention*, that reduce risks for disease before any symptoms are reported and *tertiary prevention*, that seeks to reduce the impacts of a diagnosed condition on quality of life and daily living activities. In the case of musculoskeletal disorders, recurrent and episodic symptoms can make the goals of secondary prevention difficult to define. Given that an individual reports symptoms consistent with a musculoskeletal disorder, should secondary prevention efforts focus on reducing risks for symptom chronicity, symptom recurrence, symptom-related disability, or all of these outcomes? Along a continuum of possible outcomes from minor aches and pains at one extreme to chronic, disabling conditions on the other, where should the imaginary line in the sand be drawn to discriminate primary from secondary prevention? Is it conceivable that signs of impending muscle fatigue could be detected even before symptoms occur to facilitate primary prevention? Such questions have important implications for the types of treatment chosen and resources allocated for prevention efforts. These questions have led to a highly variable list of potential risk factors, interventions, and outcome measures to reduce musculoskeletal disability across studies. For the purposes of this chapter, secondary prevention will be defined as those interventions that occur in the acute stage of illness after the onset of symptoms but before a long-term disability has developed (i.e., having less than 3 months lost work time [Dasinger et al., 1999]).

For musculoskeletal disorders, interventions that best fit our definition for secondary prevention are those that adopt one of three possible intervention strategies. The first is to promote the early detection and treatment of mild to moderate symptoms (by either the workplace, clinic, or public at large), especially among those with risk factors for chronic pain or prolonged disability. A second strategy is to reduce or accommodate functional limitations to reduce the disabling effects of pain and symptoms once they occur (e.g., by providing problem-solving strategies or job accommodations). A third form of secondary prevention is to reduce the likelihood of symptom recurrence once an acute episode of pain has subsided. All three of these outcome strategies can potentially be achieved as workplace interventions, although choice of strategy may depend on occupational and organizational characteristics.

What are the scope and nature of workplace secondary prevention efforts for musculoskeletal disorders? Fig. 1 illustrates a conceptual framework linking risk factor domains, goals of secondary prevention, and some examples of specific workplace strategies. This framework combines evidence from epidemiological studies, models of job stress, and models of ergonomic/biomechanical influences. Three general risk factor domains can be identified for work-related musculoskeletal disorders: (1) ergonomic and biomechanical factors, (2) work organization and psychosocial factors, and (3) individual psychosocial and health behavior factors. Workplace strategies to reduce ergonomic exposures among symptomatic workers typically include engineering controls, administrative controls, modified duty, and physical conditioning (Cohen et al., 1997). Workplace strategies to reduce organizational barriers include early reporting, integrated case management, facilitated return to work, and supervisor training.

Risk Factor Domain Secondary Prevention Workplace Strategies

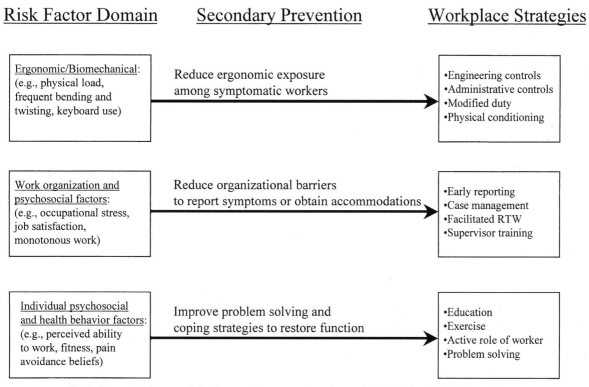

Fig. 1. Conceptual framework for the secondary prevention of musculoskeletal disorders in the workplace.

Workplace strategies to improve individual coping efforts include education, exercise, increasing the role of the worker in recovery and reintegration, and problem-solving skills training. Within the first two risk factor domains (ergonomic exposures and work organization), strategies for secondary prevention resemble those of primary prevention but are provided only for those reporting symptoms.

Research and development of disease prevention has traditionally followed a public health approach that includes the programmatic stages of *surveillance, risk identification, intervention, outcomes assessment,* and *cost/benefit evaluation*. While an extensive discussion of these components is beyond the scope of this chapter, a cursory description will provide a framework for the review of interventions that follows. *Surveillance* in the occupational environment includes continuous monitoring of both hazardous exposures and health outcomes to determine what and where problems exist, the trends of identified problems, who is at greatest risk, and when

intervention should be initiated. Attention to occupational outcomes in the surveillance of diseases is consistent with the World Health Organization's inclusion of social impacts in their conceptualization of health status (World Health Organization, 1948). Surveillance also provides a baseline for assessing the effectiveness of future interventions. *Risk identification* is accomplished through studies (both case control and cohort) that can indicate links between exposures and health outcomes and the magnitude of such associations. Once risk factors are identified, *interventions* can be subsequently developed to reduce the highest risk exposures. Their effects are measured through on-going workplace surveillance and compared in the *outcomes assessment* stage to determine their efficacy and to guide decision-making processes. Decision-making may also depend on the feasibility of intervention given limited resources. This is included in the *cost/benefit evaluation* stage, when the comparative worth of alternatives are based on net gains in improved worker/workplace health.

TABLE I

A comparison of primary and secondary prevention for work-related musculoskeletal disorders using a public health model of research and development

Stages of research and development	Comparison	
	Primary prevention	Secondary prevention
(1) Surveillance	• Develop pain- and injury-reporting methods • Assess industry prevalence rates	• Assess duration of disorder • Assess course of symptoms • Assess other impacts of pain and injury
(2) Risk identification	• Identify risk factors for pain onset	• Identify risk factors for chronicity or disability • Identify prognostic factors for poor treatment outcome
(3) Intervention	• Target all workers • Focus on reducing prevalence	• Target symptomatic workers only • Focus on disability prevention
(4) Outcomes assessment	• Evaluate interventions based on reduced rates of prevalence	• Evaluate interventions based on reduced costs or duration
(5) Benefit/cost evaluation	• Benefit/cost may be low due to high cost of large-scale interventions	• Benefit/cost improved by targeting symptomatic, at-risk workers

A comparison of these five programmatic stages for primary and secondary prevention of work-related musculoskeletal disorders is shown in Table I. Surveillance, in terms of secondary prevention, involves assessment of the impacts of injury and illness (e.g., chronic symptoms or lost workdays) in addition to incidence and prevalence. Risk factors for secondary prevention are those associated with poor prognosis, disability or chronicity. The cost/benefit ratio of secondary prevention may be improved (versus primary prevention) because interventions can target symptomatic workers only and focus on specific risk factors that contribute to disability.

Although existing studies of workplace interventions for secondary prevention of musculoskeletal disorders have been promising, this area is still in its formative stages. There are very few high-quality randomized, controlled trials on which to base conclusions at this time. Systematic analysis of ergonomic, organizational, and psychosocial interventions in the workplace and combined, integrated approaches are needed. Although there is substantial evidence that employers reporting generally more attention to workplace health and disability experience lower disability costs (Habeck et al., 1998a,b;

Salkever et al., 2000), few research studies have developed and evaluated specific secondary prevention strategies in the workplace for musculoskeletal pain and disability.

3. Justification for secondary prevention

One reason for increased efforts in secondary prevention of musculoskeletal disorders relates to the failure of primary prevention to substantially reduce prevalence rates. In addition, secondary prevention may reduce variability in course of disability and improve cost/benefit compared with primary prevention. A focus on secondary prevention, however, does not imply that primary prevention efforts should be abandoned. While primary prevention can strive to reduce the onset of new musculoskeletal disorders, secondary prevention can simultaneously focus on limiting their functional impacts, symptom progression, or recurrence in those with symptoms and/or disability. The most effective workplace programs may involve a combination of primary prevention efforts (for all workers) and secondary prevention efforts (for those experiencing symptoms).

Musculoskeletal pain and discomfort is extremely common among working-age adults world-wide; for example, lifetime prevalence rates for low back pain are estimated to be 60–80% (Frymoyer, 1988). Each year, 400,000 working adults in the U.S. experience a low back pain episode that can be attributed to physical demands of work (Silverstein et al., 1997). These prevalence rates have been relatively robust across time, geographical regions, and across many sociodemographic strata (Jin et al., 2000). Even if primary prevention efforts could significantly reduce the frequency of new cases, it is doubtful that musculoskeletal disorders could ever be effectively eradicated. Therefore, secondary prevention seems a prudent investment of intervention research and resources.

A second rationale for secondary prevention is that considerable variation exists in the course of musculoskeletal pain and disability. Lost work time and workers' compensation costs vary substantially among workers with these disorders (Webster and Snook, 1994; Hashemi et al., 1998a,b). Among companies operating within the same regions and industries, ten-fold differences in the rates of workers' compensation disability have been reported (Habeck et al., 1991). This suggests that non-medical factors, including workplace characteristics, may contribute to prolonged pain and disability among workers with musculoskeletal disorders. By targeting secondary prevention efforts to treat and restore function among potential high-risk cases early, it is theoretically possible to prevent unnecessary disability and tailor secondary prevention strategies from prognostic information. This would focus attention only on those cases likely to require intervention (Burton and Tillotson, 1991; Tousignant et al., 2000), thus potentially reducing unnecessary diagnostic and treatment modalities for low risk cases.

A third rationale for secondary prevention programs is cost. Primary prevention may require global changes in the workplace with significant budgetary allocations up front. A comparison of primary prevention risk factors identified by our group for back and upper extremities is shown in Fig. 2. In contrast, accommodating individual workers who report discomfort may be more affordable and with more significant gains per dollar spent. Employers that provide individual accommodations for workers with low back pain report that 50% of accommodations involve no cost, and another 30% cost less than $500 (Wiesel et al., 1985).

4. Surveillance in medical and disability databases

Surveillance of musculoskeletal pain and disability has helped to describe overall prevalence rates, to identify high-risk occupations or work activities, to identify specific problematic diagnoses, and to provide a basis for determining treatment effectiveness. The indemnification of lost work time by workers' compensation systems in the U.S. has provided a convenient opportunity to access both medical data (symptoms, treatment, etc.) and functional outcome data (lost days due to disability) in the same administrative databases (e.g., Webster and Snook, 1994; Feuerstein et al., 1998). Other sources of data have been from clinical records (e.g., chart review), from patient self-report surveys, or from employer records of reported illnesses and work absences (e.g., OSHA 200/300 logs).

Since 1990, prevalence of work-related low back disorders has remained relatively constant in the U.S., while disability costs have shown some decrease (Hashemi et al., 1998a). Burgeoning claim rates for work-related upper-extremity disorders in the 1980s (and concomitant disability costs) led to improved surveillance methods for tracking the prevalence of these disorders in the 1990s (Halperin and Ordin, 1996). In 1994, total costs associated with health-care costs and indemnity payments for work-related upper-extremity cumulative trauma disorders were estimated to be $563 million based on the claims costs of a large U.S. insurer (Webster and Snook, 1994). Industries involving heavy physical loads and manual materials handling (e.g., warehousing and distribution, commercial deliveries) report the highest rates of low back disorders (National Research Council and Institute of Medicine,

Back

SYMPTOMS

Upper Extremities

Huang & Feuerstein (2002)
<u>n</u> = 289 U.S. Marines in high risk jobs
<u>Symptoms since current job</u>
Age: 1.09 (1.02 – 1.16)
Family conflict: 1.30 (1.03 – 1.64)
Time pressure (3 – 15): 1.18 (1.00 – 1.38)
Interpersonal demands (1 – 7): 0.73 (0.54 – 1.00)

Huang & Feuerstein (2002)
<u>n</u> = 289 U.S. Marines in high risk jobs
<u>Symptoms since current job</u>
Family conflict: 1.27 (1.04 – 1.55)
Ergonomic exposure (0 – 152): 1.03 (1.00 – 1.05)
Time pressure (3 – 15): 1.16 (1.00 – 1.34)

Huang & Feuerstein (2002)
<u>n</u> = 289 U.S. Marines in high risk jobs
<u>Concurrent back & UE symptoms since current job</u>
Age: 1.13 (1.07 – 1.20)
Ergonomic exposure (0 – 152): 1.04 (1.01 – 1.06)
Interpersonal demands (1 – 7): 1.56 (1.05 – 2.33)
Skill discretion (10 – 50): 1.09 (1.02 – 1.15)
Cognitive demands (5-25): 1.20 (1.04 – 1.39)
Cognitive uncertainty (5-25): 1.22 (1.05 – 1.43)

Huang et al. (2002)
<u>n</u> = 289 U.S. Marines in high risk jobs
<u>Symptoms since current job</u>
↑ Ergonomic Exposure & ↑ Time Pressure: 2.61 (1.39 – 4.91)

Huang et al. (2002)
<u>n</u> = 289 U.S. Marines in high risk jobs
<u>Symptoms since current job</u>
↑ Ergonomic Exposure & ↑ Time Pressure: 2.90 (1.49 – 5.66)

Huang et al. (2002)
<u>n</u> = 289 U.S. Marines in high risk jobs
<u>Concurrent back & UE symptoms since current job</u>
↑ Ergonomic Exposure & ↑ Cognitive Demands: 2.25 (1.23 – 4.09)
↑ Ergonomic Exposure & ↓ Participatory Management: 2.50 (1.30 – 4.81)
↑ Ergonomic Exposure & ↑ Time Pressure: 2.21 (1.19 – 4.10)
↑ Ergonomic Exposure & ↑ Perceived Responsibility: 2.15 (1.14 – 4.06)
↑ Ergonomic Exposure & ↑ Cognitive Uncertainty: 2.08 (1.16 – 3.75)
↑ Ergonomic Exposure & ↑ Interpersonal Demands: 2.44 (1.35 – 4.41)

Feuerstein et al. (2002b)
<u>n</u> = 282 workers from community
<u>Symptomatic case status</u>
% time spent at VDU: 1.03 (1.01 – 1.05)
Job stress (0 – 20): 0.83 (0.72 – 0.97)
Workstyle: 1.27 (1.08 – 1.51)

Feuerstein et al. , 1997
<u>n</u> = 1398 sign language interpreters
<u>Pain intensity</u>
Work in painful way to assure high quality
Fear of developing pain at work
Move hands as fast as can
Years interpreting
Unpleasant physical conditions at work
Perceived effects on consumer
Sole contact for service
(Model R^2 = 0.34)
<u>Muscle tension</u>
Fear of developing pain at work
Work in painful way to assure high quality
Forceful/jerky moves
Perceived exertion
Constant pressure
Wrist deviate from neutral
(Model R^2 = 0.32)

Haufler et al., 2000
<u>n</u> = 124 female office workers

<u>Pain during work</u>	<u>Pain during work week</u>
Job stress	Work demands
Work support	Job stress
Workstyle	Workstyle
(Model R^2 = 0.41)	Work support
	(Model R^2 = 0.41)

Note: Figures represent odds ratios (95% confidence intervals)
unless otherwise specified

Fig. 2. Targets for primary prevention of musculoskeletal disorders.

2001); however, work-related low back pain occurs in nearly every industry and occupation. Industries reporting the highest prevalence of upper-extremity disorders are meat packing, frozen foods, fish processing, carpentry, and logging operations (Falck and Arnio, 1983; Chiang et al., 1990, 1993; Ashbury, 1995).

Surveillance has also been useful to identify specific types of musculoskeletal disorders that result in greater functional limitation and disability. For example, nerve entrapment disorders (i.e., carpal tunnel syndrome) have been associated with longer periods of disability (Feuerstein et al., 1998) and more difficulty returning to modified duty (Feuerstein et al., 2002a). This type of surveillance should become more helpful as methods for classifying and rating the severity of upper-extremity disorders become more standardized (Katz et al., 2000). For the majority of low back pain, diagnostic categories have had limited ability to predict disability outcomes except for a small minority of cases with a specifically identified organic etiology. These have been associated with a slower recovery than cases of nonspecific low back pain (Shinohara et al., 1998).

Another important aspect of surveillance has been to characterize the scope and variation in disability associated with musculoskeletal disorders. As of 1996, low back disorders accounted for approximately 15% of workers' compensation claims and 23% of costs (Hashemi et al., 1998a). The natural history of low back pain is highly variable, ranging from brief, acute, episodes that resolve without treatment to chronic or recurrent patterns that lead to prolonged disability (Burdorf et al., 1998). These variable patterns are presumably related to the difficulty of healing and reconditioning damaged soft tissues, as well as psychosocial and occupational factors (Frank et al., 1996). Occupationally attributed low back pain (OLBP) is distinct from similar non-work-related conditions, in that a sudden onset is usually reported and disability outcomes are less favorable despite more intensive treatments (Johnson et al., 1996). The substantial variation in the course of disability associated with OLBP has underscored the need to identify improved secondary

prevention strategies for reducing OLBP disability.

Although not as prevalent as back disorders, work-related upper-extremity disorders (WRUEDs) also account for a significant proportion of claims, lost time, and indemnity and health-care costs (Feuerstein et al., 1998; Hashemi et al., 1998b; Courtney and Webster, 1999). From surveillance of medical and disability databases, there is evidence that these disorders are difficult to manage clinically and administratively, with a small but significant proportion of cases experiencing delayed functional recovery (Personick and Jackson, 1993; Cheadle et al., 1994; Feuerstein et al., 1998). From a workers' compensation claims database for U.S. Federal Government employees, carpal tunnel syndrome cases with lost work time showed average days lost similar to that of back disorders (Feuerstein et al., 1998). The impact of these disorders on lost time, health-care costs, and quality of life requires innovative efforts to improve outcomes.

5. Risk factor identification for secondary prevention

Risk factors that guide secondary prevention efforts are those that correlate with illness duration and disability. A secondary prevention program that adequately addresses these risk factors after pain onset should provide optimal results. Epidemiological studies of the natural history of musculoskeletal disorders have included a variety of work and health outcomes. Among 132 epidemiological studies reviewed by the National Research Council and Institute of Medicine (2001), outcome measures included self-reported symptoms, self-reported work status, clinical evaluation, and administrative records. Several of these studies that have particular relevance to secondary prevention are those predicting disability duration (i.e., total days absent from work) or discriminating those still out of work at a designated follow-up interval (i.e., 90 days after the injury) from a list of potential prognostic variables. In the following sections, risk factors for disability associated with low back disorders (Section 5.1) and upper-extremity disorders (Section 5.2) are reviewed separately.

5.1. Risk factors for persistent low back pain and work disability

Studies that have identified prognostic factors soon after the onset of low back pain have been helpful to target secondary prevention efforts and determine who may benefit the most from specific interventions. Disability outcomes have included both lost workdays and self-report measures of function. A recent review including only those studies with early prognostic data (within 30 days of pain onset) was conducted by Shaw et al. (2001c). This review attempted to synthesize findings and identify consistent risk factors for low back disability across 22 studies of prognosis for acute occupational low back pain. Data sources for the studies included administrative records (6 studies), medical chart reviews (4 studies), patient or worker surveys (10 studies), or a combination of database and patient or worker surveys (2 studies). Sample sizes ranged from $N = 59$ to 8629. Disability outcomes were measured in terms of total days lost from work, return to work within a designated time frame (yes/no), or workers' compensation indemnity costs for lost work time. The follow-up periods for assessing return-to-work status ranged from 2 weeks to 2 years (modal follow-up period was 1 year).

Summary results of the review are shown in Table II. Significant prognostic factors included low workplace support, personal stress, shorter job tenure, prior episodes, heavier occupations with no modified duty, delayed reporting, severity of pain and functional impact, radicular findings, and extreme symptom report. These data suggest potential opportunities for secondary prevention in the workplace by improving communication with physicians, improving return to work accommodations, and applying behavioral approaches for secondary prevention.

Another method for identifying potential target areas for secondary prevention of musculoskeletal

disability is to look for variables that may explain discrepancies between musculoskeletal symptoms and perceived functional limitations among workers. In a sample of 475 soldiers with jobs identified as high-risk for low back disability, problem-solving style (problem avoidance, lack of a positive problem-solving orientation, and impulsive decision-making) was associated with higher functional limitations attributed to musculoskeletal pain (Shaw et al., 2001a). These findings suggest that secondary prevention might be improved by assisting affected workers to conceptualize low back pain as a problem that can be overcome and by using strategies to promote an active employee role in reducing risks.

A comparison of general primary prevention risk factors (those predicting onset of low back pain) with secondary prevention risk factors (those predicting duration of low back disability) is shown in Table III. As illustrated by this table, there is a substantial overlap among risk factors for pain and disability. Work-related physical factors are not only predictive of low back pain, but also longer duration of subsequent disability. Low job satisfaction, though predictive of low back pain, has had somewhat less association with disability outcomes. Individuals reporting high levels of pain and functional limitations immediately following pain onset experience longer periods of disability. These data suggest that secondary prevention should address a number of workplace factors including ergonomic exposures, managerial and co-worker support, and work characteristics.

5.2. Risk factors for persistent upper-extremity pain and work disability

Studies of risk factors that predict a longer duration of pain and disability following the onset of a WRUED have identified the importance of both ergonomic and psychosocial factors. Secondary prevention efforts in the workplace may help to address risk factors not normally addressed by traditional medical management approaches. Ergonomic factors include: repetition, awkward postures, excessive force, inadequate work/rest cycles, vibration,

TABLE II

Early risk factors (within 30 days following pain onset) related to disability duration for occupational low back pain from a review of 22 prospective studies (Shaw et al., 2002)

Risk factor for low back disability	Number of studies including this factor	Number of studies showing prospective association with disability duration[a]
Demographic factors		
Age	16	8 (50%)
Gender	16	4 (25%)
Marital status	5	1 (20%)
Body mass index	3	0 (0.0%)
Smoking	3	0 (0.0%)
Education	2	0 (0.0%)
Workplace factors		
Work environment	3	3 (100%)
Occupation/industry	9	6 (67%)
Employer size	3	2 (67%)
Physical demands	11	5 (45%)
Job tenure	6	2 (33%)
Job satisfaction	6	1 (17%)
Circumstances of injury		
Reporting lag	6	5 (83%)
Cause of injury	5	4 (80%)
History of low back pain	12	5 (42%)
Patient self-report		
Pain	9	9 (100%)
Function	7	5 (71%)
Clinical findings		
Physical exam	8	8 (100%)
Diagnosis	7	6 (86%)
Radiographic findings	3	1 (33%)
Psychosocial factors		
Pain beliefs/coping	5	5 (100%)
Stress/social support	3	3 (100%)
Psychopathology	1	1 (100%)

[a] Percentages add to greater than 100% because some studies assessed multiple domains.

and temperature extremes (National Research Council and Institute of Medicine, 2001). Occupational psychosocial factors include: high job demands, self-reported occupational stress, pain-coping style, and low perceived job support (National Research Council and Institute of Medicine, 2001). Secondary prevention that integrates medical care with reduction of workplace ergonomic risks and attention to psychosocial factors may be most helpful to reduce recurrent pain and disability.

Feuerstein et al. (2000) followed 61 individuals with WRUEDs for 1 year. At the time of study recruitment, participants completed a self-report survey of variables believed to influence disability outcomes, including demographics, symptom severity, functional limitations, ergonomic risk exposure, physical work demands, social support, mental distress, and anxiety. Participants were assessed 1, 3, and 12 months after completing the questionnaire on measures of symptoms, function, workdays lost,

TABLE III

Comparison of risk factors for primary and secondary prevention of occupational low back pain

	Primary prevention Risk factors for symptom onset	Secondary prevention Risk factors for symptom-related disability
Source	National Research Council and Institute of Medicine, 2001	Shaw et al., 2001c
Work-related physical factors	Manual material handling Frequent bending and twisting Physically heavy work Whole-body vibration	Manual material handling Physically heavy work Job tenure < 2 years Transportation and construction
Work-related psychosocial factors	Low job satisfaction Monotonous work Poor social support at work High perceived stress High perceived job demands Perceived ability to return to work	Poor social support at work High perceived stress High perceived job demands Perceived ability to return to work
Individual psychosocial factors	Pain beliefs Emotional distress Poor social support at home Behavioral coping patterns	Pain beliefs Emotional distress Poor social support at home Behavioral coping patterns Pain report at onset Functional limitations at onset

and mental health. A composite index of outcome combining these four measures determined either favorable or unfavorable outcome for each participant at each follow-up assessment. At 1 month follow-up, predictors of poorer outcome were: upper-extremity co-morbidity, pain severity, ergonomic risk exposure, low job support, and pain-coping style. At 3 months follow-up, predictors of poorer outcome were: symptom severity, job stress, and pain-coping style. At 1 year follow-up, predictors of poorer outcome were: number of prior treatments and providers, past recommendation for surgery, and pain-coping style.

In a study of 165 government workers with newly accepted workers' compensation claims for WRUEDs, Feuerstein et al. (2002a) examined self-report factors that discriminated those who were not able to resume at least modified or transitional duty jobs within the first 90 days after reporting their illness. Those on disability leave reported higher pain ratings, greater functional limitations, and greater ergonomic exposures at work.

A comparison of secondary prevention risk factors identified by our group for back and upper extremities is shown in Fig. 3. This figure focuses on the potential risk factors associated with case status, lost time, clinic visits, perceived functional limitations, and multidimensional outcome (symptoms, function, mental health, lost time from work). While these results highlight the important role of both physical and psychosocial stressors at work to improve occupational musculoskeletal outcomes, they also identify a set of specific workplace psychosocial, individual psychosocial, ergonomic factors and health behaviors associated with a range of outcomes. Inspection of this figure reveals that these variables consistently appear as risk factors for a diverse range of outcomes in both the military and community samples. While one needs to be cautious about overgeneralizing from this figure, the variables identified could assist in the de-

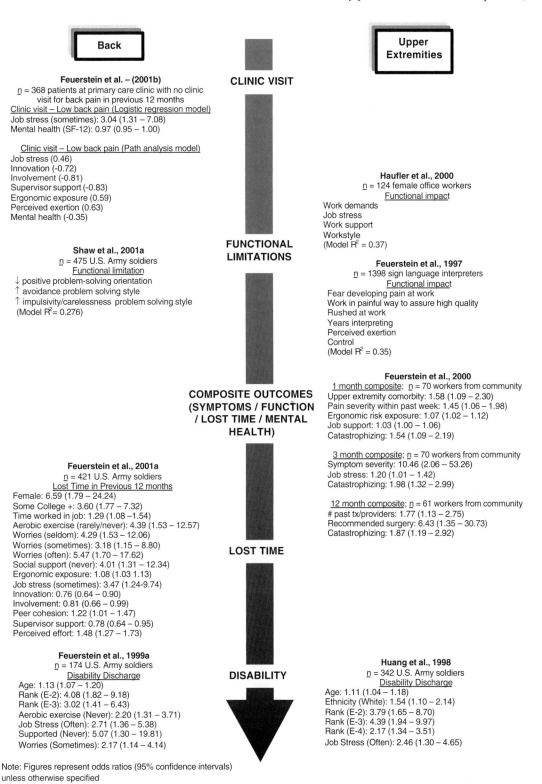

Back

Feuerstein et al. – (2001b)
n = 368 patients at primary care clinic with no clinic
visit for back pain in previous 12 months
Clinic visit – Low back pain (Logistic regression model)
Job stress (sometimes): 3.04 (1.31 – 7.08)
Mental health (SF-12): 0.97 (0.95 – 1.00)

Clinic visit – Low back pain (Path analysis model)
Job stress (0.46)
Innovation (-0.72)
Involvement (-0.81)
Supervisor support (-0.83)
Ergonomic exposure (0.59)
Perceived exertion (0.63)
Mental health (-0.35)

Shaw et al., 2001a
n = 475 U.S. soldiers
Functional limitation
↓ positive problem-solving orientation
↑ avoidance problem solving style
↑ impulsivity/carelessness problem solving style
(Model R^2 = 0.276)

Feuerstein et al., 2001a
n = 421 U.S. Army soldiers
Lost Time in Previous 12 months
Female: 6.59 (1.79 – 24.24)
Some College +: 3.60 (1.77 – 7.32)
Time worked in job: 1.29 (1.08 –1.54)
Aerobic exercise (rarely/never): 4.39 (1.53 – 12.57)
Worries (seldom): 4.29 (1.53 – 12.06)
Worries (sometimes): 3.18 (1.15 – 8.80)
Worries (often): 5.47 (1.70 – 17.62)
Social support (never): 4.01 (1.31 – 12.34)
Ergonomic exposure: 1.08 (1.03 1.13)
Job stress (sometimes): 3.47 (1.24-9.74)
Innovation: 0.76 (0.64 – 0.90)
Involvement: 0.81 (0.66 – 0.99)
Peer cohesion: 1.22 (1.01 – 1.47)
Supervisor support: 0.78 (0.64 – 0.95)
Perceived effort: 1.48 (1.27 – 1.73)

Feuerstein et al., 1999a
n = 174 U.S. Army soldiers
Disability Discharge
Age: 1.13 (1.07 – 1.20)
Rank (E-2): 4.08 (1.82 – 9.18)
Rank (E-3): 3.02 (1.41 – 6.43)
Aerobic exercise (Never): 2.20 (1.31 – 3.71)
Job Stress (Often): 2.71 (1.36 – 5.38)
Supported (Never): 5.07 (1.30 – 19.81)
Worries (Sometimes): 2.17 (1.14 – 4.14)

CLINIC VISIT

**FUNCTIONAL
LIMITATIONS**

**COMPOSITE OUTCOMES
(SYMPTOMS / FUNCTION
/ LOST TIME / MENTAL
HEALTH)**

LOST TIME

DISABILITY

**Upper
Extremities**

Haufler et al., 2000
n = 124 female office workers
Functional impact
Work demands
Job stress
Work support
Workstyle
(Model R^2 = 0.37)

Feuerstein et al., 1997
n = 1398 sign language interpreters
Functional impact
Fear developing pain at work
Work in painful way to assure high quality
Rushed at work
Years interpreting
Perceived exertion
Control
(Model R^2 = 0.35)

Feuerstein et al., 2000
1 month composite; n = 70 workers from community
Upper extremity comorbity: 1.58 (1.09 – 2.30)
Pain severity within past week: 1.45 (1.06 – 1.98)
Ergonomic risk exposure: 1.07 (1.02 – 1.12)
Job support: 1.03 (1.00 – 1.06)
Catastrophizing: 1.54 (1.09 – 2.19)

3 month composite; n = 70 workers from community
Symptom severity: 10.46 (2.06 – 53.26)
Job stress: 1.20 (1.01 – 1.42)
Catastrophizing: 1.98 (1.32 – 2.99)

12 month composite; n = 61 workers from community
past tx/providers: 1.77 (1.13 – 2.75)
Recommended surgery: 6.43 (1.35 – 30.73)
Catastrophizing: 1.87 (1.19 – 2.92)

Huang et al., 1998
n = 342 U.S. Army soldiers
Disability Discharge
Age: 1.11 (1.04 – 1.18)
Ethnicity (White): 1.54 (1.10 – 2.14)
Rank (E-2): 3.79 (1.65 – 8.70)
Rank (E-3): 4.39 (1.94 – 9.97)
Rank (E-4): 2.17 (1.34 – 3.51)
Job Stress (Often): 2.46 (1.30 – 4.65)

Note: Figures represent odds ratios (95% confidence intervals)
unless otherwise specified

Fig. 3. Targets for secondary prevention of musculoskeletal disorders.

velopment of future secondary prevention programs. Of course, such programs will need to be determined using appropriate research designs.

6. Interventions for secondary prevention

Based on the evidence that multiple risk factors may contribute to musculoskeletal disability, a number of workplace secondary prevention strategies have been implemented and evaluated in recent years. As illustrated in Fig. 1, workplace strategies have been developed from at least three general secondary prevention themes: (1) reducing ergonomic exposures among symptomatic workers, (2) reducing organizational barriers to report symptoms or obtain accommodations, and (3) improving problem solving and coping strategies to restore function. In the following section, we describe workplace interventions to reduce disability associated with work-related musculoskeletal disorders and some of the preliminary results from these efforts.

6.1. Physical workplace and equipment modifications

Occupational risk factors may be far more important for evaluating disability risk than for predicting the onset of pain (Andersson, 1991). For those at computer workstations, useful accommodations to reduce upper-extremity discomfort might include improving computer keyboards, altering chair or desk height, adding a telephone headset or voice-activated software, or rounding desk edges. For workers performing manual materials handling tasks, possible upper-extremity accommodations might include workstation reconfiguration, improved hand tools, non-vibratory gloves, providing additional work space, increased job rotation, or more frequent breaks (Shaw et al., 2000). Part of the challenge of returning workers to their regular duty work is to identify and eliminate physical risk factors that presumably contributed to the onset of symptoms. A subsequent exposure to the same work demands may exacerbate or maintain symptoms after a return to work.

An ergonomic intervention program was one of several components to a large-scale effort to reduce upper-extremity disability at Johns Hopkins University in 1992 (Bernacki et al., 2000). The ergonomic program for any employee reporting symptoms included a worker self-report ergonomic survey and a work site inspection provided by a trained industrial hygienist. The elements of the ergonomic survey were (1) to document repeated, sustained, and forceful exertions, (2) to document awkward postures, (3) to summarize ergonomic stressors and risk factors, (4) to provide information on ergonomic principles on a one-to-one basis, (5) to document and report results of the ergonomic survey, and (6) to monitor the implementation of corrective actions. Following initiation of the ergonomic intervention program in 1992, the prevalence rate of reported upper-extremity disorders declined 80% over the subsequent 7-year period. At the same time, employee requests for ergonomic evaluations (to assess work areas that supervisors or employees felt were potentially hazardous) increased 400%, highlighting a potential need to assess the continued cost-effectiveness of this approach. Controlled trials of such ergonomic interventions are needed to rule out the possibility that other factors may be responsible for such dramatic changes in the prevalence of upper-extremity disorders within a single organization.

Back belts have grown in popularity for use as an ergonomic accommodation for low back pain, with the expectation that this would decrease impairment or disability or prevent a recurrence of pain. However, there is little evidence supporting their use for secondary prevention, and this practice has not reduced prevalence rates of acute low back pain among workers (Jellema et al., 2001). Four randomized trials comparing back belt and no back belt conditions (Walsh and Schwartz, 1990; Reddell et al., 1992; Alexander et al., 1995; Van Poppel et al., 1998) found no beneficial effects on low back prevalence, pain severity, and sick leave due to low back pain. Based on this evidence, use of a back belt is not a sufficient accommodation for low back pain, and use of the device may actually give workers a false sense of security.

Other ergonomic interventions for work-related musculoskeletal discomfort have been effective when closely integrated with clinical care. In a randomized clinical trial, Loisel et al. (1997) compared four treatment groups for subacute (4 weeks) work-related low back pain: clinical intervention, occupational intervention, combined clinical/occupational intervention, and a (usual care) control group. The *occupational intervention* included two components: (1) referral to an occupational physician; and (2) a participatory ergonomics evaluation conducted by an ergonomist and coordinated with union and employer representatives. The *clinical intervention* included a visit to a back pain specialist, regular attendance at a back care education school, and a multidisciplinary work rehabilitation program. Return to work required fewer days in the combined clinical/occupational intervention group when compared with the control group (odds ratio = 2.41), but benefits of the other two groups (occupational intervention only, clinical intervention only) were not significantly better than the control condition. The researchers concluded that both clinical and occupational factors need to be addressed in order to influence disability duration for work-related low back pain.

Randomized trials of various workplace modifications for secondary prevention of musculoskeletal disability are needed to make clearer inferences about their effectiveness. Several studies that have reported no benefits of workplace modification (e.g., Shi, 1993; Daltroy et al., 1997) have been discounted by others for being either low-quality or providing insufficient statistical analyses (Maher, 2000). Also, the process by which workplace modifications are planned and implemented may be critical to success of this secondary prevention strategy. Ergonomic accommodations that do not involve the joint participation of workers or lack the collaboration of clinical care providers may fall short.

6.2. Providing modified duty

One of the most common methods for easing return to work after a musculoskeletal disorder is to recommend temporary alternate or modified duty work (Mueller, 1999; Strunin and Boden, 2000). This intervention can be conceptualized as either organizational (i.e., setting up a modified duty program within an organization) or individual (i.e., modifying an individual's work to reduce ergonomic exposures). In the case of occupational low back pain, there is evidence to suggest that this step may increase the likelihood that workers will ultimately resume their normal work activities (Wiesel et al., 1994; Yassi et al., 1995), and thus prevent longer-duration disability.

Modified duty provisions are based on the substantial evidence from several disciplines linking ergonomic exposures to upper-extremity disorders (National Research Council and Institute of Medicine, 2001). This evidence suggests that modifying work activities, in addition to making physical changes to the workplace, may reduce upper-extremity symptoms. Permanent redesign of jobs and workstations may be recommended for workers who experience delayed recovery or recurrent symptoms (Harris, 1997). For those with milder symptoms, temporary alternate or modified work may reduce workplace ergonomic exposure while allowing time for spontaneous recovery or to exercise the affected limbs and increase tolerance gradually. For workers who have experienced a significant episode of work-related pain and disability (i.e., persistent pain, multiple medical treatments, and significant work absence), modified duty work may be an opportunity to gradually restore functional self-efficacy with the assurance that protections are in place to limit maximal physical demands.

The viability of modified duty may depend on a variety of workplace and individual factors. Providing modified duty accommodations to workers with musculoskeletal disorders has been particularly challenging for smaller employers (Kenny, 1999) and for employers without proactive return to work programs (Habeck et al., 1991). For some physically demanding occupations or industries it may be found that work loads cannot be lightened sufficiently to accommodate a worker recovering from a musculoskeletal disorder; for example, longer-duration disability after acute low back pain has been reported for construction (Oleinick et al., 1996; McIntosh et al., 2000), transportation (Gluck and Oleinick, 1998), and manual materials handling trades (Gluck and Oleinick, 1998). For these occupations, reduced work hours or alternate duty positions may be necessary as an alternative to modified duty. Other industry-specific barriers to job modification may result from wage scale requirements or labor union agreements limiting job rotation or from public safety concerns (e.g., transportation workers). Therefore, efforts to provide better workplace accommodation need to involve all key stakeholders.

A review of empirical studies on the benefits of workplace accommodation, including modified or temporary alternate duty, graded work exposure and work trials showed that return-to-work rates were doubled among workers offered such options (Krause et al., 1998). Furthermore, this review concluded that accommodated work reduced the number of lost workdays by 50%. Surveys comparing manufacturing companies' policies have shown that modified duty programs are associated with having fewer workers' compensation claims (Habeck et al., 1998a,b). Earlier work by these investigators also observed lower rates of workers' compensation claims in companies that provided temporary alternate or modified work and created an environment where employees participated in problem-solving and decision-making within company operations (Habeck et al., 1991).

After the initial treatment of symptoms, employers may disagree with employees about the perceived need for modified or alternate duty or physical accommodations. Among a sample of Florida workers with occupational back pain and greater than 4 weeks' work absence, only half were offered modifications to their original jobs, and only half the employers provided special equipment needs requested by the worker or treating physician (Strunin and Boden, 2000). Among workers with disabilities in general (including both work-related and non-work-related injury and illness), reasonable accommodation is the most common area of dispute between employees and their employers (Huang and

Feuerstein, 1998). Although corporate policies and procedures appear to impact disability rates, there have only recently been attempts to examine these policies from the perspective of workers (McLellan et al., 2001). The success of a modified duty transition requires the joint cooperation and agreement of the worker, treating physician, and employer.

6.3. Group education, physical conditioning, and exercise

One approach proposed to prevent recurrences of low back pain has been to provide education and physical conditioning to workers. This type of intervention, originally adopted by physical therapists (Hayne, 1984), can be provided or hosted by employers. Back schools or back rehabilitation programs introduce proper lifting technique and body mechanics based on accepted ergonomic principles, often with practical training in simulated work environments. Specific instructions include bending the knee and hip joints, avoiding twisting, and using short lever arms. Typical programs provide biweekly meetings consisting of both didactic presentations and exercise for a period of 10–15 weeks following diagnosis.

The efficacy of these programs has been controversial (Cohen et al., 1994), with some studies reporting fewer back pain recurrences (e.g., Lonn et al., 1999; Glomsrod et al., 2001; Soukup et al., 2001) and others reporting no reduction in recurrences or lost work time (e.g., Leclaire et al., 1996). From a review of six randomized trials of education programs, Maher (2000) found moderate evidence that education is ineffective to reduce the prevalence of low back pain and limited evidence that education is further ineffective to reduce the costs of work-related low back pain. Discrepancies between studies may relate to the choice of comparable control groups (no treatment control group versus standard care control group) and to the intensity of treatment provided. For example, in the randomized clinical trial by Lonn et al. (1999) that showed positive results among workers reporting a prior episode of low back pain, the back study group received extensive instruction (20 1-h lessons over 13 weeks), and the control group was provided no systematic attention or information. The cost effectiveness of this more intensive approach (20 lessons) relative to return to work benefits has not been reported.

Although back school programs have been shown to improve participants' knowledge of ergonomic exposures and proper exercise technique (Leclaire et al., 1996), the superiority (and cost effectiveness) of this approach over other secondary prevention strategies has not been convincingly supported. A limiting factor may be that workers typically participate in these programs in clinical settings away from work where there may be limited influence over employer accommodation. Educational programs provided or hosted by employers that include workplace accommodation might be more successful and can be less constrained by time and distance.

In comparison with workplace educational programs which have received little research support, workplace exercise programs may have potential benefits for secondary prevention of low back disability. These programs can be easily incorporated into employers' work wellness programs and can be provided early in the course of a developing musculoskeletal problem (i.e., before medical attention is needed). Several randomized trials of exercise versus no-treatment controls have shown reductions in the severity of low back pain (Linton et al., 1989; Gundewall et al., 1993) and reductions in sick leave after low back pain (Linton et al., 1989; Kellet et al., 1991; Gundewall et al., 1993). The presumed mechanism for this benefit is that exercise increases blood flow in damaged tissues and aids in healing; however, there is no direct evidence of this effect. Future studies are needed to assess whether exercise programs reduce costs associated with OLBP or whether this intervention approach is cost-effective (Maher, 2000).

6.4. Case management intervention

Case management (CM) has played an increasingly important role in workers' compensation benefits (Salazar, 1999), although such services have often been limited to monitoring of the claims process and surveillance of medical treatment. For the secondary prevention of work-related pain and disability, nurse case managers may be able to intervene by improving communication between medical providers and employers and facilitating accommodations needed for a modified or full duty release. These secondary prevention efforts may reduce disability duration, reduce risk of recurrence, and improve musculoskeletal function.

The authors are currently conducting a randomized, controlled trial of CM services for individuals with WRUEDs (Feuerstein and Miller, 1998). In this study, randomly selected nurse case managers from a national workers' compensation system participate in a 2-day training workshop on Integrated Case Management (ICM). The focus of the ICM approach is to better engage workers in their recovery and return-to-work process through collaborative problem-solving and accommodation. After the training, workers with newly adjudicated claims for WRUEDS are randomly assigned to either workshop (ICM) nurses or usual case managers.

The ICM approach to WRUEDs was developed based on a literature review, consultation with experts in management of upper-extremity disorders, clinical experience of the authors in musculoskeletal rehabilitation, a chart review of WRUED cases, a review of Federal claims data (Feuerstein et al., 1998), and consultations with the U.S. Department of Labor, Office of Workers' Compensation Programs (OWCP, the host agency). The process involved conceptualization of an eight-step CM process, creation of an ICM Provider Manual (Feuerstein et al., 1999b), intensive review and revision with the host agency, and consultations with key stakeholders (labor unions and employing agencies) (for more details of the ICM approach, see Shaw et al., 2001b).

Volunteer nurse case managers were provided instruction in the ICM approach in a 16-h 2-day training workshop. This workshop included a combination of didactic presentations, case simulations and hands-on exercises. Site trainers included a health psychologist, an ergonomist or rehabilitation engineer, a staff nurse from the regional OWCP office, and a senior claims representative from the National OWCP office. Case managers were informed at the initial training session that project staff would be available by telephone, e-mail, and internet site throughout the course of the 3-year project to provide a consultation/sounding board for discussing strategies on individual cases, providing suggestions, and receiving feedback. During the follow-up period, volunteer Federal workers with compensable WRUEDs and lost work time would be randomized to receive either the ICM or 'usual care' CM and would be periodically assessed in terms of work status, symptoms, and function.

Although longitudinal disability data are still being collected for the ICM study, some preliminary analyses have shown that nurses can be trained in the ICM approach and that they modify their practice behaviors following the training. Both ergonomic assessment and problem-solving skills training are activities that appear to be acceptable and of interest to workers' compensation case managers. Among a randomly selected group of case managers, course ratings for the workshop indicated high satisfaction with the course itself and moderate to high levels of confidence to apply these skills in the management of subsequent WRUED claims (Shaw et al., 2001b).

Nurse case managers who attended the ICM workshop recommended more employer accommodations than control case managers for workers preparing to return to work (Lincoln et al., 2002). Following the training, 101 claimants with compensable upper-extremity disorders were randomly assigned to case mangers with and without training. Overall, 208 accommodations were recommended and 155 of these were implemented (75%). Claimants of trained nurses received 1.5 times as many recommendations for accommodations as claimants managed by nurses not trained in the process and 1.4 times as many accommodations were implemented, although differences between the two groups in implementation rates were modest (Lincoln et al., 2002). Trained nurses were more likely to recommend accommodations addressing workstation layout, computer-related improvements, furnishings, accessories, and lifting/carrying aids while the untrained nurses were more likely to suggest light duty.

This finding indicates that the training was associated with a change in the practice behavior of case managers regarding the workplace accommodation process. More studies are needed to identify similar ways to provide stronger liaisons between medical providers and employers for more effective work site accommodations of carpal tunnel syndrome and other persistent musculoskeletal disorders.

6.5. Optimizing supervisor role for secondary prevention

Effective management practices of supervisors may reduce the risk of delayed functional recovery or symptom recurrence. Supervisors can contribute to secondary prevention efforts by their prompt, knowledgeable, and confidential response to musculoskeletal pain in the workplace. A supervisor can provide modified work, interpret corporate policies, facilitate access to corporate and medical resources, monitor the worker's health and function, and communicate a positive message of concern and support (Gates, 1993). Supervisors may fail to communicate regularly with workers after the filing of a claim because of other management and production demands, as well as concerns that this may interfere with confidential medical and/or legal activities. Negative employer responses, including a lack of employer contact, have been cited by several authors as important correlates of prolonged disability (Akabas et al., 1992; Shrey, 1996).

In 1980, the American Biltrite Company (400 workers) instituted a sensitivity training program for management that focused on early reporting of musculoskeletal pain, positive acceptance and empathy for affected workers, and providing modified duty work. The program resulted in a 50% reduction in claims with lost work time and a ten-fold decrease in workers' compensation costs for low back disorders (Fitzler and Berger, 1982, 1983). Another study (Wood, 1987) provided hospital managers with training that emphasized frequent communications with employees (every 10 days), communicating a positive message ('Your job is waiting for you'), and providing modified duty work assignments. This program resulted in a five-fold reduction in low back claims exceeding 125 days lost work time.

From the original work by Wood (1987), Linton (1991) developed a more specific, 1-day training course for immediate supervisors in how to help employees return to work after treatment for OLBP. In addition to providing information about musculoskeletal pain and treatment, the course encouraged supervisors (1) to hold a formal meeting with employees upon return to work to assess the need for temporary accommodations, (2) to maintain contact with employees who are on sick leave, and (3) to schedule regular follow-up meetings with employees after a return to work to prevent a recurrence of symptoms. Although outcomes of worker disability or worker satisfaction were not available, supervisors rated the course as highly useful and the proposed changes feasible to implement (Linton, 1991).

In a more recent study, a supervisor training program was conducted as part of a pilot program in the State of New Hampshire (McLellan et al., 2001). One hundred eight supervisors from seven employers participated. The overall goal of the program was to enhance communication between physicians, employers, claims adjusters, and workers to improve occupational health and safety. The supervisor training component (a single 1.5-h workshop) was intended to reduce disability by facilitating a proactive, supportive, and knowledgeable response to occupational pain and symptoms among workers. Specific recommendations for supervisor intervention included meeting privately with workers, validating health concerns, using supportive language, and making recommendations for seeking additional resources or medical care.

Data from convenience samples of workers reporting symptoms before and after the supervisor training indicated some potential benefits of the program. Prior to the supervisor training sessions, 105 workers with work injuries and illnesses completed a questionnaire about their previous experiences with supervisors. Approximately half were identified by reviewing the company's OSHA and first aid logs from the prior year. The remaining half were workers who, when surveyed confidentially, recalled a prior

work-related health problem that had not been formally reported. In the survey, workers described the nature of the injury or illness and whether they had been generally satisfied with their supervisors' responses (yes/no). They then answered 11 questions describing details of the interaction (e.g., 'Did your supervisor blame you for your injury? [yes/no],' and 'Did your supervisor talk with you privately and confidentially? [yes/no]'). In the 12 months after the supervisor workshop, a sample of 23 workers who experienced new work injuries or illnesses were asked to complete identical information.

In the pre-intervention retrospective survey of workers, 73 of 105 workers reported an interaction with a supervisor pertaining to work-related discomfort or injury. Injuries or illnesses reported to supervisors were primarily arm/hand (43.8%) or back (37.0%), and most problems were described as gradual onset (56.2%). In the post-intervention sample of workers ($N = 25$), types of injuries/illnesses were similar. All 11 items describing supervisor interactions improved, and three of these ('talked with you privately,' 'provided opportunity to speak with doctor or nurse', and 'blamed you for your injury') reached statistical significance (Chi-square test of contingency, $p < 0.05$). Overall satisfaction with the supervisor's response improved from 71.8% in the pre-intervention sample to 80.0% in the post-intervention sample, but this change did not reach statistical significance ($p > 0.05$). This pilot program demonstrated that a brief training intervention, when accompanied by management support, may achieve demonstrable impacts on supervisor responses to work-related musculoskeletal problems; however, controlled trials are needed.

7. Future directions

The accumulated evidence on secondary prevention of musculoskeletal disorders in the workplace seems to indicate a potential for these approaches to reduce disability and recurrence. Specifically, efforts to reduce ergonomic risk factors through modified duty or physical accommodation appear to be most successful when developed with direct input from workers and their physicians. Exercise programs to relieve musculoskeletal discomfort appear to be more effective than either worker education programs or personal protective devices (i.e., back belts). Finally, the direct influence of case managers and supervisors to facilitate a 3-way communication between workers, their treating physicians, and their employers represents an opportunity for secondary prevention. From the preliminary results of a variety of intervention strategies, the theme of integrating care and facilitating communication among various parties emerges repeatedly.

A major challenge for workplace intervention has been to address psychosocial factors, both organizational and individual, that repeatedly rank as important risk factors for prolonged pain and disability. Cognitive behavioral and other psychotherapeutic strategies have been shown to be beneficial as a clinical treatment for *subacute*, as well as *chronic* low back pain (Linton and Andersson, 2000), but can psychosocial factors (both individual and organizational) be routinely addressed in the workplace? We believe that this needs to be the case if these approaches are to be implemented.

Linton (1995) has provided a review of psychologically based strategies in secondary prevention for low back pain. These include goal-setting with employees, including involvement of family and workplace, focusing on coping strategies, and training all members of the treatment team to be aware of psychosocial factors that may influence recovery. Also, intervention efforts in the workplace should strive to reduce the sometimes negative stigma attached to musculoskeletal disorders, and to take seriously all symptom reports of workers. A basic tenet of this approach is that avoiding disability is a collaborative decision made by the employee, employer, and physician. In the acute stage immediately following symptom onset, individuals may develop a so-called sick role, where reinforcement of pain behavior and learned helplessness may reduce efforts to gradually increase activity and cope with obstacles to recovery (Linton et al., 1984). This can be further exacerbated by delays in treatment, exclusion of the worker from the planning process, unnecessary medical diagnostics and intervention, and lack of communication between the treatment team. Although clinical intervention with a psychologist is common for chronic pain conditions, this treatment may be neither cost-effective, necessary, nor acceptable to individuals immediately following the onset of pain. However, some attention to potential psychological factors in the acute stage may be helpful to supervisors, treating physicians, and case managers to avoid a chronic progression of disability.

One clear need for future research in secondary prevention is to conduct controlled trials comparing various methods of intervention. The Hawthorne effect (wherein employees report benefits of *any* changes positively advanced by their employer) and other threats to internal validity are particularly problematic among workplace intervention studies. However, the challenges of performing carefully controlled trials of health intervention in work settings are numerous, including sometimes tenuous labor–management relations, rapidly changing organizational structures, potential cross-contamination between groups, cost control concerns, and difficulties of providing intervention for only some worker groups within a larger company. Nevertheless, controlled trials of accommodation and intervention based upon the past five to ten years of empirical research on risk factors should provide a stronger basis for recommending these strategies to employers.

References

Akabas, S.H., Gates, L.B. and Galvin, D.E. (1992) Disability management: A complete system to reduce costs, increase productivity, meet employee needs, and ensure legal compliance. American Management Association, New York.

Alexander, A., Woolley, S.M., Bisesi, M. et al. (1995) The effectiveness of back belts on occupational back injuries and worker perception. Prof. Saf., 40: 22–27.

Andersson, G.B.J. (1991) Concepts in prevention. In: M.H. Pope et al. (Eds.), Occupational Low Back Pain. Mosby Year Book, St. Louis, pp. 211–216.

Ashbury, F.D. (1995) Occupational repetitive strain injuries and gender in Ontario, 1986 to 1991. J. Occup. Environ. Med., 37: 479–485.

Bernacki, E.J., Guidera, J.A., Schaefer, J.A. and Tsai, S. (2000)

A facilitated early return to work program at a large urban medical center. J. Occup. Environ. Med., 42: 1172–1177.

Burdorf, A., Naaktgeboren, B. and Post, W. (1998) Prognostic factors for musculoskeletal sickness absence and return to work among welders and metal workers. Occup. Environ. Med., 55(7): 490–495.

Bureau of Labor Statistics (2001) Case and demographic characteristics for workplace injuries and illnesses involving days away from work – 1999. U.S. Department of Labor, Washington, DC.

Burton, A.K. and Tillotson, K.M. (1991) Prediction of the clinical course of low-back trouble using multivariable models. Spine, 16: 7–14.

Cheadle, A., Franklin, G., Wolfhagen, C., Savarino, J., Liu, P.Y., Salley, C. and Weaver, M. (1994) Factors influencing the duration of work-related disability: A population-based study of Washington State workers' compensation. Am. J. Public Health, 84: 190–196.

Chiang, H., Chen, S., Yu, H. and Ko, Y. (1990) The occurrence of carpal tunnel syndrome in frozen food factory employees. Kao Hsiung J. Med. Sci., 6: 73–80.

Cohen, A.L., Gjessing, C.C., Fine, L.J., Bernard, B.P. and McGlothlin, J.D. (1997) Elements of ergonomics programs: A primer based on workplace evaluations of musculoskeletal disorders (DHHS [NIOSH] Publication No. 97-117). National Institute for Occupational Safety and Health, Washington, DC.

Cohen, J.E., Goel, V., Frank, J.W., Bombardier, C., Peloso, P. and Guillemin, F. (1994) Group education interventions for people with low back pain. An overview of the literature. Spine, 19: 1214–1222.

Courtney, T.K. and Webster, B.S. (1999) Disabling occupational morbidity in the United States. J. Occup. Environ. Med., 41: 60–69.

Daltroy, L., Iversen, M., Larson, M., Lew, R., Wright, E., Ryan, J., Zwerling, C., Fossel, A. and Llang, M. (1997) A controlled trial of an educational program to prevent low back injuries. N. Engl. J. Med., 337: 322–328.

Dasinger, L.K., Krause, N., Deegan, L.J., Brand, R.J. and Rudolph, L. (1999) Duration of work disability after low back injury: A comparison of administrative and self-reported outcomes. Am. J. Ind. Med., 35: 619–631.

Falck, B. and Arnio, P. (1983) Left-sided carpal tunnel syndrome in butchers. Scand. J. Work Environ. Health, 9: 291–297.

Feuerstein, M. and Miller, V.I. (1998) Enhanced Case Management Intervention for Workers Covered Under the Federal Employees Compensation Act [Grant Proposal to the Robert Wood Johnson Foundation, Workers' Compensation Health Initiative].

Feuerstein, M., Carosella, A.M., Burrell, L.M., Marshall, L. and DeCaro, J. (1997) Occupational upper extremity symptoms in sign language interpreters: Prevalence and correlates of pain, function, and work disability. J. Occup. Rehabil., 7: 187–205.

Feuerstein, M., Miller, V.L., Burrell, L.M. and Berger, R. (1998) Occupational upper extremity disorders in the federal work force: Prevalence, health care expenditures, and patterns of disability. J. Occup. Environ. Med., 40: 546–555.

Feuerstein, M., Berkowitz, S.M. and Huang, G.D. (1999a) Predictors of occupational low back disability: Implications for secondary prevention. J. Occup. Environ. Med., 41: 1024–1031.

Feuerstein, M., Miller, V.I., Shaw, W.S., Wood, P.W., Berger, R.H., Lincoln, A.E. and Hickey, P.F. (1999b) Integrated Case Management for work-related upper extremity disorders: Provider manual. Unpublished manual, Georgetown University, Washington, DC.

Feuerstein, M., Huang, G.D., Haufler, A.J. and Miller, J.K. (2000) Development of a screen for predicting clinical outcomes in patients with work-related upper extremity disorders. J. Occup. Environ. Med., 42: 749–761.

Feuerstein, M., Berkowitz, S.M., Haufler, A.J., Lopez, M.S. and Huang, G.D. (2001a) Working with low back pain: Workplace and individual psychosocial determinants of limited duty and lost time. Am. J. Ind. Med., 40: 627–638.

Feuerstein, M., Huang, G.D., Clark, C. and Lopez, M. (2001b) Predictors of recovery from low back pain in primary care patients. Presented at the VA Guidelines Working Group Meeting, Uniformed Services University of the Health Sciences, Bethesda, MD.

Feuerstein, M., Shaw, W.S., Lincoln, A.E., Miller, V.I. and Wood, P.M. (2002a) Work-related upper extremity disorders: Factors associated with a return to modified duty. Journal of Occupational and Environmental Medicine. Submitted.

Feuerstein, M., Nicholas, R., Huang, G.D., Pransky, G., Haufler, A. and Robertson, M. (2002b) Workstyle: Scale development and validation. In preparation.

Fitzler, S.L. and Berger, R.A. (1982) Attitudinal change: The Chelsea Back Program. Occup. Health Saf., 51: 24–26.

Fitzler, S.L. and Berger, R.A. (1983) Chelsea Back Program: One year later. Occup. Health Saf., 52: 52–54.

Frank, J.W., Brooker, A., DeMaio, S.E., Kerr, M.S., Maetzel, A., Shannon, H.S., Sullivan, T.J., Norman, R.W. and Wells, R.P. (1996) Disability resulting from occupational low back pain: Part II: What do we know about secondary prevention? A review of the scientific evidence on prevention after disability begins. Spine, 21: 2918–2929.

Frymoyer, J.W. (1988) Back pain and sciatica. N. Engl. J. Med., 318(5): 291–300.

Gates, L.B. (1993) The role of the supervisor in successful adjustment to work with a disabling condition: Issues for disability policy and practice. J. Occup. Rehabil., 93(3): 179–190.

Glomsrod, B., Lonn, J.H., Soukup, M.G., Bo, K. and Larsen, S. (2001) Active Back School, prophylactic management for low back pain: Three-year follow-up of a randomized, controlled trial. J. Rehabil. Med., 33: 26–30.

Gluck, J.V. and Oleinick, A. (1998) Claim rates of compensable back injuries by age, gender, occupation, and industry. Spine, 23: 1572–1587.

Gundewall, B., Liljeqvist, M. and Hansson, T. (1993) Primary prevention of back symptoms and absence from work: A prospective randomized study among hospital employees. Spine, 18: 587–594.

Habeck, R.V., Leahy, M.J., Hunt, H.A., Chan, F. and Welch, E.M. (1991) Employer factors related to workers' compensation claims and disability management. Rehabil. Couns. Bull., 34: 210–226.

Habeck, R.V., Hunt, H.A. and VanTol, B. (1998a) Workplace factors associated with preventing and managing work disability. Rehabil. Couns. Bull., 42: 98–143.

Habeck, R.V., Scully, S.M., VanTol, B. and Hunt, H.A. (1998b) Successful employer strategies for preventing and managing disability. Rehabil. Couns. Bull., 8(42): 144–160.

Halperin, W.E. and Ordin, D.L. (1996) Closing the surveillance gap. Am. J. Ind. Med., 31: 479–480.

Harris, J.S. (Ed.) (1997) Occupational Medicine Practice Guidelines: Evaluation and Management of Common Health Problems and Functional Recovery in Workers. OEM Press, Beverly Farms, MS.

Hashemi, L., Webster, B.S. and Clancy, E.A. (1998a) Trends in disability duration and cost of workers' compensation low back claims (1988–1996) J. Occup. Environ. Med., 40(12): 1110–1119.

Hashemi, L., Webster, B.S., Clancy, E.A. and Courtney, T.K. (1998b) Length of disability and cost of work-related musculoskeletal disorders of the upper extremity. J. Occup. Environ. Med., 40: 261–269.

Haufler, A.J., Feuerstein, M. and Huang, G.D. (2000) Job stress, upper extremity pain and functional limitations in symptomatic computer users. Am. J. Ind. Med., 38: 507–515.

Hayne, C.R. (1984) Back school and total back care program. Physiotherapy, 40: 14–17.

Huang, G.D. and Feuerstein, M. (1998) Americans with Disabilities Act litigation and musculoskeletal-related impairments: Implications for work re-entry. J. Occup. Rehabil., 8: 91–102.

Huang, G.D., Feuerstein, M. (2002) Targeting work organization factors in work-related musculoskeletal outcome interventions. Paper presented at the 23rd Annual Meeting of the Society of Behavioral Medicine, Washington, DC.

Huang, G.D., Feuerstein, M., Berkowitz, S.M. and Peck, C.A. (1998) Occupational upper extremity-related disability: Demographic, physical, and psychosocial factors. Mil. Med., 163: 552–558.

Huang, G.D., Feuerstein, M., Kop, W., Schor, K. and Arroyo, F. (2002) Individual and combined impacts of ergonomic and work organization factors in work-related musculoskeletal symptoms. Under review.

Jellema, P., van Tulder, M.W., van Poppel, M.N.M., Nachemsonm, A.L. and Bouterm, L.M. (2001) Lumbar supports for prevention and treatment of low back pain: A systematic review within the framework of the Cochrane Back Review Group. Spine, 26: 377–386.

Jin, K., Sorock, G.S., Courtney, T., Liang, Y., Yao, Z., Matz, S., Ge, L. (2000) Risk factors for work-related low back pain in the People's Republic of China. Int. J. Occup. Environ. Health, 6: 26–33.

Johnson, W.G., Baldwin, M.L. and Burton Jr., J.F. (1996) Why is the treatment of work-related injuries so costly? New evidence from California. Inquiry, 33: 53–65.

Katz, J.N., Stock, S.R., Evanoff, B.A., Rempel, D., Moore, J.S., Franzblau, A. and Gray, R.H. (2000) Classification criteria

and severity assessment in work-associated upper extremity disorders: Methods matter. Am. J. Ind. Med., 38: 369–372.

Kellet, K., Kellet, D. and Nordholm, L. (1991) Effects of an exercise program on sick leave due to back pain. Phys. Ther., 71: 283–293.

Kenny, D.T. (1999) Employers' perspectives on the provision of suitable duties in occupational rehabilitation. J. Occup. Rehabil., 9(4): 267–276.

Krause, N., Dasinger, L.K. and Neuhauser, F. (1998) Modified work and return to work: A review of the literature. J. Occup. Rehabil., 8: 113–140.

Leclaire, R., Esdaile, J.M., Suissa, S., Rossignol, M., Proulx, R. and Dupuis, M. (1996) Back school in a first episode of compensated acute low back pain: A clinical trial to assess efficacy and prevent relapse. Arch. Phys. Med. Rehabil., 77: 673–679.

Lincoln, A.E., Feuerstein, M., Shaw, W.S., Miller, V.I. and Wood, P.M. (2002) Impact of case manager training on worksite accommodations in workers' compensation claimants with upper extremity disorders. J. Occup. Environ. Med., 44: 237–245.

Linton, S.J. (1991) The manager's role in employees' successful return to work following back injury. Work Stress, 5: 189–195.

Linton, S.J. (1995) Developing psychologically based secondary prevention programs for low back pain. Orthop. Phys. Ther. Clin. N. Am., 4(3): 403–413.

Linton, S.J. and Andersson, T. (2000) Can chronic disability be prevented? A randomized trial of a cognitive-behavioral intervention and two forms of information for patients with spinal pain. Spine, 25: 2825–2831.

Linton, S.J., Melin, L. and Gotestam, K.G. (1984) Behavioral analysis of chronic pain and its management. Prog. Behav. Modif., 18: 1–42.

Linton, S.J., Bradley, L.A., Jensen, I., Spangfort, E. and Sundell, L. (1989) The secondary prevention of low back pain: A controlled study with follow-up. Pain, 36: 197–207.

Loisel, P., Abenhaim, L., Durand, P., Esdaile, J.M., Suissa, S., Gosselin, L., Simard, R., Turcotte, J. and Lemaire, J. (1997) A population-based, randomized clinical trial on back pain management. Spine, 22: 2911–2918.

Lonn, J.H., Glomsrod, B., Soukup, M.G., Bo, K. and Larsen, S. (1999) Active back school: Prophylactic management for low back pain. Spine, 24: 865–871.

Maher, C.G. (2000) A systematic review of workplace interventions to prevent low back pain. Aust. J. Physiother., 46: 259–269.

McIntosh, G., Frank, J.W., Hogg-Johnson, S., Bombardier, C. and Hall, H. (2000) Prognostic factors for time receiving workers' compensation benefits in a cohort of patients with low-back pain. Spine, 25: 147–157.

McLellan, R.K., Pransky, G. and Shaw, W.S. (2001) Disability management training for supervisors: A pilot intervention program. J. Occup. Rehabil., 11: 33–41.

Mueller, J.L. (1999) Returning to work through job accommodation: A case study. AAOHN J., 47(3): 120–129.

National Research Council (1998) Work-Related Musculoskeletal Disorders: A Review of the Evidence. National Academy Press, Washington, DC.

National Research Council and Institute of Medicine (2001) Musculoskeletal Disorders and the Workplace: Low Back and Upper Extremities. National Academy Press, Washington, DC.

Oleinick, A., Gluck, J.V. and Guire, K. (1996) Factors affecting first RTW following a compensable occupational back injury. Am. J. Ind. Med., 30: 540–555.

Personick, M.E. and Jackson, E.C. (1993) Recuperation time for work injuries, 1987–1991. Mon. Labor Rev., 16: 33–34.

Reddell, C.R., Congleton, J.J. and Huchingson, R.D. et al. (1992) An evaluation of a weight-lifting belt and back injury prevention training class for airline baggage handlers. Appl. Ergon., 23: 319–329.

Salazar, M.K. (1999) The occupational health nurse as case manager. AAOHN J., 47: 347.

Salkever, D.S., Goldman, H., Purushothaman, M. and Shinogle, J. (2000) Disability management, employee health and fringe benefits, and long-term-disability claims for mental disorders: an empirical exploration. Milbank Q., 78: 79–113.

Shaw, W.S., Feuerstein, M., Miller, V.I., Lincoln, A.E., Berger, R.H. and Wood, P.M. (2000) Ergonomics and workplace accommodation to improve outcomes in a large workers' compensation system. Proceedings of the RESNA 2000 Annual Conference, USA, 20, pp. 587–591.

Shaw, W.S., Feuerstein, M., Haufler, A.J., Berkowitz, S.M. and Lopez, M.S. (2001a) Working with low back pain: Problem-solving orientation and function. Pain, 93: 129–137.

Shaw, W.S., Feuerstein, M., Lincoln, A.E., Miller, V.I. and Wood, P.M. (2001b) Case management services for work related upper extremity disorders. AAOHN J., 49: 378–389.

Shaw, W.S., Pransky, G. and Fitzgerald, T.E. (2001c) Early prognosis for low back disability: Intervention strategies for health care providers. Disabil. Rehabil., 23: 815–828.

Shi, L. (1993) A cost-benefit analysis of a California county's back injury prevention program. Public Health Rep., 108: 204–211.

Shinohara, S., Okada, M., Keira, T., Ohwada, M., Niitsuya, M. and Aizawa, Y. (1998) Prognosis of accidental low back pain at work. Tohoku J. Exp. Med., 186: 291–302.

Shrey, D.E. (1996) Disability management in industry: The new

paradigm in injured worker rehabilitation. Disabil. Rehabil., 18: 408–414.

Silverstein, B.A., Stetson, D.S., Keyserling, W.M. and Fine, L.J. (1997) Work-related musculoskeletal disorders: Comparison of data sources for surveillance. Am. J. Ind. Med., 31: 600–608.

Soukup, M.G., Lonn, J., Glomsrod, B., Bo, K. and Larsen, S. (2001) Exercises and education as secondary prevention for recurrent low back pain. Physiother. Res. Int., 6: 27–39.

Strunin, L. and Boden, L.I. (2000) Paths of reentry: Employment experiences of injured workers. Am. J. Ind. Med., 38: 373–384.

Tousignant, M., Rossignol, M., Goulet, L. and Dassa, C. (2000) Occupational disability related to back pain: Application of a theoretical model of work disability using prospective cohorts of manual workers. Am. J. Ind. Med., 37: 410–422.

Van Poppel, M.N.M., Koes, B.W. and van der Ploeg, T. et al. (1998) Lumbar supports and education for the prevention of low back pain in industry. Occup. Environ. Med., 54: 841–847.

Walsh, N.E. and Schwartz, R.K. (1990) The influence of prophylactic orthoses on abdominal strength and low back injury in the workplace. Am. J. Phys. Med. Rehabil., 69: 245–250.

Webster, B.S. and Snook, S.H. (1994) The cost of 1989 workers' compensation low back claims. Spine, 19: 1111–1116.

Wiesel, S.W., Feffer, H.L. and Rothman, R.H. (1985) Industrial Low Back Pain. The Michie Company, Charlottesville, VA, pp. 602–641.

Wiesel, S.W., Boden, S.D. and Feffer, H.L. (1994) A quality-based protocol for management of musculoskeletal injuries. A ten-year prospective outcome study. Clin. Orthop., 301: 164–176.

Wood, D.J. (1987) Design and evaluation of a back injury prevention program within a geriatric hospital. Spine, 12: 77–82.

World Health Organization (1948) Constitution of the World Health Organization. WHO Basic Documents, Geneva.

Yassi, A., Tate, R., Cooper, J.E., Snow, C., Vallentyne, S. and Khokhar, J.B. (1995) Early intervention for back-injured nurses at a large Canadian tertiary care hospital: an evaluation of the effectiveness and cost benefits of a two-year pilot project. Occup. Med. (Lond.), 45(4): 209–214.

New Avenues for the Prevention of Chronic Musculoskeletal Pain and Disability
Pain Research and Clinical Management, Vol. 12
Edited by S.J. Linton

CHAPTER 15

The stepped care approach to chronic back pain

Benjamin H.K. Balderson * and Michael Von Korff

Center for Health Studies, Group Health Cooperative, Seattle, WA 98101, USA

Abstract: Stepped care provides a framework for allocating limited resources to the greatest effect on a population basis, while individualizing care. To illustrate the application of stepped care in the prevention of chronic musculoskeletal pain this chapter explores the utilization of a stepped care model for the provision of care in chronic back pain. Examining previous research on the treatment of chronic back pain three intervention steps are identified. Step 1 addresses fear–avoidance beliefs via education and reassurance to reduce such beliefs and the development of activity limitations. Step 2 directly addresses common activity limitations via education, reassurance and gradual return to activities guided by goal setting, problem solving and exercise. Step 3 efforts are reserved for the small but significant group of back pain patients who evidence work disability. In such cases treatment efforts focus on work performance and return to work, including identifying and treating mental health difficulties such as depression that may interfere with treatment efforts. Stepped care is exemplified with approaches being used in an ongoing intervention trial. Future research efforts in the area are suggested to develop stepped care as an approach to preventing disability associated with back pain.

1. Introduction

A stepped care approach guides care based on the observed outcome of each patient. It provides a framework allocating limited resources to the greatest effect on a population basis, while individualizing care. Stepped care is not an intervention in and of itself. Rather it is an approach to sequencing interventions so the intensity, complexity and cost of care are guided by each patient's need. A stepped care approach initiates care with the least expensive, intensive and restrictive treatment deemed sufficient to meet the patient's needs, increasing treatment intensity until a favorable outcome has been achieved (Donovan and Marlatt, 1993). Thus, stepped care seeks to optimize care at both the individual and population level by providing each patient the level and kind of care needed to achieve a favorable outcome, no more and no less. Stepped care approaches have been advocated for the treatment of a wide range of chronic conditions (Von Korff and Tiemens, 2000) including chronic back pain (Von Korff, 1999; Von Korff and Moore, 2001).

2. Levels of prevention

Preventive measures have typically been defined at three levels. Primary prevention refers to preventing the occurrence of the illness. Secondary prevention

---
* Correspondence to: B. Balderson, Center for Health Studies, Group Health Cooperative, 1730 Minor Avenue, Suite 1600, Seattle, WA 98101, USA. Tel.: +1 (206) 287-2803; Fax: +1 (206) 287-2871; E-mail: balderson.b@ghc.org

refers to limiting the expression and duration of the illness once it has occurred. Tertiary prevention refers to limiting the effects of the illness by diminishing the disability and handicap the illness produces (Perrin and MacLean, 1988). Stepped care, as it is currently conceptualized, provides a continuum of responses to an evolving chronic illness that encompasses both secondary and tertiary prevention.

3. Guiding stepped care by outcome

While there is increasing consensus that the primary outcome of back pain management is disability, intermediate outcomes that precede or contribute to disability may also be targeted using a stepped care approach. Drawing on data from studies conducted by our research group (Von Korff et al., 1993, 1998; Moore et al., 2000) patients' needs were identified and used to help guide the construction of a stepped care approach. In the case of back pain, simple and brief educational interventions may be sufficient to address fear–avoidance beliefs and assure resumption of normal activities for most patients (Step 1). However, some back pain patients continue to have residual activity limitations despite reassurance. These patients may benefit from being stepped

up to brief, structured interventions that increase physical exercise, support resumption of normal activities, and/or provide supervised exposure to the feared activity. A more intensive rehabilitative intervention may be appropriate for patients at risk of chronic work role disability, one that targets return to work and work role performance (Step 3). At Step 3, identification and treatment of co-morbid psychological illness that may interfere with rehabilitative efforts (e.g., major depression) may be beneficial in improving functional outcomes. This suggested stepped care approach for back pain is summarized in Table I.

4. A model of step care for chronic lower back pain

4.1. Step 1: identify and address patient worries, support self-care

Fear–avoidance is believed to be an important determinant of disability among back pain patients (Turk et al., 1983; Vlaeyen et al., 1995; Crombez et al., 1999). Fear–avoidance in back pain is characterized by beliefs that activity and movement will contribute to back pain and increase risk of re-injury. It is hy-

TABLE I

A stepped care approach for managing back pain in primary care

Level of care	Targeted patients	Objectives	Provider
Step 1	All back pain patients	Identify and address specific patient worries, encourage return to normal activities.	Primary care clinicians supported by minimal educational interventions.
Step 2	Back pain patients with activity limitations continuing at 6–8 weeks	Help patients identify difficulties, set functional goals and define and carry out plans to achieve their goals. Provide support for resumption of activities and exercise.	Case manager (e.g., nurse, physical therapist) in individual or group format, supported by self-care educational materials.
Step 3	Back pain patients with significant disability in work and/or family roles, patients with co-morbid mental illness which may impede recovery efforts	Interventions to restore work and family role function. Graded exercise program. Treatment of co-morbid mental illness if present.	Case manager and/or referral for rehabilitation. Psychological treatment (if indicated) in primary or specialty care.

TABLE II

Percent of primary care back pain patients reporting specific worries about back pain and activity limitations 2 months after a primary care back pain visit

Worries about back pain (n = 226)	
The wrong movement might cause a serious problem with my back.	64%
Avoiding unnecessary movements is the safest way to prevent back pain from worsening.	51%
My body is indicating that something is dangerously wrong.	50%
I might become disabled for a long time due to back pain.	47%
I am unable to do all the things normal people do because it is too easy to be injured.	44%
I am afraid of injuring myself if I exercise.	31%
My back pain may be due to a serious disease.	19%
Activity limitations (n = 481)	
Doing less housework.	45%
Difficulty standing for short periods of time.	38%
Difficulty walking short distances.	26%
Decreased sexual activity.	24%
Doing no housework.	23%

Data source: Von Korff et al., 1998; Moore et al., 2000.

pothesized that these beliefs lead to reduced activity and a subsequent increase in disability. Two months after seeking care for back pain, a large proportion of primary care back pain patients continue to have significant worries regarding back pain, movement and re-injury (see Table II). For example, almost two-thirds of surveyed patients continued to have concerns that a wrong movement might cause a serious problem with their back, and half believed that avoiding certain movements was the safest way to prevent back pain from worsening. It is easy to see how such perceptions could result in limiting activities and lead to increased disability. (Von Korff et al., 1998; Moore et al., 2000).

Recent randomized controlled trials of brief interventions have found significant benefits of addressing fear–avoidance beliefs and encouraging resumption of normal activities. For example, Burton et al. (1999) found that an educational booklet addressing fear–avoidance beliefs reduced fears and yielded a short-term reduction in disability. Increasing the intensity of such educational measures have proven even more beneficial. Von Korff and colleagues found in two randomized trials that brief group-format interventions addressing worries and concerns and advice to stay active reduced worry about back pain and reduced activity limitations

among primary care back pain patients. These effects were sustained at a 1-year follow-up (Von Korff et al., 1998; Moore et al., 2000; Von Korff and Moore, 2001). Addressing fear–avoidance beliefs early on constitutes an initial secondary prevention measure leading to a reduction in disability.

4.2. Example

We are currently fielding a randomized controlled trial that includes a brief intervention to address the patient's worries and concerns. Our present study intervenes with patients continuing to have moderate to high levels of self-reported disability 2 months after a primary care visit for back pain. In an effort to combine patient-centered care with a structured approach to soliciting worries based in common concerns, we have developed the following simple format. First, patients are asked open-ended questions to solicit current worries or concerns regarding their back pain. These worries are then explored so that the practitioner has a better understanding of the patient's concerns and how it motivates avoidance of activity. Next, patients are assessed for common worries similar to those listed in the upper half of Table II. We have found that this results in recognition of underlying concerns often not mentioned to other health-care providers. After identified worries are explored, the patient is provided with relevant information, delivered in a way that is sensitive to how ready they are to receive this type of information. The patient is encouraged to discuss this information further in an effort to promote understanding and integration into the patient's personal belief system. Finally, the patient is given written information to take home that addresses common concerns. These materials are intended to reinforce the initial discussion and to provide information that can be shared with family members.

4.3. Step 2: address activity limitations, support gradual activation and self-care

It is common for back pain patients to report continuing activity limitations two months after seeking care. As shown in the lower half of Table II, the percentage reporting doing no or less housework, decreased sexual activity, difficulty with walking or standing for short periods ranged from 23 to 45% (Von Korff et al., 1998; Moore et al., 2000). These kinds of activity limitations, while not indicative of total disability, suggest that many patients experience sustained decrements in quality of life due to back pain. Thus, in line with the hypothesized hierarchy of disability, a large percentage of people report fear–avoidance beliefs and a smaller but still significant percentage of patients report of activity limitations.

Burton et al. (1999), comparing two educational books, found that both books resulted in greater improvement on the Roland Disability Questionnaire when compared to a usual care group. However, there were no significant differences between the two educational groups in Roland scores. More intensive educational, activating approaches have shown significant effects on Roland disability scores at follow-up (Von Korff et al., 1998; Moore et al., 2000; Von Korff and Moore, 2001). Rossignol et al. (2000) also found that care coordination efforts that encouraged activation, yielded significant between-group differences in disability scores at a 6-month follow-up. Malmivaara et al. (1995) showed that advice to avoid bed rest and to continue routine activity as normally

as possible resulted in better functional outcomes than either advice to rest in bed for two days or back mobilizing exercises implemented during acute care. Moffett et al. (1999) comparing patients in usual care with patients assigned a physical therapist utilizing a structured exercise program, incorporating cognitive-behavioral principles and aims to increase activation and self-reliance, found significant between-group differences favoring the later group on the Roland Disability Questionnaire at a 12-month follow-up. Frost et al. (1995) compared a group of individuals advised to stay active to individuals who in addition to advice also had structured exercise and cognitive-behavioral intervention. They found that the combined advice–exercise group did significantly better on the Oswestry at 6-month and 2-year follow-up.

4.4. Example

In our current randomized control trial we are addressing common activity limitations by several approaches. It has been suggested that in efforts to support self-care of chronic illness, patient-centered approaches may be more successful than directive advice (Anderson, 1995). Thus, we allow the patient's aspirations and preferences to guide session content and goals. We begin by reassuring patients regarding common fears (see Step 1 above). Next, we assess activity limitations common to patients with back pain, assessing difficulties in work, household, self-care, social and recreational activities. Activities the patient may fear or avoid are directly addressed, providing education, reassurance regarding activity and exploring what is feared about the activities. Patients are led through an effort to establish which activity limitations have the most impact on their quality of life and what specific activities they wish to work on. Based on the patients' selected activity goal they are guided through weekly goal setting aimed at gradual activation. This goal-setting technique is integrated with physical therapy, which provides suggested exercises, stretches and body mechanics directly relevant to the patient's personal goals. Thus, this effort is a practitioner-guided, patient-centered approach to care addressing common activity limitations, guided by the patient's concerns and functional goals.

4.5. Step 3: address work disability, identify and treat clinical depression

Examining work disability, a smaller but significant minority of primary care patients (approaching 10%) reported significant work role disability or reported missing days from work due to back pain (Von Korff et al., 1993). Under stepped care, more complex problems require more complex and intense intervention efforts. Brief educational interventions have shown limited effects on work disability (Roland and Dixon, 1989). Brief activating interventions, capable of addressing common activity limitations, may not be sufficient to address significant work disability (Rossignol et al., 2000; Von Korff and Moore, 2001). However, it is less clear what might be an adequate intervention to address work disability.

For example, Malmivaara et al. (1995) found that advice to stay active was sufficient to find between-group differences in days off work when compared to a bed-rest group or an exercise group. Although this study gives a good indication of what may work in acute phases of back pain, advice alone may not be sufficient in chronic or recurrent pain populations. Indahl et al. (1995, 1998) found that advice to stay active, addressing body mechanics and fear of movement, resulted in return to work and reduced sicklisting when compared to a usual care group. Modification of this intervention by Hagen et al. (2000) also found significant changes in return to work and days of sickness compensation when compared to usual care. Linton and Anderson (2000) found that an educational pamphlet and a series of information packets to reduce injury fears were both less effective in decreasing the number of sick days than a cognitive-behavioral group combined with structured exercise.

These findings are encouraging, particularly given that the reviewed studies generally follow the lines that increasing intervention intensity enhances success in addressing work disability. However, there are some studies that do not show that increasing intensity or adding treatment components results in reduced work disability. For example, a complex multimodal cognitive-behavioral treatment program compared to usual care, examined by Haldorsen et al. (1998), did not find significant between-group differences in return to work despite significant changes in hypothesized intermediate variables such as work ability. Thus, it is not safe to assume that simply increasing intensity or changes in intermediate variables such as work ability will guarantee an increased rate of return to work.

4.6. Example

In our current randomized control trial we treat work disability as an important and high-priority activity limitation. In essence, treating work disability similar to other activity limitations but we attempt to increase its salience by having patients focus on activity limitations at work and guiding them toward setting return-to-work goals. Patients are provided education on how return to work relates to long-term health outcomes, reassuring patients regarding worries they may have about return to work. Next we assess specific activity difficulties or limitations they may be having at work and, where possible, provide education and reassurance. Patients are encouraged to set goals to increase work abilities. In this intervention, a physical therapist assesses current abilities in light of work duties and, if appropriate, tries to increase work abilities via training in body mechanics, activity pacing, stretching, exercise and gradual activation through weekly patient established goals. Often weekly goals set by patients are aimed at gradually increasing abilities by building strength via recommended exercises and slowly increasing time at work. Thus, the intervention seeks to increase a patient's motivation and confidence regarding return to work rather than the practitioner being highly directive in prescribing return-to-work activities. Hence, the intervention is guided by the goals set by the patient but patients are typically guided towards setting return to work as their highest priority.

Further, patients are screened for major depression. For those reporting symptoms of depression, treatment options are discussed with the option of referring the patient to appropriate treatment. This helps to address mental health problems that may impede progress of back pain treatment.

5. Future research

Although promising, the use of stepped care as an intervention model for back pain needs further research. As outlined above, our group is currently conducting a trial testing a theory-driven stepped care intervention for improving back pain outcome. This intervention is intended to limit disability rather than to prevent back pain. Our current intervention trial utilizes two kinds of providers, a doctorate in clinical psychology and a physical therapist. Efforts to further integrate this model into routine care may make it more feasible and readily adaptable by health care systems. Step 1 efforts to provide education, address fear–avoidance beliefs, and reassure patients may be appropriately addressed in the primary care visit. More intensive efforts at Step 2 and Step 3 of activating patients and reducing limitations may be more appropriately addressed in Physical Therapy, Behavioral Health, or Occupational Medicine.

Other areas needing further research are the timing of prevention efforts and targeting populations. The effectiveness of stepped care interventions may be enhanced by focusing on specific target populations and timing of intervention in relation to the onset of work disability. As the mechanisms of disability and how it develops are better understood, stepped care may be a useful framework for providing the optimal level of care to improve back pain outcome at both the patient and population level.

References

Anderson, R.M. (1995) Patient empowerment and the traditional medical model: a case of irreconcilable differences?. *Diabetes Care*, 18: 412–415.

Burton, A.K., Waddell, G., Tillotson, K.M. and Summerton, N. (1999) Information and advice to patient with back pain can have a positive effect: a randomized controlled trial of a novel educational booklet in primary care. Spine, 25: 115–120.

Cherkin, D., Deyo, R.A., Battie, M., Street, J. and Barlow, W. (1998) A comparison of physical therapy, chiropractic manipulation, and provision of an educational booklet for the treatment of patients with low back pain. N. Engl. J. Med., 339: 1021–1029.

Crombez, G., Vlaeyen, J.W.S., Heuts, P.H.T.G. and Lysens, R. (1999) Pain-related fear is more disabling than pain itself: Evidence on the role of pain-related fear in chronic back pain disability. Pain, 80: 329–339.

Donovan, D.M. and Marlatt, G.A. (1993) Recent developments in alcoholism behavioral treatment. Recent Dev. Alcohol., 11: 397–411.

Fordyce, W.E. (1987) Prevention of reinjury. Ergonomics, 30: 457–462.

Frost, H., Klaber Moffett, J.A., Moser, J.S. and Fairbank, J.C. (1995) Randomised controlled trial for evaluation of fitness programme for patients with chronic low back pain. Br. Med. J., 310: 151–154.

Hagen, E.M., Eriksen, H.R. and Ursin, H. (2000) Does early intervention with a light mobilization program reduce long-term sick leave for low back pain? Spine, 25: 1973–1976.

Haldorsen, E.M., Kronholm, K., Skouen, J.S. and Ursin, H. (1998) Multimodal cognitive behavioral treatment of patients sicklisted for musculoskeletal pain: a randomized controlled study. Scand. J. Rheumatol., 27: 16–25.

Indahl, A., Velund, L. and Reikeraas, O. (1995) Good prognosis for low back pain when left untampered: a randomized clinical trial. Spine, 20: 473–477.

Indahl, A., Haldorsen, E.H., Holm, S., Reikeras, O. and Ursin, H. (1998) Five-year follow-up study of a controlled clinical trial using light mobilization and an informative approach to low back pain. Spine, 23: 2625–2630.

Linton, S.J. and Anderson, T. (2000) Can chronic disability be prevented? A randomized trial of a cognitive-behavior intervention and two forms of information for patients with spinal pain. Spine, 25: 2825–2831.

Ljunggren, A.E., Weber, H., Kogstad, O., Thom, E. and Kirkesola, G. (1997) Effect of exercise on sick leave due to low back pain: a randomized, comparative, long-term study. Spine, 22: 1610–1616.

Malmivaara, A., Hakkinen, U., Aro, T., Heinrichs, M.-L., Koskenniemi, L., Kuosma, E., Lappi, S., Paloheimo, R., Servo, C. and Vaaranen, V. (1995) The treatment of acute low back pain — bed rest, exercises, or ordinary activity? N. Engl. J. Med., 332(6): 351–355.

Moffett, J.K., Torgerson, D., Bell-Syer, S., Jackson, D., Llewlyn-Phillips, H., Farrin, A. and Barber, J. (1999) Randomized controlled trial of exercise for low back pain: clinical outcomes, costs and preferences. Br. Med. J., 319: 279–283.

Moore, J.E., Von Korff, M., Cherkin, D., Saunders, K. and Lorig, K. (2000) A randomized trial of a cognitive–behavioral program for enhancing back pain self-care in a primary care setting. Pain, 88: 145–153.

Perrin, J.M. and MacLean Jr., W.E. (1988) Children with chronic illness: the prevention of dysfunction. Pediatr. Clin. North Am., 35: 1325–1337.

Roland, M. and Dixon, J. (1989) Randomized controlled trial of an education booklet for patients presenting with back pain in general practice. J. R. Coll. Gen. Pract., 39: 244–246.

Rossignol, M., Abenhaim, L., Seguin, P., Neveu, A., Collet, J.P., Ducruet, T. and Shapiro, S. (2000) Coordination of primary health care for back pain. A randomized controlled trial. Spine, 23: 251–259.

Turk, D.C., Meichenbaum, D. and Genest, M. (1983) Pain and Behavioral Medicine: A Cognitive Behavioral Perspective. Guilford Press, New York, NY.

Vlaeyen, J.W.S., Kole-Snijders, A.M.J., Boeren, R.G.B. and van Eek, H. (1995) Fear of movement/(re)injury in chronic low back pain and its relation to behavioral performance. Pain, 62: 363–372.

Von Korff, M. (1999) Pain management in primary care: an individualized stepped care approach. In: R. Gatchel and D. Turk (Eds.), Psychosocial Factors in Pain: Evolution and Revolutions. Guilford Press, New York, NY, pp. 360–373.

Von Korff, M. and Moore, J.E. (2001) Stepped care for back pain: activating approaches for primary care. Ann. Intern. Med., 134: 911–917.

Von Korff, M. and Tiemens, B. (2000) Individualized stepped care of chronic illness. West. J. Med., 172: 133–137.

Von Korff, M., Deyo, R.A., Cherkin, D. and Barlow, W. (1993) Back pain in primary care: outcomes at one year. Spine, 18: 855–862.

Von Korff, M., Moore, J.E., Lorig, K., Cherkin, D.C., Saunders, K., Gonzales, V.M., Laurent, D., Rutter, C. and Comite, F. (1998) A randomized trial of layperson-led self-management group intervention for back pain patients in primary care. Spine, 23: 2608–2615.

New Avenues for the Prevention of Chronic Musculoskeletal Pain and Disability
Pain Research and Clinical Management, Vol. 12
Edited by S.J. Linton
© *2002 Elsevier Science B.V. All rights reserved*

CHAPTER 16

Educational and informational approaches

A. Kim Burton [1,*] and Gordon Waddell [2]

[1] *Spinal Research Unit, University of Huddersfield, Huddersfield HD1 3DH, UK*
[2] *Glasgow Nuffield Hospital, Glasgow, UK*

Abstract: This chapter reviews and discusses written educational material for back pain, and provides empirical evidence about the information and advice that should be given to patients with back pain. Traditional educational material about back pain has been based on a biomedical model, often without considering its impact on patients. From a biopsychosocial perspective, such traditional information and advice can convey negative messages about back pain with damaging effects on patients' beliefs and behaviours. However, carefully selected and presented information and advice about back pain in line with current management guidelines *can* have a positive effect on patients' beliefs and clinical outcomes. Written educational material is just one way of achieving this and, whilst its effect size may be small, its very low per-patient cost may render it highly cost-effective. Nevertheless, there is considerable scope for refinement of the messages and their method of delivery within the whole scope of health care, and the contribution of innovative educational interventions for back pain deserves serious further scientific investigation.

1. Background

The emergence of the concept of evidence-based medicine, and the attendant increased 'openness' of medical practice, has fostered an increasing interest in patient information. The quantity of patient-information material, covering most medical conditions, is now vast and available in multimedia format including pamphlets, books, videos, and Internet sites. However, this material is of widely varying quality (Coulter, 1998), much of it simply representing the views of individuals or interest groups without any firm evidence base. Over recent years health educationalists have begun to address this problem by investigating the nature and effectiveness of patient education.

The Toronto Statement on the Relationship Between Communication and Practice and Outcomes (Simpson et al., 1991) listed a number of key issues. It was recognised that communication problems in medicine are both important and common, and that patient anxiety, dissatisfaction and uncertainty are related to a lack of information; suitable explanations can diminish anxiety and psychological distress, and the quality of information is related to positive health outcomes; greater participation by the patient can improve satisfaction and outcomes. Whilst the concern was predominantly with the clinical contact between doctor and patient, it is reasonable to assume that the same principles apply to information provided in other ways.

The field of health informatics is huge and com-

---

* Correspondence to: A. Kim Burton, Spinal Research Unit, University of Huddersfield, 30 Queen Street, Huddersfield HD1 2SP, UK. Tel.: +44 (1484) 535200; Fax: +44 (1484) 435744; E-mail: kim@spineresearch.org.uk

plex, and serves a number of purposes: health promotion and disease prevention, encouragement of self-care to reduce inappropriate service use, presentation of treatment options to ensure appropriateness of (and satisfaction with) treatment decisions, and improvement in effectiveness of clinical care. Poor information, or even worse mis-information, can adversely affect health behaviour and health outcomes (Coulter et al., 1998). However, the primary focus for most clinical patient information seems to have been on shared decision-making and satisfaction with care rather than direct attempts to influence outcomes, and studies evaluating patient information have tended to concentrate on matters such as acceptability, comprehensibility, accuracy, comprehensiveness and currency, through techniques such as patient focus groups (Coulter et al., 1998; Scotland's Working Backs Partnership, 2000).

Patient information is frequently used as part of a multi-modal approach to a health problem, and it then becomes difficult to determine what proportion of any effect is due to the educational component and how much is due to other aspects of the intervention. Simply mailing an information booklet on minor illness has been investigated recently through two randomised trials in the UK (Heaney et al., 2001; Little et al., 2001b). Both studies included over 4000 general-practice patients randomised between the booklet and various controls, with the intention of investigating the influence of information that encouraged self-management of 40 common illnesses on consultation rates. The booklet, *What should I do?* was developed in The Netherlands and translated into English. One trial (Heaney et al., 2001) found no effect on health care services from either the experimental booklet or a similar control. The other trial (Little et al., 2001b) found a small reduction in consultation rates for some illnesses together with an increased level of confidence in managing illness among patients receiving the experimental booklet. Both studies, though, concluded that this strategy had limited use in attempting to reduce the number of consultations for minor self-limiting illness. This finding should not be surprising, since it is somewhat unlikely that receiving information about illness at a time when the patients

were not ill would affect future behaviour (Fitzmaurice, 2001). Delivery of information at the time of consultation may be an entirely different matter, and may have a variety of positive influences on health or health care. Nevertheless, the acquisition of self-management skills may depend on patients' 'readiness to change' (as has been shown for cognitive behavioural therapy; Dijkstra et al., 2001).

It is not possible adequately to review the entire field of information and education here, or even that for musculoskeletal disorders; the range of approaches, target audiences, and environments is simply too diverse. Instead, the focus is on information in the field of low back pain. Even with this limitation, the amount of material and implementation strategies is unwieldy so, following a general introduction, this review will largely be limited to written material intended to influence clinical and occupational outcomes.

2. Introduction

The primary prevention of back pain may transpire to be an unrealistic goal (Burton, 1997), and a recent systematic review has found that evidence to support the possibility of prevention is limited to strategies using exercise (Linton and van Tulder, 2001). Accepting that prevention of the incidence of back pain is at best limited, it is logical to transfer attention to consideration of the costly consequences of back pain, these being disability, work absence and chronicity (Burton, 1997). The progressive rise in disability due to back pain in the latter half of the 20th century, in the absence of increased prevalence rates, is a clear indication that traditional clinical management is at best suboptimal and at worst adds to iatrogenic disability (Burton, 1997; Waddell, 1998). A novel approach, that takes account of the biopsychosocial model (Waddell, 1987) and established psychosocial risk factors for chronicity (Kendall et al., 1997; Pincus et al., 2002), proposes that interventions should focus on interventions designed to reduce (or remove) 'obstacles to recovery' (Burton and Main, 2000; Main and Burton, 2000).

The proposed conceptual framework is based on identification of 'flags' (or markers) for those factors that have a detrimental influence on outcomes, and include clinical 'yellow flags' (e.g. psychological distress, dysfunctional beliefs, inadequate coping strategies), occupational 'blue flags' (perceived features of work, e.g. high demand/low control, poor social support, lack of job satisfaction, perceptions about the safety of return to work), and occupational 'black flags' (e.g. sickness policy, management style, benefit systems; Main and Burton, 2000). A basic management strategy for back pain, that takes account of obstacles to recovery, would be to provide a psychosocial preventative approach to the individual, promoting self-help, establishing confidence and reducing unnecessary apprehension (Burton and Main, 2000). Among numerous clinical interventions that could accommodate this approach, provision of appropriate information and advice should be seen as central. Whilst the basic content of the information will be the same, the means of implementation will vary depending on such issues as the target group, the site of delivery and cost implications.

There is now compelling and consistent evidence that back pain should not be treated with rest, but should be managed by protocols that include advice to stay active (Waddell et al., 1997). This is reflected in all national clinical guidelines for the management of low back pain which consistently recommend activity as opposed to rest (Koes et al., 2001). Whilst physicians' recommendations still vary widely and reflect personal attitudes as well as patients' clinical symptoms (Rainville et al., 2000), some measure of adoption of the 'activity versus rest' concept by primary care physicians is emerging (Frankel et al., 1999). Interestingly, dissemination of the same messages to patients (using multimedia approaches) can significantly shift patients' beliefs in a positive direction (Buchbinder et al., 2001; WorkingBacks Scotland, unpublished data). Specific education of physicians (as opposed to guidelines dissemination) can improve perceived physician knowledge, confidence, and patient-reassuring behaviour in the treatment of low back pain (Cherkin et al., 1991b), but that did not result in significant improvements in

patient satisfaction or clinical outcomes (Cherkin et al., 1991a). It may be that direct education of the patients themselves is actually a more promising route for influencing outcomes.

It has been questioned whether family doctors' management matched guidelines (Little et al., 1996) and whether health services for back pain have actually changed (Underwood et al., 1997). However, some recent surveys demonstrate that family doctors are now more aware of the guidelines, and there is a shift from prescription of rest to advice on staying active (Frankel et al., 1999; Schers et al., 2000). Two recent controlled trials show that guidelines can be implemented in primary care and can improve clinical outcomes for back pain (Rossignol et al., 2000; McGuirk et al., 2001).

Written advice about back pain in the form of booklets or pamphlets is the easiest and least expensive direct approach, and has generated a plethora of publications. This review aimed to explore the scientific evidence on written education for back pain. A systematic search of the literature revealed seven controlled trials of written material that had been designed to have a specific influence on clinical and/or work outcomes. Numerous other trials where an educational component (non-written) was built into a multi-modal intervention were excluded from the review. An additional trial of a multimedia public educational campaign was, however, included because it was based primarily on the messages of a patient booklet and included distribution of that written material. Whilst all the studies had the common element of written material designed to educate the patient about low back pain, they varied in terms of subject populations, method of delivery and educational material. All but two of the trials were of randomised design.

3. Trials of written material for back pain

3.1. Roland and Dixon (1989)

3.1.1. Study details
A randomised controlled trial (RCT) in five primary-care group practices in the UK. Low back pain pa-

tients (with no restriction on duration of symptoms) were randomised to receive either an experimental booklet or no booklet, together with usual care. Patients were randomised at first consultation for that episode, and those randomised to the booklet (an earlier version of *The Back Book*) received it at that time from the doctor. The main outcomes concerned clinical referral patterns and work loss over the 1-year follow-up period, and a mailed questionnaire at 1 year was used to establish patient reactions.

3.1.2. Educational material
The booklet comprised 21 pages in A5 format. The messages betray its vintage; following a brief anatomical introduction, it gave a strong message that rest for severe pain will speed recovery. However, it was said that back pain is rarely due to serious disease. There was considerable practical advice on daily activities (mostly concerned with reducing physical stress), and some back-specific exercises and relaxation are recommended. Despite the insistence on rest, there was a central self-help message with a subliminal message not to bother the doctor unless the pain is not improving. The language was simple and unambiguous with partly humorous, partly instructive illustrations.

3.1.3. Results
The booklet had no immediate effect on consultation rates for back pain, but between 2 weeks and 1 year significantly fewer in the booklet group consulted with back pain (36% versus 42%). There was no significant influence on work loss, but referral rates (for physiotherapy and to hospital) were less in the booklet group (almost reaching statistical significance at the 5% level). Almost all patients said they had read the booklet, and 84% said they found it useful. Scores on a test of knowledge of back pain were significantly higher in the booklet group. It was concluded that the booklet had some effect in altering both the knowledge and behaviour of patients with back pain.

3.2. Symonds et al. (1995)

3.2.1. Study details
A prospective controlled trial of a psychosocial pamphlet in industry. In a quasi-experimental design a pamphlet (*Back pain — do not suffer needlessly*) was broadcast to all employees (not just those with back pain) at one factory, whilst a traditional nonspecific 'good posture' pamphlet was broadcast in one control factory, and a second control had no intervention. The pamphlets were distributed at baseline and again at 4 months. Outcomes were measured at 12 months using questionnaires for beliefs about the inevitable consequences of back pain, and company records for work absence.

3.2.2. Educational material
The experimental pamphlet, an A4-size card folded in three, was peer reviewed and piloted before the trial. The fear–avoidance model was used as the theoretical basis for the messages, the main aim of which was to encourage early activity by emphasising that early return to work is not detrimental to recovery. The dichotomy between 'coper' and 'avoider' was used to highlight that individuals who confronted and carried on with life when experiencing back pain would benefit more than avoiders, who faced becoming disabled. The pamphlet was designed to change passive beliefs and attitudes towards back pain, using blunt, positive messages written in simple language. For example: 'Usually back pain has a simple cause and often gets better quickly of its own accord'; 'The *avoider* believes that hurting always means further damage — it does not'; 'The *coper* deals with the pain by being positive and taking little time off work'. There was no anatomical information, no diagnostic labelling, and no illustrations. It was hypothesised that the pamphlet would reduce what was termed 'extended absence' (absence beyond that initially prescribed by a doctor (1–2 weeks)) and beliefs about the inevitable consequences of back pain.

3.2.3. Results

In the company whose employees received the experimental pamphlet, a significant reduction occurred in the number of spells with extended absence and in the number of days of absence (70% and 60%, respectively) compared with extrapolated values. A concomitant positive shift in beliefs concerning the locus of pain control and the inevitable consequences of low back pain was found. The employees at the factory receiving the traditional pamphlet experienced a statistically significant negative shift in inevitability beliefs.

3.3. Cherkin et al. (1996)

3.3.1. Study details

In a large Health Maintenance Organisation (primary care), back pain patients were randomised to receive usual care, an educational booklet, or a 15-min session with a nurse (plus booklet). Outcome measures included satisfaction with care, perceived knowledge, participation in exercise, functional status, symptom relief, and health care usage assessed at 1, 3, 7 and 52 weeks after the intervention.

3.3.2. Educational material

The experimental booklet (*Back in action — a guide to understanding your low back pain and learning what you can do about it*) was developed especially for this trial. It comprised 17 pages and was similar in size to A4 folded in three. It comprised somewhat conventional biomedical information based on current scientific knowledge, addressed patients' concerns about causation, prognosis, the role of imaging and referrals, and suggested actions to promote recovery, although it also emphasised the value of return to normal activities as soon as possible. Two pages of traditional anatomy introduced the text, followed by question/answer sections on expectations and treatment. Advice was given about communicating with the employer to facilitate work return, and active exercise was advocated along with a self-completion exercise progress log. Cartoon illustrations were used to illustrate some points. The nurse-led educational intervention was given by nurses who had had about 16 h training (including 4 h relevant reading and an interactive session). In a 20-min educational session the nurse verbally presented the same messages as the booklet and also gave the booklet to the patient. This was followed by a telephone call after 3 days to give further reassurance and answer questions.

3.3.3. Results

The nurse intervention resulted in higher patient satisfaction and higher perceived knowledge than usual care or booklet-only groups; self-reported exercise was higher after 1 week (97% versus 65%) although this was not maintained on longer-term follow-up. There were no significant differences among the groups in worry, symptoms, functional status, or health care use at any follow-up point. It was concluded that the findings challenged the value of educational approaches in reducing functional impact or health care use related to back pain.

3.4. Cherkin et al. (1998)

3.4.1. Study details

Acute back pain patients in primary care were randomly allocated to physical therapy (McKenzie method), chiropractic manipulation, or an educational booklet, which was really used as an ineffective control in view of the findings of the previous study (Cherkin et al., 1996). Outcomes (bothersomeness, dysfunction, work loss and cost of care) were assessed over a 2-year period.

3.4.2. Educational material

The educational booklet (*Back in action — a guide to understanding your low back pain and learning what you can do about it*) was that used in Cherkin et al. (1996).

3.4.3. Results

The chiropractic and physical therapy groups had marginally improved symptoms at 4 weeks compared with the booklet group. Differences in physical dysfunction among the groups were small, and approached significance only at 1 year, with greater dysfunction in the booklet group compared with the others. There were no differences between the groups for days of reduced activity, days off work or recurrences of back pain. More patients receiving physical therapy were satisfied with their care than in the booklet group (75% versus 30%), but the costs for the booklet group were about one third of those for the other groups. It was concluded that physical therapy and chiropractic had only marginally better outcomes than those receiving the booklet; but whether the extra cost is justifiable was open to question.

3.5. Burton et al. (1999)

3.5.1. Study details
Primary care patients with acute or recurrent back pain were randomised to receive one of two booklets; a novel evidence-based booklet (*The Back Book*) or a traditional booklet (*Handy Hints*). The trial design was double-blind with questionnaire follow-up at 2 weeks, 3 months and 1 year. The analysis focused on clinically important changes in beliefs and self-rated disability.

3.5.2. Educational material
The starting point for development of *The Back Book* was the original booklet of the same name used by Roland and Dixon (1989), and also incorporated the messages and concepts introduced in the pamphlet of Symonds et al. (1995). It was produced by a multi-author team covering the major disciplines involved in back care; the information from the previous material was updated and supplemented by reference to the scientific evidence base. Following peer review it was piloted on primary care patients. The final version was linked to the Royal College of General Practitioners' Clinical Guidelines for the Management of Acute Low Back Pain, 1996 (Royal College of General Practitioners, 1996), published by a UK government publisher and made available commercially (Roland et al., 1996). The main aim of the booklet was to change beliefs and behaviour, which is quite different from imparting information (Cedraschi et al., 1996). The 23-page A5-sized format

presented its simple messages in an uncompromising style; there was no attempt to give anatomical detail and no specific exercises were advocated; illustrations were general depictions of activity, and the text was sprinkled with post-it notes emphasising the main messages (e.g. 'Use it or loose it', 'Bed rest is bad for backs'). Pilot studies showed that this approach was well accepted by patients and capable of shifting beliefs about back pain (Burton et al., 1996). In view of this being the only randomised trial comparing two booklets giving very different messages (traditional and novel), their main concepts are summarised in Table I. It was hypothesised that the experimental booklet would have an effect on disability (through shifting fear–avoidance beliefs) but not on pain.

3.5.3. Results
Compared with the control group, patients receiving the experimental booklet showed a substantial and statistically significant early improvement in beliefs, which was maintained at 1 year. A greater proportion of patients with an initially high fear–avoidance beliefs score who received the experimental booklet had clinically important improvement in fear–avoidance beliefs about physical activity at 2 weeks, followed by a clinically important improvement in self-rated disability at 3 months. There was no effect on pain. There were insufficient patients off work to draw any conclusions about the effect of the booklet on return to work. It was concluded that carefully selected and presented information and advice about back pain can have a positive effect on patients' beliefs and clinical outcomes. Looking at clinically important effects in individual patients can provide further insights into the management of back pain.

3.6. Hazard et al. (2000)

3.6.1. Study details
A pamphlet was mailed at random to workers filing a back-related report of injury within 11 days of the event. The control group received no pamphlet, but both groups received usual care. Outcomes, measured as back pain, work status, health care use,

TABLE I

Comparison of the main messages given in the experimental and control booklets in Burton et al. (1999)

The Back Book (experimental intervention)	*Handy hints* (control booklet)
There is no sign of any serious disease.	Imparts information rather than tackling beliefs/behaviours.
The spine is strong. There is no suggestion of any permanent damage. Even when it is very painful that does not mean that there is any serious damage to your back: hurt does not mean harm.	Traditional biomedical concepts of spinal anatomy, injury and damage. (Implicit messages that the spine is easily damaged, that medicine should diagnose and treat the problem, but there is often permanent damage.)
Back pain is a symptom that your back is simply not moving and working quite as it should. It is unfit or out of condition.	Avoid activity when in pain; your GP may advise bed rest.
There are a number of treatments that can help to control the pain, but lasting relief then depends on your own effort.	Describes further investigations and surgery. (Reinforces the message that back pain is a medical problem, and that there is little the patient can do.)
Recovery depends on getting your back moving and working again and restoring normal function and fitness. The sooner you get active, the sooner your back will feel better.	Concentrates on pain rather than activity. (Implicit message that restoring activity and function must await relief of pain.)
Positive attitudes are important. Do not let your back take over your life. 'Copers' suffer less at the time, get better quicker and have less trouble in the long term.	Encourages patient to be passive.

and pamphlet impact were assessed at three and six months through telephone interviews. The setting of this study differed from all the other studies reviewed here in that these were entirely workers compensation patients and the pamphlet was posted from the compensation board.

3.6.2. Educational material

The pamphlet (*Good news about low back pain*) was an A4-size sheet folded in three. Developed by compiling information from recent publications, its central goal was encouraging self-care and quick return to activities and work. Similar in style to the Symonds et al. (1995) pamphlet, the presentation was essentially short bullet-point statements, along with a section on 'danger' signs. There was no anatomical information, and no illustrations were included. However, although the advice and messages were to some extent comparable to the Burton et al. (1999) booklet there was much less attempt to challenge and change dysfunctional beliefs.

3.6.3. Results

The pamphlet had no statistically significant impact on pain severity or reduction, health care visits, or work absence. Over 50% of pamphlet recipients thought that it had provided useful information. Whilst one third thought it helped them recover, only 11% thought it had helped them return to work more quickly (yet they did not actually have any less work loss). It was concluded that a psychosocial pamphlet did not prevent post-injury pain, health care use or work absence in this study population.

3.7. Linton and Andersson (2000)

3.7.1. Study details

Acute or subacute back pain patients (from primary care and newspaper advertisements), who perceived themselves at risk for developing a chronic problem, were randomised to receive a six-session cognitive behavioural intervention or one of two forms of information (a pamphlet or a more extensive information package comprising six instalments) which were used as controls for the main intervention. All groups continued to receive usual care. The key self-reported outcomes at 1 year were absenteeism and health care usage, along with pain, function, fear–avoidance beliefs and cognitions.

3.7.2. Educational material

The pamphlet was a direct translation of the Symonds et al. (1995) pamphlet into Swedish. The cognitive behavioural intervention comprised six structured group sessions organised to activate participants and promote coping. The extensive informational package comprised six packets of traditional information based on a back school approach.

3.7.3. Results

All groups reported benefit. The risk for long-term sick leave was significantly and substantially lowered for the cognitive behavioural intervention, and these participants demonstrated significantly reduced physician/therapist visits compared with the other groups. All three groups tended to improve in terms of pain, fear–avoidance beliefs, and cognitions. Whether or not the general improvements seen in all groups would have occurred without the interventions could not be answered. Approximately a quarter of the pamphlet group reported the information to be very helpful. It was concluded that this may represent an encouraging benefit given the low cost and time saving, but the improvements were small compared to the cognitive behavioural group.

3.8. Buchbinder et al. (2001)

3.8.1. Study details

This study was a controlled quasi-experimental trial of a population-based, state-wide public health intervention. In essence, it built on the concepts introduced by Symonds et al. (1995) in that psychosocial messages were broadcast to a general population rather than a clinical back pain population. The intervention was implemented over 2.5 years in Victoria, Australia, with a neighbouring state acting as the control. Outcomes were beliefs about the inevitable consequences of back pain (elicited by telephone

surveys of the general population, and by postal surveys of general practitioners), incidence of workers' financial compensation claims for back pain, rate of days compensated, and medical payments for back pain and other claims (taken from the insurer's claims database).

3.8.2. Educational material

The entire public health campaign was based on the messages in *The Back Book* (Roland et al., 1996). The multimedia campaign comprised prime time television commercials featuring international and national medical experts, and national sporting and television personalities, who endorsed the benefits of staying active, not resting for prolonged periods, and remaining at work, supplemented by radio and printed advertisements, billboards, posters, seminars, workplace visits, and publicity articles. *The Back Book* was made widely available in 13 languages, whilst doctors in Victoria were provided with evidence-based guidelines that promoted the same messages as the rest of the campaign. The intensity of the campaign varied during the study period, and ceased some months before the evaluation.

3.8.3. Results

In Victoria, population beliefs about back pain became statistically significantly more positive between successive surveys, but there was no such change in the control state. Beliefs about back pain also improved among doctors. There was a concomitant decline in the number of claims for back pain, rates of days compensated, and medical payments for claims over the duration of the campaign.

3.9. Little et al. (2001a)

3.9.1. Study details

Sequential patients attending general practitioners with low back pain were randomised to receive either a booklet, verbal exercise advice from the doctor, booklet plus advice, or neither. All groups were given advice to keep as mobile as possible, to minimise bed rest and take simple analgesics. The primary outcome was ascertainment of pain and function by a telephone call during the first week and after the third week. In addition, satisfaction and knowledge were measured.

3.9.2. Educational material
The 10-page booklet (*Back Home*) was professionally printed in one-third A4 size. The messages covered the traditional biomedical subjects of anatomy and physical causes, not all of which were strictly evidence-based (e.g. sitting was given as a 'major cause of pain'); the strength of the spine was emphasised along with the limited role of radiographs, and a good prognosis was noted. The predominant focus was practical hints (with simple illustrations) on how to perform normal activities of daily living. An active management approach was, though, incorporated into the traditional messages with advice to minimise bed rest, keep mobile, and progressively increase activity/exercise. Return to work whilst symptomatic was mildly encouraged, but 'great care' was recommended with bending, sitting and lifting. The verbal advice from the doctor was to take exercise as soon as the pain allowed, and to aim for regular aerobic exercise in the longer term.

3.9.3. Results
Compared with the control, during the first week there were modest reductions in pain/function by provision of either the booklet or advice to exercise, but much less effect was found for the combination of booklet and exercise advice. There was no significant difference between the groups by week 3, when 58% reported being back to normal. Satisfaction was increased in booklet and exercise groups, and the booklet also increased knowledge. It was concluded that it may not be helpful to provide detailed information booklet and advice together, where the amounts and formats of the information differ.

3.10. Summary of review

It is difficult to draw wide-ranging conclusions from these studies. The results presented reveal considerable discrepancy over the effectiveness of written material about back pain, which probably derive from methodological differences as well as the material tested.

The study populations studied varied between patients in primary care (Roland and Dixon, 1989; Cherkin et al., 1996, 1998; Burton et al., 1999; Linton and Andersson, 2000; Little et al., 2001a), workers compensation patients (Hazard et al., 2000b), working non-patients (Symonds et al., 1995), and a general population that included patients (Buchbinder et al., 2001). Consequently the method of delivery varied: for some the booklets were broadcast to a population (Symonds et al., 1995; Buchbinder et al., 2001) or were simply mailed (Hazard et al., 2000b), whilst the remainder were given by a clinician at consultation (Roland and Dixon, 1989; Cherkin et al., 1996, 1998; Burton et al., 1999; Linton and Andersson, 2000; Little et al., 2001a).

The outcome variables were not consistent across studies. Some concerned clinical outcomes (Cherkin et al., 1996, 1998; Burton et al., 1999; Linton and Andersson, 2000; Little et al., 2001a), whilst others also involved psychometric change (Symonds et al., 1995; Burton et al., 1999; Linton and Andersson, 2000; Buchbinder et al., 2001), and some concerned work-related and/or health care outcomes (Roland and Dixon, 1989; Symonds et al., 1995; Hazard et al., 2000b; Buchbinder et al., 2001). The chosen outcome points also varied. One study considered only short-term outcomes (1 and 3 weeks; Little et al., 2001a), whilst two considered long-term outcomes (2 years[+]; Cherkin et al., 1998; Buchbinder et al., 2001). The remainder mainly assessed 12-months outcomes, though some included interim points (Cherkin et al., 1996; Burton et al., 1999; Hazard et al., 2000b), in one of which short-term outcomes were not maintained (Cherkin et al., 1996).

The format of the publications (which might influence the intensity of the messages) was not consistent: three studies used a brief pamphlet (Symonds et al., 1995; Hazard et al., 2000b; Linton and Andersson, 2000); six studies used a substantial booklet (Roland and Dixon, 1989; Cherkin et al., 1996, 1998; Burton et al., 1999; Buchbinder et al., 2001; Little et al., 2001a), but in one of these, the booklet was only a part of a much larger intervention (Buchbinder et al., 2001).

The method of control varied also: some studies compared different types of written material (Symonds et al., 1995; Burton et al., 1999) whilst others compared written material with another form of intervention (Cherkin et al., 1996, 1998; Linton and Andersson, 2000; Little et al., 2001a), and four studies compared the educational effect with 'usual care' (Roland and Dixon, 1989; Hazard et al., 2000b; Buchbinder et al., 2001; Little et al., 2001a).

There were however similarities. All the studies were well conducted and included adequate numbers, though two were a quasi-experimental design (Symonds et al., 1995; Buchbinder et al., 2001). The messages in all studies were ostensibly rather similar in that they promoted activity and self-care, though one older booklet included a message to rest (Roland and Dixon, 1989), whilst four were overtly psychosocial and specifically tackled fear–avoidance beliefs (Symonds et al., 1995; Burton et al., 1999; Linton and Andersson, 2000; Buchbinder et al., 2001).

Three interventions that were particularly effective (Symonds et al., 1995; Burton et al., 1999; Buchbinder et al., 2001) shared not only their messages but also the literary style and uncompromising manner in which they were presented. Yet the Swedish application of this concept (Linton and Andersson, 2000) did not produce the same clear-cut result, even if it did influence beliefs to some extent. The success of the early trial (Roland and Dixon, 1989) is somewhat counter-intuitive; perhaps the patients selected information that suited them from the somewhat mixed messages offered. The booklet in the other successful trial (Little et al., 2001a) also presented somewhat mixed messages, but the study design meant that it was presented under a background of physician advice to stay active and minimise bed rest. Of the interventions that were not successful, two used a booklet that was informative in nature rather than directed specifically at changing beliefs, and was somewhat traditional in style and content (Cherkin et al., 1996, 1998), whilst another used a

particularly brief pamphlet that was also informative in nature (Hazard et al., 2000b).

From the available evidence it would seem that educational interventions can have a psychosocial influence that has the potential to influence both clinical and work-related outcomes, but it is likely that this is highly dependent on the quality and clarity of the messages, and the style in which they are presented. The effect size is likely to be modest at best, but placed in the population context has the potential to offer substantial rewards.

4. Other musculoskeletal disorders

No controlled trials of written educational material directed at musculoskeletal disorders outside the field of back pain were found. However, a booklet for whiplash-associated disorders, *The Whiplash Book* (Waddell et al., 2001), has recently been produced. Whilst this new booklet has not yet been subjected to a randomised trial, pilot studies have shown that it has a statistically significant effect in shifting beliefs about whiplash in a positive direction and it is well accepted by patients, the vast majority of whom said they found the (active management) messages helpful (T. McClune et al., Huddersfield, unpublished data).

A version of the Symonds et al. (1995) back pain pamphlet has been written to address upper-limb disorders, and is currently being evaluated in an occupational health study; however no data on efficacy are yet available (S. Bartys et al., Huddersfield, personal communication).

5. Discussion

A recent review of clinical guidelines for the management of back pain in primary care (Koes et al., 2001) found that consistent recommendations are early and gradual activation, avoidance of bed rest and recognition of psychosocial factors for chronicity. Patient advice and information is seen to play an important role: patients should be reassured that they do not have a serious disease, that the prognosis is generally favourable (although recurrence is not unusual), and that activity is safe and desirable (Koes et al., 2001). Just how this information is to be imparted is generally not specified, though three guidelines do recommend specific patient educational material: the USA guidelines (Agency for Health Care Policy and Research, 1994a) were published together with an accompanying booklet for patients (Agency for Health Care Policy and Research, 1994b), whilst in the UK primary care guidelines (Royal College of General Practitioners, 1999) and occupational health guidelines (Carter and Birrell, 2000) both recommend the same booklet (Roland et al., 1996).

There is now an extensive theoretical and scientific base for modern management approaches to back pain, but it is only recently that there is emerging empirical evidence that a simple written educational intervention, either in routine primary care or at a population level, can have a positive effect on patient beliefs and outcomes. The successful interventions represent a major departure from the traditional orthopaedic and physiotherapy information and advice, and instead focus on patients' beliefs and on what they themselves should do about their back pain. Preparing and developing effective educational booklets, though, is no easy matter; it should not be assumed that simply producing a 'home-grown' booklet or pamphlet will have any clinical influence. In fact, the evidence suggests that it is particularly difficult to determine and present the messages that are important and acceptable to patients, and also effective in changing beliefs and behaviours.

It must be recognised that written educational material is a weak intervention; and simply handing patients a small booklet without any other attempt to influence their management is likely to be suboptimal. Educational experts advise that a co-ordinated approach, in which physicians and therapists all give the same information and advice, and use educational material to reinforce that message, is likely to have a more powerful effect (Grimshaw and Russell, 1993). Such an integrated management package for back pain (which involves training family doctors and their staff in an 'active management' approach supplemented by prescription of an evidence-based booklet) is presently being explored in the UK BEAM trial, which is due to report its results in 2002 (*www.york.ac.uk/org/ukbeam/ukbeam*). The need for care in this sort of approach is highlighted by Little et al. (2001a), who showed that a mismatch between the amount, content, and format of the information when delivered in both written and verbal form can be less effective than either delivery method alone. The exciting concept of public health educational campaigns to influence behaviours among people with back pain (Scotland's Working Backs Partnership, 2000; Buchbinder et al., 2001) certainly deserves further research attention. It is quite possible that it may be easier to educate patients who then change doctors' behaviour rather than vice versa!

Demonstrating that educational materials have an influence on return to work and health care usage is problematic. Because many primary care patients do well, return to work, and do not seek further health care, manageable trials may have insufficient statistical power to test any effect on work loss or subsequent health care. The success of the one primary care trial that showed an effect on health care usage (Roland et al., 1996) has not yet been replicated. In view of the multiple social and other influences on work loss, changing such a 'hard' outcome is likely to be more difficult than a softer outcome such as self-reported disability (Scheer et al., 1995; Deyo et al., 1998). It has been shown that perceived educational needs of back-injured workers may differ from those of their health care professionals and their employers or insurers, suggesting that even when there is good evidence to support the truth of an information statement, there may be an issue over whether it should be included in a brochure (Hazard et al., 2000a). Furthermore, we would suggest that a booklet in isolation is unlikely to have much impact on work absence and that only complete management strategies that get all the players onside is likely to have any significant impact (Frank et al., 1998; Carter and Birrell, 2000; Waddell and Burton, 2000). Indeed, there is recent evidence that this is the case (Buchbinder et al., 2001), but there is doubtless scope for improving such strategies.

This review provides empirical evidence about the information and advice that should be given to patients with back pain, which forms an integral part of the more active strategy of management recommended in current guidelines. It supports the premise that the information and advice that health professionals give to patients, whether deliberately or inadvertently, may be a potent element of the health care intervention. Traditional information and advice about back pain has been based on a biomedical model and too often given without considering its impact on patients. From a biopsychosocial perspective, that traditional information and advice often conveyed negative messages about back pain with damaging effects on patients' beliefs and behaviours. All doctors and therapists need to be more aware of, and consider much more carefully, what they say to patients and the impressions they give. What is said may be less important than how it is said; what matters most is the message the patient takes away from the consultation.

6. Conclusion

The most important clinical message from this review is that carefully selected and presented information and advice about back pain in line with current management guidelines *can* have a positive effect on patients' beliefs and clinical outcomes. Written educational material is just one way of achieving this and, whilst its effect size may be small, its very low per-patient cost may render it highly cost-effective. Nevertheless, there is considerable scope for refinement of the messages and their method of delivery within the whole scope of health care, and the contribution of innovative educational interventions for back pain deserves serious further scientific investigation.

References

Agency for Health Care Policy and Research (1994a) Acute low-back problems in adults. Clinical Practice Guideline Number 14. U.S. Government Printing Office, Washington, DC.

Agency for Health Care Policy and Research (1994b) Understanding Acute Low Back Problems: Patient Guide (Consumer Version, Clinical Practice Guideline Number, 14). U.S. Department of Health and Human Services, Rockville, MD.

Buchbinder, R., Jolley, D. and Wyatt, M. (2001) Population based intervention to change back pain beliefs and disability: three part evaluation. BMJ, 322: 1516–1520.

Burton, A.K. (1997) Back injury and work loss: Biomechanical and psychosocial influences. Spine, 22: 2575–2580.

Burton, A.K. and Main, C.J. (2000) Obstacles to recovery from work-related musculoskeletal disorders. In: W. Karwowski (Ed.), International Encyclopedia of Ergonomics and Human Factors. Taylor and Francis, London, pp. 1542–1544.

Burton, A.K., Waddell, G., Burtt, R. and Blair, S. (1996) Patient educational material in the management of low back pain in primary care. Bull. Hosp. Joint Dis., 55: 138–141.

Burton, A.K., Waddell, G., Tillotson, K.M. and Summerton, N. (1999) Information and advice to patients with back pain can have a positive effect: a randomized controlled trial of a novel educational booklet in primary care. Spine, 24: 2484–2491.

Carter, J.T. and Birrell, L.N. (2000) Occupational health guidelines for the management of low back pain at work — principal recommendations. Faculty of Occupational Medicine, London.

Cedraschi, C., Reust, P., Lorensi-Cioldi, F. and Vischer, T.L. (1996) The gap between back pain patients' prior knowledge and scientific knowledge and its evolution after a back school teaching programme: a qualitative evaluation. Patient Educ. Couns., 27: 235–246.

Cherkin, D., Deyo, R.A. and Berg, A.O. (1991a) Evaluation of a physician education intervention to improve primary care for low-back pain II: Impact on patients. Spine, 16: 1173–1178.

Cherkin, D., Deyo, R.A., Berg, A.O., Bergman, J.J. and Lishner, D.M. (1991b) Evaluation of a physician education intervention to improve primary care for low-back pain I: Impact on physicians. Spine, 16: 1168–1172.

Cherkin, D.C., Deyo, R.A., Street, J.H., Hunt, M. and Barlow, W. (1996) Pitfalls of patient education. Limited success of a program for back pain in primary care. Spine, 21: 345–355.

Cherkin, D.C., Deyo, R.A., Battie, M., Street, J. and Barlow, W. (1998) A comparison of physical therapy, chiropractic manipulation, and provision of an educational booklet for the treatment of patients with low back pain. N. Engl. J. Med., 339: 1021–1029.

Coulter, A. (1998) Evidence based patient information. Br. Med. J., 317: 225–226.

Coulter, A., Entwistle, V. and Gilbert, D. (1998) Informing patients. An assessment of the quality of patient information materials. Kings Fund, London.

Deyo, R.A., Battié, M., Beurskens, A.J.H.M., Bombardier, C., Croft, P., Koes, B., Malmivaara, A., Roland, M., Von Korff, M. and Waddell, G. (1998) Outcome measures for low back pain research: A proposal for standardized use. Spine, 23: 2003–2013.

Dijkstra, A., Vlaeyen, J.W.S., Rijnen, H. and Nielson, W. (2001) Readiness to adopt the self-management approach to cope with chronic pain in fibromyalgic patients. Pain, 90: 37–46.

Fitzmaurice, D.A. (2001) Written information for treating minor illness. BMJ, 322: 1193–1194.

Frank, J., Sinclair, S., Hogg-Johnson, S., Shannon, H., Bombardier, C., Beaton, D. and Cole, D. (1998) Preventing disability from work-related low-back pain. New evidence gives new hope — if we can just get all the players onside. Can. Med. Assoc. J., 158: 1625–1631.

Frankel, B.S.M., Moffett, J.K., Keen, S. and Jackson, D. (1999) Guidelines for low back pain: changes in GP management. Fam. Pract., 16: 216–222.

Grimshaw, J.M. and Russell, I.T. (1993) Effect of clinical guidelines on medical practice: a systematic review of rigorous evaluations. Lancet, 342: 1317–1322.

Hazard, R.G., Reid, S. and Clark, A.A. (2000a) Educating back-injured workers: what should we be teaching. Work, 15: 159–166.

Hazard, R.G., Reid, S., Haugh, L.D. and McFarlane, G. (2000b) A controlled trial of an educational pamphlet to prevent disability after occupational low back injury. Spine, 25: 1419–1423.

Heaney, D., Wyke, S., Wilson, P., Elton, R. and Rutledge, P. (2001) Assessment of impact of information booklets on use of healthcare services: randomised controlled trial. BMJ, 322: 1218.

Kendall, N.A.S., Linton, S.J. and Main, C.J. (1997) Guide to assessing psychosocial yellow flags in acute low back pain: Risk factors for long-term disability and work loss. Accident Rehabilitation and Compensation Insurance Corporation of New Zealand and the National Health Committee, Wellington.

Koes, B.W., van Tulder, M.W., Ostelo, R., Burton, A.K. and Waddell, G. (2001) Clinical guidelines for the management of low back pain in primary care: an international comparison. Spine, 26: 2504–2513.

Linton, S.J. and Andersson, T. (2000) Can chronic disability be prevented? A randomized trial of a cognitive–behavior intervention and two forms of information for patients with spinal pain. Spine, 25: 2825–2831.

Linton, S.J. and van Tulder, M.W. (2001) Preventive interventions for back and neck pain problems: What is the evidence. Spine, 26: 778–787.

Little, P., Smith, L., Cantrell, T., Chapman, J., Langridge, J. and Pickering, R. (1996) General practitioners' management of acute back pain: a survey of reported practice compared with clinical guidelines. BMJ, 312: 485–488.

Little, P., Roberts, L., Blowers, H., Garwood, J., Cantrell, T., Langridge, J. and Chapman, J. (2001a) Should we give detailed advice and information booklets to patients with back pain? A randomized controlled factorial trial of a self-management booklet and doctor advice to take exercise for back pain. Spine, 26: 2065–2072.

Little, P., Somerville, J., Williamson, I., Warner, G., Moore, M., Wiles, R., George, S., Smith, A. and Peveler, R. (2001b) Randomised controlled trial of self management leaflets and booklets for minor illness provided by post. BMJ, 322: 1214.

Main, C.J. and Burton, A.K. (2000) Economic and occupational influences on pain and disability, in Pain management. In: C.J. Main and C.C. Spanswick (Eds.), An Interdisciplinary Approach. Churchill Livingstone, Edinburgh, pp. 63–87.

McGuirk, B., King, W., Govind, J., Lowry, J. and Bogduk, N (2001) Safety, efficacy, and cost effectiveness of evidence-based guidelines for the management of acute low back pain in primary care. Spine, 26: 2615–2622.

Pincus, T., Burton, A.K., Vogel, S. and Field, A.P. (2002) A systematic review of psychological factors as predictors of chronicity/disability in prospective cohorts of low back pain. Spine, 27: E109–120.

Rainville, J., Carlson, N., Polatin, P., Gatchel, R.J. and Indahl, A. (2000) Exploration of physicians' recommendations for activities in chronic low back pain. Spine, 25: 2210–2219.

Roland, M. and Dixon, M. (1989) Randomized controlled trial of an educational booklet for patients presenting with back pain in general practice. J. R. Coll. Gen. Pract., 39: 244–246.

Roland, M., Waddell, G., Klaber-Moffett, J., Burton, K., Main, C. and Cantrell, T. (1996) The Back Book. The Stationery Office, Norwich (www.clicktso.com).

Rossignol, M., Abenhaim, L., Seguin, P., Neveu, A., Collet, J.-P., Ducruet, T. and Shapiro, S. (2000) Coordination of primary health care for back pain: A randomized controlled trial. Spine, 25: 251–259.

Royal College of General Practitioners (1996) Clinical Guidelines for the Management of Acute Low Back Pain RCGP, London.

Royal College of General Practitioners (1999) Clinical Guidelines for the Management of Acute Low Back Pain Royal College of General Practitioners (www.rcgp.org.uk), London.

Scheer, S.J., Radack, K.L. and O'Brien Jr., D.R. (1995) Randomized controlled trials in industrial low back pain relating to return to work, Part 1. Acute interventions. Arch. Phys. Med. Rehabil., 76: 966–973.

Schers, H., Braspenning, J., Drijver, R., Wensing, M. and Grol, R. (2000) Low back pain in general practice: reported management and reasons for not adhering to the guidelines in the Netherlands. Br. J. Gen. Pract., 50: 640–644.

Scotland's Working Backs Partnership (2000) WorkingBacks Scotland, www.workingbacksscotland.com

Simpson, M., Buckman, R., Stewart, M., Maguire, P., Lipkin, M., Novack, D. and Till, J. (1991) Doctor–patient communication: the Toronto consensus statement. Br. Med. J., 303: 1385–1387.

Symonds, T.L., Burton, A.K., Tillotson, K.M. and Main, C.J. (1995) Absence resulting from low back trouble can be reduced by psychosocial intervention at the work place. Spine, 20: 2738–2745.

Underwood, M.R., Vickers, M.R. and Barnett, A.G. (1997) Availability of services to treat patients with acute low back pain. Br. J. Gen. Pract., 47: 501–502.

Waddell, G. (1987) A new clinical model for the treatment of low back pain. Spine, 12: 632–644.

Waddell, G. (1998) The Back Pain Revolution. Churchill Livingstone, Edinburgh.

Waddell, G. and Burton, A.K. (2000) Occupational health guidelines for the management of low back pain at work — Evidence review. Faculty of Occupational Medicine, London.

Waddell, G., Feder, G. and Lewis, M. (1997) Systematic reviews of bed rest and advice to stay active for acute low back pain. Br. J. Gen. Pract., 47: 647–652.

Waddell, G., Burton, K. and McClune, T. (2001) The Whiplash Book. The Stationery Office, Norwich (www.clicktso.com).

New Avenues for the Prevention of Chronic Musculoskeletal Pain and Disability
Pain Research and Clinical Management, Vol. 12
Edited by S.J. Linton

CHAPTER 17

Early rehabilitation: the Ontario experience

Sandra J. Sinclair [1,2,3,*] and Sheilah Hogg-Johnson [1,2,3]

[1] *Institute for Work and Health, Toronto, ON, Canada*
[2] *Department of Public Health Sciences, University of Toronto, Toronto, ON, Canada*
[3] *School of Rehabilitation Science, McMaster University, Toronto, ON, Canada*

Abstract: Because musculoskeletal disorders ranked first as the cause of chronic health problems, long-term disability, and consultations with a health professional in the province of Ontario in 1990, a secondary prevention program was initiated. The purpose of this chapter is to describe the circumstances under which this early, active, intervention program for work-related musculoskeletal disorders was established and subsequently evaluated. A community clinical program was launched where early, active intervention based on a sport's medicine model was offered by providers throughout the province. However, our evaluation indicated that it did not yield the benefits anticipated in terms of time on wage replacement benefits, total costs, health-related quality of life, functional status or pain. In the context of a review of the more recent literature we suggest that the concept of early intervention is quite variable both temporally and with regard to type of care provided. Appropriately matching interventions with stage in recovery, is an approach which may prove more effective.

1. Introduction

Over the past 20 years the approach to the management of musculoskeletal work-related injuries has changed dramatically. Through the early 1980s, a still standard prescription for the rehabilitation of low back pain, the single-most common musculoskeletal problem, was bed rest and activity avoidance, followed by passive modalities of heat/cold to relieve pain and muscle spasm, and the gradual introduction of abdominal strengthening exercise. Although a few studies were beginning to suggest the success of a more active treatment approach, early, active, intervention was still relatively untested, when the workplace injury insurance program in Ontario, Canada (Kaegi, 1989) began in 1986, to explore this approach to medical rehabilitation. This initiative represented an early attempt at the systematic integration of evidence on treatment effectiveness into the design of an innovative program of care.

In this chapter, we describe the circumstances under which this early, active, intervention program for work-related musculoskeletal disorders (WMSD) was initiated and subsequently evaluated. Program design limitations are discussed in light of the then current evidence. In the context of a review of the more recent literature we suggest that the concept of early intervention is quite variable both temporally and with regard to type of care provided. Appropri-

---
*Correspondence to: Sandra J. Sinclair, Institute for Work and Health, 481 University Avenue, 8th Floor, Toronto, ON M5G 2E9, Canada. Tel.: +1 (416) 927-2027, ext. 2102; Fax: +1 (416) 927-4167; E-mail: ssinclair@iwh.on.ca

ately matching interventions with stage in recovery, is an approach which may prove more effective. Finally, recent initiatives undertaken in Ontario to improve the evidence-based management and treatment of work-related musculoskeletal injuries, particularly low back pain, are noted.

2. Background

2.1. Burden of illness

Musculoskeletal disorders are a significant cause of burden of illness in Canada as in other countries (Nachemson and Jonsson, 2000). Based on data from the Health and Activity Limitation Survey, conducted in 1986 in Canada, about one million adult Canadians are estimated to have a physical disability attributed to a musculoskeletal condition at a prevalence rate of 50.1/1000 adults (Reynolds et al., 1992). The most common type of disabling musculoskeletal disease was arthritis/rheumatism (27.1/1000) followed by back problems (16.2/1000), trauma (i.e. fracture) (3.6/1000) and other bone problems (0.6/1000) (Reynolds et al., 1992).

In the province of Ontario, musculoskeletal disorders ranked first as the cause of chronic health problems, long-term disability, and consultations with a health professional, and ranked second as the cause for restricted activity days and for the use of both prescription and non-prescription drugs as reported in the 1990 Ontario Health Survey (Badley et al., 1994). While back and neck disorders specifically are only a component of the musculoskeletal system, this sub-grouping of musculoskeletal disorders ranks in the top three against other body systems on the above morbidity indicators (except prescription drug use) in the Ontario adult population (Badley et al., 1994).

Estimates from the 1994 National Population Health Survey (Moore et al., 1997) show musculoskeletal problems with the highest morbidity costs due to long-term disability accounting for $13.5 billion in 1993, roughly one third the total annual value

of productivity loss in Canada. Musculoskeletal problems also ranked third in terms of the costs of short-term disability (Moore et al., 1997). In terms of overall cost of illness in Canada in 1993, musculoskeletal conditions ranked second highest preceded only by cardiovascular conditions (Moore et al., 1997).

2.2. Management of work-related musculoskeletal disorders in Ontario in the 1980s

A significant proportion of the burden of musculoskeletal pain and disability is seen in the workplace, with back conditions constituting approximately 30%, and upper-extremity musculoskeletal problems over 20% of all lost time workers' compensation claims (Beaton, 1995).

In Canada, payment for health care and wage replacement benefits for work-related injuries and disability are covered by the 12 monopolistic provincial and territorial workers' compensation boards. Of the approximately 380,000 claims for wage replacement benefits (i.e. lost time claims) in Canada in 1999, over 100,000 were from Ontario, exceeded only by Quebec at over 116,000 (Association of Workers' Compensation Boards of Canada, 2000).

Through the first half of the 1980s the Ontario Workers' Compensation Board [1] (WCB) found, as did many compensation systems, that they were facing a rapidly increasing lost time injury rate, and an increase in the duration of these claims on wage replacement benefits, particularly for musculoskeletal disorders.

By the middle of the decade, the WCB was managing approximately 250,000 claims each year for injuries requiring time off work (Kaegi, 1989). Well over 50% of these claims were for musculoskeletal conditions, with back problems, as the single-most common complaint. These back-related claims accounted for approximately 40% of the total annual benefit costs (Workers' Compensation Board, 1990).

[1] The Workers' Compensation Board of Ontario was renamed the Workplace Safety and Insurance Board (WSIB) in 1998.

The marked increase in claims incidence and duration led to increased employer costs for workers' compensation coverage, causing pressure from the employer community for better management strategies.

Potentially contributing to the increased duration of work absence were the long delays in access to rehabilitation programs. Waiting times of 4–6 weeks before the start of physiotherapy treatment were not uncommon (Workers' Compensation Board, 1988a). As a result injured workers were not receiving treatment early on, and it was suggested that they consequently remained off work becoming increasingly deconditioned. Timely access to rehabilitation was but one of a number of areas of medical care where the worker and unions were dissatisfied with the programs available through the WCB (McCombie, 1984).

From the perspective of the compensation board, there was concern that rehabilitation programs provided for the general population, which focused on returning patients to a level at which they could carry out activities of daily living, might not be sufficient to return injured workers to the pressures and demands of full-time employment. The WCB believed that the "medical rehabilitation services it provided or purchased must have the goal of returning the injured worker to productive work and active participation in the workplace" (Kaegi, 1989).

Although the compensation board ran its own in-patient rehabilitation hospital (Downsview Rehabilitation Centre — DRC) its programs, though highly regarded, were geared for the tertiary rehabilitation of severe and traumatic injury cases, and for individuals with chronic recurring musculoskeletal problems. These programs did not address the needs of most workers with acute and subacute non-traumatic work-related musculoskeletal conditions. Moreover, external reviews of DRC in 1983 and 1986, undertaken under the auspices of the WCB and the Ministry of Labour, respectively, raised questions about DRC's ongoing role and about the appropriateness of a workplace injury insurance program having direct involvement in the delivery of health care services (Workers' Compensation Board, 1988b). Clearly, there were pressures from several

directions to improve the approach and access to medical rehabilitation for injured workers.

Evidence about the effectiveness of new active approaches to the management of musculoskeletal conditions, particularly low back problems, was emerging from several sources. With musculoskeletal conditions constituting well over half of the lost time injury cases, this appeared an appropriate avenue to explore. Although the work of the Quebec Task Force (Spitzer et al., 1987) was not published until 1987, there were earlier indications of the direction and recommendations which would emerge. The work of Nachemson (1983, 1985) pointed to the success of activation programs, in acute, subacute and chronic low back pain. Earlier work by Bergquist-Ullman and Larsson (1977) showed the positive effects of education combined with a work site evaluation on return to work outcomes. Mayer et al. (1987) in the U.S., showed positive effects in low back pain cases of aggressive exercise and education, with 87% of the treatment group working at 2-year follow-up, compared with only 41% of the non-treatment comparison group. Deyo's work on the use of bed rest (1986) published in the New England Journal of Medicine, demonstrated that minimal bed rest was better than longer-term inactivity in returning low back pain patients to normal activities with no greater complaints of symptoms.

Based on these findings, as well as the reported successes of early return to activity used by sports medicine physicians in the treatment of athletes (Saal, 1987), in late 1986, the WCB established a small number of pilot programs across the province. These pilot sites were to test and refine a new model of active rehabilitation and education for those workers with work-related musculoskeletal injuries still off work after 3 weeks (Kaegi, 1989).

The success of the Board's own pilot program (Mitchell and Carmen, 1990) in reducing duration of wage loss and overall claims costs, despite higher rehabilitation expenditures, for those workers attending the pilot program, in comparison to a retrospectively matched group of workers who did not attend the program, provided powerful additional evidence for the direction of a new province-wide program.

3. The Community Clinic program

This new program was introduced in 1988 (Workers' Compensation Board, 1988b, 1989) to be delivered by up to 100 independently operated community clinics across the province with whom the Workers' Compensation Board had established fee-for-service contracts. The programs which were to provide preferred access to injured workers with work-related musculoskeletal injuries focused on early intervention, activation, and education. There were essentially two program phases. The first, was a 2-week daily program with sessions lasting up to 2 h to relieve pain and begin movement around the injured area; the second phase, if necessary, was a 4–6-week program which included individualized physiotherapy, education regarding injury prevention and management, and a fitness component. These sessions were to last 3–4 h per day, with patients actively involved in the process of getting well through setting their own goals and assisting in planning their own programs. Treating physicians were encouraged to refer patients early, within 2 (van Schoor, 1989) to 5 days (Kaegi, 1989), but no later than 70 days post-injury. It was anticipated at the time of program development that over 50% of workers entering the program would recover in the first 2 weeks (Workers' Compensation Board, 1989) and therefore would not need to participate in the second phase of the program.

The Community Clinic (CC) program was nested within a new three-tiered medical rehabilitation strategy whose guiding principles included: ready and timely access to high-quality multidisciplinary, well co-ordinated medical care for injured workers; delivered in a caring community setting; with the goal of returning the injured worker to work (Workers' Compensation Board, 1988b).

4. Evaluation of the CC program

By 1993, when the formal evaluation of the CC program was initiated, it was well established with over 100 participating clinics treating approximately 20,000 workers per year at an annual cost of $20

million (Cdn.). Because of the widespread availability of the program and its overall acceptance by all parties a randomized study design was not possible.

A longitudinal prospective cohort study, with repeat measures over a 1-year follow-up was conducted involving over 1500 workers with WMSD, 36% of whom attended the CC program. The study design and the results for the 885 low back pain patients in the sample are fully described elsewhere (Sinclair et al., 1997). The study showed that program attenders were not systematically different from non-attenders on over 70 demographic, injury descriptor and work-related variables measured at baseline, and that there was no advantage to the program in comparison to usual care based on duration of wage replacement benefits, functional status, health-related quality of life or pain measures. Both attender and non-attender groups improved significantly over time, but there was no statistically significant difference in rate of improvement over the 1-year follow-up, although the health care costs for attenders were significantly higher than for non-attenders ($1000 Cdn. per patient on average, which was similar to the average cost per case in the CC program).

Results of the study were released to the WCB, as program sponsors in mid-1995 (Institute for Work and Health, 1995; Erdeljan et al., 1995) and included the following recommendations from the researchers:

- the need to reconsider the merits of an intensive intervention within the first 4 weeks following absence from work due to WMSD;
- the need to consider the development of more intensive treatment modules for workers with WMSD still off work 6–10 weeks after injury;
- the need to consider an enhanced link and communication between treatment programs and the workplace.

Subsequently, the WCB modified the eligibility criteria for the CC program to include only those workers off work for 4 weeks or more. However, regular (less intensive) physiotherapy and chiropractic care, covered and paid for by WCB, remained available prior to that time.

By the following year, an expert clinical panel had been struck by the WCB to develop new evidence-based program guidelines for the management of acute and subacute low back pain which considered the findings from the substantially increased body of literature, published in the decade since the formulation of the original CC program.

5. Differences between pilot study and the CC program

Clearly, the results from the evaluation of the CC program differed significantly from the results of the earlier and positive pilot program evaluation. There are a number of potential explanations for this.

From a methodological perspective, although both the studies included comparison groups, the CC evaluation, as a prospective longitudinal cohort, involving baseline interview data as well as WCB administrative data, had the capacity to demonstrate if clinic attenders and non-attenders were similar to begin with on a wide range of potentially confounding variables. The pilot evaluation on the other hand, was a cohort with a retrospectively matched comparison group, based on administrative data only, with very limited ability to adjust for baseline differences on prognostic factors especially markers of clinical severity.

The two programs also varied in three significant areas: intake screening; attendance eligibility; and workplace contact. In the pilot study, the referral of potential program attenders was screened by the single medical consultant overseeing the program. Clearly this was not feasible in a fully functioning province-wide program. During the pilot study, cases were only accepted for referral after 21 days off work, up to 70 days after injury. When the program was expanded as the CC program, referral was encouraged as early as 2 days after injury, this despite the fact that there was no evidence to suggest the increased benefit of an intensive intervention of this type within the first 3 weeks other than the sports medicine model which focused on highly motivated semi-professional and professional athletes. While

athletes can be viewed as 'workers' in their sport, the underlying fitness level, motivation and context of the injured worker and the injured athlete returning to the work environment are very different. Without proven screening strategies to identify those individuals who might benefit from an early intensive intervention it is difficult to show effectiveness, particularly given the favorable natural history of WMSD. A third program element which varied substantially between the pilot and CC programs, was in the communication which took place between the treatment facility and the workplace around activity restrictions at discharge and return to work circumstances. While this type of communication generally took place during the pilot study, it was not considered an element of the fully implemented CC program and it was not supported by WCB.

It may also be of relevance to note, that in the development of the program, the WCB espoused the position that "medical rehabilitation services must have the goal of returning the injured worker to work" (Kaegi, 1989). However, the community clinics themselves were not in a position to indicate if a worker was ready to return to work, since the overall medical management remained the responsibility of the worker's primary care physician. Workers, on program completion, were referred back to their own physician, and it was left to the physician to make the decision regarding suitability for return to work.

What effect this lack of responsibility around the 'return to work' recommendation or process had on the program is unclear and whether this may in part have influenced the different outcomes of the pilot study and CC program results is further uncertain. In the full-scale implementation of the program, these differences may have been important.

The evidence available at the time promoted fitness, active graded programs and education and these were the components of the program (Bergquist-Ullman and Larsson, 1977; Nachemson, 1983, 1985; Deyo et al., 1986). The importance of such instrumental factors as (1) the link with the workplace, (2) the role of patient reassurance in the early stages of recovery rather than daily treatment, (3) the distinction between a treatment program of activity versus the resumption of regular activity, or (4) the timing of introduction of any intervention, which later research confirmed, were not fully appreciated. Do the results from the evaluation of the CC program suggest that *early* intervention for WMSD is ineffective? It is worth considering this in light of more recent studies.

6. When is early and what interventions are effective?

There have been many proponents of 'early' care for work-related musculoskeletal conditions. But what is meant by 'early' and what type of care or guidance is recommended varies considerably from study to study. For some, 'early' means immediately after injury or onset of symptoms, within a day or two (Zigenfus et al., 2000) for others it means after 8–12 weeks of sick leave (Hagen et al., 2000), while still others use 'early' to describe any situation in which a worker goes back to work before he/she is ready to do his/her regular job (Williams, 1991).

It is perhaps more informative to think of three stages in the recovery of an episode of WMSD (Frank et al., 1996; Hogg-Johnson et al., 1998). The acute phase lasting from 0 to 4 weeks following onset is characterized by a favorable natural history with many cases of WMSD resolving during this period. Typically, between 50% and 60% of lost time WMSD claims end within 4 weeks (Waddell, 1998). On the other hand, the subacute phase between 4 and 12 weeks after onset is characterized by a slower rate of resolution, and possible secondary complications or responses on the part of the worker related to prolonged absence from work. By 12 weeks, many experts now believe that early chronic pain has set in (Frank et al., 1996).

It is critical that any type of care or intervention offered early is respectful of the favorable natural history. One trap that the clinician or researcher may fall into is to observe that injured workers treated earlier tend to get better more quickly than those workers treated later and therefore to conclude that it is better to treat earlier rather than later. How-

ever, in this scenario, timing of treatment may be strongly confounded with severity of injury. Many patients receiving earlier care would likely have recovered spontaneously without the treatment offered. The favorable natural history in the early stages, if not properly accounted for, can lead people to draw questionable conclusions. A useful measure which helps to illustrate this point is called the Number Needed to Treat (NNT) (Jaeschke et al., 1995); a measure of treatment efficiency. The NNT is based on the number of additional patients (or claimants) one would need to treat with a new treatment, as compared to some standard treatment, in order to ensure one additional success over and above what would be achieved with the standard treatment (Frank et al., 1996). The higher the NNT is, the less efficient the treatment. For acute low back pain, the NNT is a function of, among other things, the timing of the treatment with the highest values (and therefore less efficiency) in the early stages and a gradual reduction in NNT (and therefore greater efficiency) over time (Frank et al., 1996). Treatment efficiency, though, must be balanced with treatment effectiveness, and it is also apparent that it is more difficult to find beneficial treatment programs for chronic WMSD than it is for acute or subacute WMSD.

Two published studies (Ehrmann-Feldman et al., 1996; Zigenfus et al., 2000) have concluded that the earlier physiotherapy is started, the better the patient will do, but both have compared timing of treatment in an observational study design with inadequate control for a priori differences in the comparison groups. The conclusions are suspect because of the study design used.

Programs or courses of action offered within the acute stage of injury appear to be successful only under certain circumstances, for instance, when the course of action is geared more toward early involvement rather than intervention (Ryan et al., 1995; Van Doorn, 1995). Boschen (1989) made this insightful distinction, and stressed the importance of getting *involved* with the injured worker as early as possible — but not necessarily *intervening* at that early time. Boschen (1989) specified that the goal of early involvement should be: "to arrest this process of identity change before the disabled worker discontinues the view of him or herself as a worker". Involvement might include offering reassurance, assessing long-term risk, and promoting maintenance of regular activities (Pope, 1987; McKinney, 1989; Haig et al., 1990; Linton et al., 1993; Borchgrevink et al., 1998; The Back Letter, 1998). This message, the importance of reassurance and promotion of return to regular activities, closely matches the recommendations of the guidelines for care of acute low back pain released in various jurisdictions in the 1990s (Agency for Health Care Policy and Research, 1994; Waddell et al., 1996; Accident Rehabilitation and Compensation Insurance Corporation and the New Zealand National Advisory Committee on Health and Disability, 1997). As per the screening tool for yellow flags provided with the New Zealand guidelines, other successful early programs have included some type of assessment or prognostic screening tool up front to gear the program toward the individual needs of the patients or workers at greater risk of chronicity (Cooper et al., 1996, 1997; Yassi et al., 1995; Linton and Andersson, 2000; McIntosh et al., 2000). In many of these cases, the work site was involved either by being the site of the intervention, or the initiator of the program. The CC program, on the other hand, while offered to workers in the acute stage of injury did not involve contact with the work site and did not include any screening mechanism to target workers at higher risk of chronicity. Other study results published shortly before completion of the CC evaluation had similar negative findings for similar scenarios. Malmivaara et al. (1995) showed no benefit to extension exercises or bed rest of 2 days duration, compared with advice to continue ordinary activity as tolerated and training offered within 3 weeks of onset, while Faas et al. (1995) showed increased median time lost for the group receiving physiotherapy-directed flexion exercises during the acute stage of injury.

On the other hand, comprehensive programs targeting injured workers at the subacute stage of injury have been generally more successful (Lindstrom et al., 1992a,b; Loisel et al., 1994, 1997; Hagen et al., 2000). Although the interventions in these three

studies are all initiated at approximately 6–8 weeks sick leave, only Hagen et al. (2000) refer to this as an 'early' intervention. The investigators in the other two studies referred to the timing of their program as during the subacute stage. By this stage, many less severe, more transient cases of WMSD have resolved, and the natural history for those still experiencing pain and disability is no longer as favorable. The Sherbrooke Model (Loisel et al., 1994, 1997), integrated medical and occupational aspects of the injury and involved the workplace in finding solutions. The program by Lindstrom et al. (1992a,b) was set within a work site, and included physiotherapy, mobilization, graded activity geared toward the participant's job and a visit to the workstation. The intervention described by Hagen et al. (2000) for workers with at least 8–12 weeks of sick leave for low back pain was less involved than the other two described here, but it included reassurance about a favorable prognosis and advice to remain active. Similarly, Indahl et al. (1995) demonstrated the benefits of an intervention which included reassurance and instructions to mobilize through light activity for low back pain patients with at least 8 weeks of sick leave.

A key message here is that we cannot easily separate out the *when* something is done from *what* is done, nor for that matter from *where* it takes place and any program of care or intervention for WMSD must carefully marry the timing, nature and site of the intervention (Frank et al., 1996; Hogg-Johnson et al., 1998).

7. Current status

On an annual basis, the Ontario WSIB now spends about $250 (Cdn.) million for health services for workers. In 1998 they began a process to redefine their health care model, consistent with their goal of providing quality health care at the right time for injured and ill workers to restore them to maximum function possible (Workplace Safety and Insurance Board, 2000a).

As in the mid-1980s back injuries was one of the first problems for which a comprehensive new program was developed as part of the process of re-definition. The Program of Care for Acute Low Back Injuries (Workplace Safety and Insurance Board, 2000b) was developed to incorporate the scientific evidence and best practices guidelines with respect to health care interventions into the assessment and treatment of injured workers. This program is now being piloted in Ontario.

8. Conclusions

It would be easy to dismiss the CC program as a good idea badly interpreted, or as a failed experiment, but that would be shortsighted. It did not yield the benefits anticipated (in terms of time on benefits, total costs, health-related quality of life, functional status or pain). But, in the mid-1980s, the Ontario WCB demonstrated great foresight and leadership in the movement toward evidence-based care by developing a medical rehabilitation program for acute and subacute WMSD based on the emerging evidence at the time. They carried through with the evidence-based approach by putting a mechanism in place for the evaluation of that program. By implementing and evaluating the CC program, a key piece of information was added to the accumulating evidence, thus advancing what is known about the best care for WMSD. Perhaps the results of the CC evaluation are all the more important because the results were not what was expected. Indeed, the investigators themselves were rather surprised that the clinics had so little impact, given their cost and the apparent 'common sense' of the sports medicine approach, involving early active rehabilitation and patient engagement/education. On further reflection, though, it seemed clear that the key ingredient missing from the clinics was any meaningful tie to the workplace, or even a legitimization of the clinics' role in helping to negotiate modified work suited to the injured workers' capabilities. In fact, the program's focus of early intensive intervention, of a rather fixed 4–6-week period, available to all injured workers but without a specified link to the workplace, flies in the face of what we know now to be

best practice. Ironically, the CC program may well have competed with return to work per se, especially for less severely injured soft-tissue injury cases.

A critical message which is highlighted in the Ontario experience is a need to be careful neither to sweepingly promote 'early' as better, nor to dismiss early as not the right time...the devil is in the details...when is early?...what is done early? and who is involved? Rather there is a need to consider the context in which we apply evidence in the design of any program of care.

However, the details of the program itself are probably less important when we consider more generally what can be learned from this experience about the challenges of moving from evidence to application. We need very good evidence carefully interpreted when addressing complex problems like the management of work-related musculoskeletal conditions. We need to evaluate and be prepared as policy makers, clinicians or researchers when interventions do not have the results we expect or want. Finally, we need to revise and update programs as new or clearer evidence emerges.

References

Accident Rehabilitation and Compensation Insurance Corporation and the New Zealand National Advisory Committee on Health and Disability (1997) New Zealand Acute Low Back Pain Guide, Accident Rehabilitation and Compensation Insurance Corporation and the National Advisory Committee on Health and Disability, Wellington.

Agency for Health Care Policy and Research (1994) Clinical Practice Guideline 14: Acute Low Back Problems in Adults. US Department of Health and Human Services, Rockville, MD.

Association of Workers' Compensation Boards of Canada (2000) Work Injuries and Diseases. National Work Injuries Statistics Program. Canada 1997–1999, 5th ed. Association of Workers' Compensation Boards of Canada.

Badley, E.M., Rasooly, I. and Webster, G.K. (1994) Relative importance of musculoskeletal disorders as a cause of chronic health problems, disability, and health care utilization: findings from the 1990 Ontario Health Survey. J. Rheumatol., 21(3): 505–514.

Beaton, D.E. (1995) Examining the clinical course of work-related musculoskeletal disorders of the upper extremities using the Ontario Workers' Compensation Board administrative database. MSc Thesis, University of Toronto, Toronto, ON.

Bergquist-Ullman, M. and Larsson, U. (1977) Acute low back pain in industry. A controlled prospective study with special reference to therapy and confounding factors. Acta Orthop. Scand. (Suppl.), 170: 1–117.

Borchgrevink, G.E., Kaasa, A., McDonagh, D., Stiles, T.C., Haraldseth, O. and Lereim, I. (1998) Acute treatment of whiplash neck sprain injuries: a randomized trial of treatment during the first 14 days after a car accident. Spine, 23(1): 25–31.

Boschen, K.A. (1989) Early intervention in vocational rehabilitation. Rehabil. Couns. Bull., 32: 254–265.

Cooper, J.E., Tate, R.B., Yassi, A. and Khokhar, J. (1996) Effect of an early intervention program on the relationship between subjective pain and disability measures in nurses with low back injury. Spine, 21: 2329–2336.

Cooper, J.E., Tate, R. and Yassi, A. (1997) Work hardening in an early return to work program for nurses with back injury. Work, 8: 149–156.

Deyo, R.A., Diehl, A.K. and Rosenthal, M. (1986) How many days of bed rest for acute low back pain? A randomized clinical trial. N. Engl. J. Med., 315(17): 1064–1070.

Ehrmann-Feldman, D., Rossignol, M., Abenhaim, L. and Gobeille, D. (1996) Physician referral to physical therapy in a cohort of workers compensated for low back pain. Phys. Ther., 76(2): 150–157.

Erdeljan, S., Hogg-Johnson, S., Kralj, B., Lee, D., Mondloch, M., Cole, D., Frank, J. and Sinclair, S. (1995) Evaluation of the WCB Community Clinic Program. The Early Claimant Cohort Analysis: Technical Appendix. Institute for Work and Health, Toronto, ON.

Faas, A., Van Eijk, J.T.M., Chavannes, A.W. and Gubbels, J.W. (1995) A randomized trial of exercise therapy in patients with acute low back pain: efficacy on sickness absence. Spine, 20(8): 941–947.

Frank, J.W., Brooker, A.S., DeMaio, S., Kerr, M.S., Maetzel, A., Shannon, H.S., Sullivan, T.J., Norman, R.W. and Wells, R. (1996) Disability resulting from occupational low back pain part II: What do we know about secondary prevention? A review of the scientific evidence on prevention after disability begins. Spine, 21(24): 2918–2929.

Hagen, E.M., Eriksen, H.R. and Ursin, H. (2000) Does early intervention with a light mobilization program reduce long-term sick leave for low back pain? Spine, 25(15): 1973–1976.

Haig, A.J., Linton, P., McIntosh, M., Moneta, L. and Mead, P.B. (1990) Aggressive early medical management by a specialist in physical medicine and rehabilitation: effect on lost time due to injuries in hospital employees. J. Occup. Med., 32(3): 241–244.

Hogg-Johnson, S.A., Cole, D.C., Cote, P. and Frank, J.W. (2000) Staging treatment interventions following soft tissue injuries. In: T.J. Sullivan (Ed.), Injury: the New World of Work. UBC Press, Vancouver, pp. 201–218.

Indahl, A., Velund, L. and Reikeraas, O. (1995) Good prognosis for low back pain when left untampered: A randomized clinical trial. Spine, 20(4): 473–477.

Institute for Work and Health (1995) Report to the Ontario Workers' Compensation Board on the Evaluation of the Community Clinic Program in the Rehabilitation of Workers with Soft Tissue Injury. Toronto, ON.

Jaeschke, R., Guyatt, G., Shannon, H., Walter, S., Cook, D. and Heddle, N. (1995) Assessing the effects of treatment: measures of association. Can. Med. Assoc. J., 152: 351–357.

Kaegi, E. (1989) New Approaches to Medical and Vocation Rehabilitation, 75th Anniversary Symposium, Workers' Compensation Board of Ontario, Toronto, ON.

Lindstrom, I., Ohlund, C., Eek, C., Wallin, L., Peterson, L.E. and Nachemson, A.L. (1992a) Mobility, strength, and fitness after a graded activity program for patients with subacute low back pain — a randomized prospective clinical study with a behavioral therapy approach. Spine, 17(6): 641–652.

Lindstrom, I., Ohlund, C., Eek, C., Wallin, L., Peterson, L.E., Fordyce, W.E. and Nachemson, A.L. (1992b) The effect of graded activity on patients with subacute low back pain: a randomized prospective clinical study with an operant-conditioning behavioral approach. Phys. Ther., 72(4): 279–293.

Linton, S.J. and Andersson, T. (2000) Can chronic disability be prevented? A randomized trial of a cognitive–behavior intervention and two forms of information for patients with spinal pain. Spine, 25(21): 2825–2831.

Linton, S.J., Hellsing, A.-L. and Andersson, D. (1993) A controlled study of the effects of an early intervention on acute musculoskeletal pain problems. Pain, 54(3): 353–359.

Loisel, P., Durand, P., Abenhaim, L., Gosselin, L., Simard, R., Turcotte, J. and Esdaile, J.M. (1994) Management of occupational back pain: the Sherbrooke model. Results of a pilot and feasibility study. Occup. Environ. Med., 51: 597–602.

Loisel, P., Abenhaim, L., Durand, P., Esdaile, J.M., Suissa, S., Gosselin, L., Simard, R., Turcotte, J. and Lemaire, J. (1997) A population-based, randomized clinical trial on back pain management. Spine, 22(24): 2911–2918.

Malmivaara, A., Hakkinen, U., Aro, T., Heinrichs, M.-L., Koskenniemi, L., Kuosma, E., Lappi, S., Paloheimo, R., Servo, C. and Vaaranen, V. (1995) The treatment of acute low back pain — bed rest, exercises, or ordinary activity? N. Engl. J. Med., 332(6): 351–355.

Mayer, T.G., Gatchel, R.J., Mayer, H., Kishino, N.D., Keeley, J. and Mooney, V. (1987) A prospective two-year study of functional restoration in industrial low back injury: an objective assessment procedure. J. Am. Med. Assoc., 258(13): 1763–1767.

McCombie, N. (1984) Justice for injured workers; a community responds to government reform. Can. Commun. Law J., 7: 136–173.

McIntosh, G., Frank, J., Hogg-Johnson, S., Bombardier, C. and Hall, H. (2000) Prognostic factors for time receiving workers' compensation benefits in a cohort of patients with low back pain. Spine, 25(2): 147–157.

McKinney, L.A. (1989) Early mobilisation and outcome in acute sprains of the neck. Br. Med. J., 299: 1006–1008.

Mitchell, R.I. and Carmen, G.M. (1990) Results of a multicenter trial using an intensive active exercise program for the treatment of acute soft tissue and back injuries. Spine, 15(6): 514–521.

Moore, R., Mao, Y., Zhang, J. and Clarke, K. (1997) Economic burden of illness in Canada, 1993. Health Canada, Ottawa, ON.

Nachemson, A. and Jonsson, E. (2000) Neck and Back Pain: The Scientific Evidence of Causes, Diagnosis, and Treatment. Lippincott Williams and Wilkins, Philadelphia, PA.

Nachemson, A.L. (1983) Work for all: for those with low back pain as well. Clin. Orthop., 179: 77–85.

Nachemson, A.L. (1985) Advances in low-back pain. Clin. Orthop. Rel. Res., 200: 266–278.

Pope, M.H. (1987) The biomechanical basis for early care programmes. Ergonomics, 30(2): 351–358.

Reynolds, D.L., Chambers, L.W., Badley, E.M., Bennett, K.J., Goldsmith, C.H., Jamieson, E., Torrance, G.W. and Tugwell, P. (1992) Physical disability among Canadians reporting musculoskeletal diseases. J. Rheumatol., 19(7): 1020–1030.

Ryan, W.E., Krishna, M.K. and Swanson, C.E. (1995) A prospective study evaluating early rehabilitation in preventing back pain chronicity in mine workers. Spine, 20(4): 489–491.

Saal, J.A. (1987) General principles and guidelines for the rehabilitation of the injured athlete. Physical Medicine and Rehabilitation: State of the Art Reviews, vol. 1, no. 4, pp. 523–535.

Sinclair, S.J., Hogg-Johnson, S.A., Mondloch, M.V. and Shields, S.A. (1997) The effectiveness of an early active intervention program for workers with soft tissue injuries: the Early Claimant Cohort study. Spine, 22(24): 2919–2931.

Spitzer, W.O., LeBlanc, F.E., Dupuis, M., Abenhaim, L., Belanger, A.Y., Bloch, R., Bombardier, C., Cruess, R.L., Drouin, G., Duval-Hesler, N., Laflamme, J., Lamoureux, G., Nachemson, A.L., Page, J.J., Rossignol, M., Salmi, L.R., Salois-Arsenault, S., Suissa, S. and Wood-Dauphinee, S. (1987) Scientific approach to the assessment and management of activity-related spinal disorders: a monograph for clinicians. Report of the Quebec task force on spinal disorders. Spine, 12(7S): s4–s55.

The Back Letter (1998) Whiplash: is early return to activity the key? The Back Letter, 13(3): 27.

Van Doorn, J.W.C. (1995) An early intervention program with 1-year follow-up. Acta Orthop. Scand. (Suppl.), 263(66): 2–64.

Van Schoor, J.T. (1989) Rehabilitation of the injured worker. Can. Fam. Physician, 35: 2297–2300.

Waddell, G. (1998) The Back Pain Revolution. Churchill Livingstone, Edinburgh.

Waddell, G., Feder, G., McIntosh, A., Lewis, M. and Hutchinson, A. (1996) Clinical guidelines for the management of acute low back pain. Royal College of General Practitioners, London.

Williams, J.R. (1991) Employee experiences with early return to work programs. AAOHN J., 39(2): 64–69.

Workers' Compensation Board of Ontario (1988a) MRS Strategy Report, Board of Directors, Minute #3.

Workers' Compensation Board of Ontario (1988b) Medical Rehabilitation Strategy: Feasibility Study Report.

Workers' Compensation Board of Ontario (1989) Medical Rehabilitation Strategy: Progress Report, Board of Directors Minute #5.

Workers' Compensation Board of Ontario (1990) Annual Report 1990.

Workplace Safety and Insurance Board (2000a) Program of Care for Acute Low Back Injuries: Background.

Workplace Safety and Insurance Board (2000b) Program of Care for Acute Low Back Injuries: Pilot.

Yassi, A., Tate, R., Cooper, J.E., Snow, C., Vallentyne, S. and Khokhar, J.B. (1995) Early intervention for back-injured nurses at a large Canadian tertiary care hospital: an evaluation of the effectiveness and cost benefits of a two-year pilot project. Occup. Med., 45(4): 209–214.

Zigenfus, G.C., Yin, J., Giang, G.M. and Fogarty, W.T. (2000) Effectiveness of early physical therapy in the treatment of acute low back musculoskeletal disorders. J. Occup. Environ. Med., 42(1): 35–39.

New Avenues for the Prevention of Chronic Musculoskeletal Pain and Disability
Pain Research and Clinical Management, Vol. 12
Edited by S.J. Linton

Cognitive behavioral therapy in the prevention of musculoskeletal pain: description of a program

Steven J. Linton [*]

Department of Occupational and Environmental Medicine, Örebro University Hospital, S-701 85 Örebro, Sweden

Abstract: This chapter presents a description of a cognitive behavioral program designed as a preventive intervention. This group treatment focuses on yellow flags, i.e. the psychological risk factors identified, and it offers an intervention that addresses these. After a description of the six-session group intervention, three randomized controlled trials are summarized. These studies demonstrate that the intervention indeed helps to prevent the development of long-term disability. The results underscore the need for a psychologically oriented intervention early on as secondary prevention. The program presented may be one way of altering health-care routines to better accommodate the needs of patients with musculoskeletal pain.

1. Introduction

Although psychological factors are believed to be central in the development of a chronic back pain problem, there have been relatively few attempts to prevent chronic disability with psychological techniques. Still, if psychological risk factors enhance the development of a chronic problem (Kendall et al., 1998; Linton, 2000b,c), then psychological interventions might be of real value. This chapter describes the application of a cognitive behavioral approach applied as secondary prevention. The intervention attempts to address the psychological factors identified and thus assists patients in making changes that will enhance their ability to deal with the problem.

Once patients at risk are identified it is a true challenge to provide an effective intervention that will prevent the development of chronic disability. Often medically oriented interventions are the only available resources. However, to directly address the psychological factors (e.g. avoidance to engage in activities, mood, and stress) found to increase the risk for developing long-term disability, psychological methods may be advantageous. The purpose of this chapter is to describe our program for providing cognitive behavior group interventions and to provide an overview of some first results.

2. The cognitive behavioral intervention

In order to provide a replicable secondary preventive intervention from a psychological perspective, a program was developed that builds on experiences from

[*] Correspondence to: S.J. Linton, Department of Occupational and Environmental Medicine, Örebro University Hospital, S-701 85 Örebro, Sweden. Tel.: +46 (19) 602-2456; Fax: +46 (19) 120-404; E-mail: steven.linton@orebroll.se

earlier programs provided for chronic pain patients (Compas et al., 1998; Morley et al., 1999; Linton, 2000d; van Tulder et al., 2000). Rather than provide the same intervention, we focused on the risk factors and the developmental process described in Chapter 6. Thus, the intervention has, from the beginning, been focused on *prevention* and not simply pain treatment.

2.1. Goals

The course has several goals, but the overriding aim is for each person to develop her/his own coping program. We ask that all skills be tried and tested so that participants can develop a tailored program that best suits each person's needs.

From a provider's point of view we hope to prevent pain-related disability, the need for health-care service, in addition to improving quality of life. In short, an aim is to prevent pain-related absenteeism and the need for back pain-related health-care. A natural goal is to improve the patient's quality of life so that they feel and function better. This includes factors such as pain intensity, stress levels and participating in everyday activities. We realize that back pain is recurrent and therefore we do not intend to eliminate all back pain, but rather to decrease recurrences and reduce their impact.

A final goal is that each member should have fun! Learning should be enjoyable and as will be seen below, considerable effort is extended so that participants are really engaged in the program. Humor is used and even homework assignments are given to tickle the funny bone.

2.2. Strategies for behavioral change

The interventions we offer participants involve coping that in turn require the person to alter current cognitions and behaviors. Simply put, the preventive intervention is based on changing beliefs and behavior. For example, beliefs about the relationship between pain and activity ("*The more I do, the more it will hurt*") or beliefs about stress ("*I must do everything asked of me and exactly on time*") may

need to be revised. Likewise, behaviors may need to be changed, e.g. increasing activity levels or being able to say 'no' to certain demands. The question becomes *how* this might be accomplished; we have employed several strategies.

First, the program is designed to actively engage the participant. Rather than a passive 'school' approach, active participation is prompted and then reinforced. Discussions, for example, involve *every* patient, i.e. a table round. Problem solving exercises are done in pairs to promote discussion and the results are reported by each pair. In the skills training module, each participant is encouraged to attempt to learn each skill and then apply it at home/work during the week. Homework assignments are individualized to accommodate idiosyncrasies. Above all, each person is given the charge of developing his or her own personal coping program.

Second, restricted amounts of information are used to prime behavioral changes. It appears that information may have an impact in certain situations since it challenges beliefs. However, health information is normally a rather weak method for modifying behavior. Thus, while we use modern information, we severely limit this part of the session so that more potent behavioral change methods will have sufficient time to operate.

A third strategy is behavioral tests. In this technique a patient's negative or inappropriate beliefs are examined and then a test is performed to see if the belief is actually true. For patients we conceptualize this as learning through experience. Thus, we ask patients to 'test' each skill they learn to assess its possible value for them. This is one basis for participants to select the skills for their personal coping program.

Problem solving is a fourth strategy utilized throughout to promote engagement and enhance maintenance. It is the first skill taught! Further, this skill is honed in a special problem-based learning module where pairs of patients are asked to read a case study and then to solve various 'problems' the patient is having.

Fifth, the group leader is taught to shape new thoughts and behaviors by reinforcing successive approximations of good coping behavior. Positive reinforcement, e.g. in the form of encouragement, is contingently provided when participants correctly approximate a goal behavior. Thus, gradual change is encouraged.

To maximize engagement and maintenance, another strategy is to enhance each patient's self-efficacy; that is the patient's belief that he/she can impact on their pain and its course. This is logical since many patients have low self-efficacy levels and as the participant, in fact, is changing his/her health behavior. While therapists are facilitators, it is *not* the therapist that causes the change. For example, we might ask a person who has successfully completed a homework assignment (e.g. practiced relaxation and decreased pain) to tell the entire group how he/she has accomplished this, to share the 'secret' of their success.

Finally, as mentioned above, enjoyment is used provoked to enhance learning, engagement, maintenance and pleasure. It is an important strategy to ensure that every participant feels he/she has learned something during each session. People should have the opportunity to laugh and to receive social support. Not in the least, encouragement should be contingently delivered in a rich schedule so that participants may feel good about their accomplishments.

2.3. Organization of the sessions

The intervention encompasses a six-session structured program where participants meet in groups of six to ten people, six times, once a week for 2 h. A manual guides therapy in order to standardize the intervention (Linton, 2000a). Therapists to date have had previous training in behavior therapy and in addition they have received special training in administering this intervention.

In turn, each session has several parts. First, an introduction to the session is provided lasting about 15 min. During the first session this deals mainly with helping participants feel comfortable and getting to know one another. Information about the course is provided. For the remaining sessions, this time is used to set the tone for the session as well as to

review homework. Next, a short presentation (maximum 15 min) is given by the therapist to introduce the topic of the session and to provide modern scientific facts. The third part of the session is problem solving (30 min) where pairs solve problems from a case study. Fourth, skills training is provided (30 min) to give participants the opportunity to learn or improve upon their coping skills. Homework assignments are discussed and the session is evaluated during the final 15 min of the session.

As seen in Table I, each session focuses on a particular area of relevance and participants develop a personal coping program. Controlling pain intensity and participating in activities are examples of topics. In addition, topics center on problems encountered at work, at home and during leisure. Various coping skills are taught that may be applied to real

TABLE I

An overview of the content of the CBT intervention (reprinted from *Spine*)

Session	Focus	Skills
1.	Causes of pain and the prevention of chronic problems	Problem solving Applied relaxation Learning and pain
2.	Managing your pain	Activities, maintain daily routines Scheduling activities Relaxation training
3.	Promoting good health, controlling stress at home and at work	Warning signals Cognitive appraisal Beliefs
4.	Adapting for leisure and work	Communication skills Assertiveness Risk situations Applying relaxation
5.	Controlling flare-ups	Plan for coping with flare-up Coping skills review Applied relaxation Own program
6.	Maintaining and improving results	Risk analysis Plan for adherence Own program finalized

life situations. While some skills involve pain control, many skills are oriented towards activity and function. These skills range from problem solving, and graded activity, to social and stress management skills. To enhance application individualized homework assignments have been designed so that every participant may try every technique. Participants might be asked to practice applied relaxation at work or develop a list of priorities for leisure time activities. Finally, participants develop their own individual coping program based on the techniques they believe are most effective for their problem. The last two sessions deal with finalizing the participant's program and dealing with possible flare-ups and setbacks.

3. Research results

This program has been applied in various settings and three randomized, controlled trials have been reported in the literature. This section contains a summary of those studies.

3.1. Intervention with a high risk group

Since the intervention was designed as secondary prevention for those at risk for developing a persistent problem, our first study investigated the utility of this approach for participants with high scores on a screening measure of yellow flags (Linton and Andersson, 2000). We envisioned that participants might be representative of patients seeking care at a primary care service. Although these patients had higher scores on the Örebro Screening Questionnaire for Pain (Chapter 13), they nevertheless were at an early stage as none had long-term sick absenteeism, and health-care utilization at baseline was low. To assess outcome in a randomized trial, we compared people receiving our program with two other groups. These comparison groups received 'treatment as usual' and in addition, modern written advice about dealing with their back pain.

Participants were recruited via primary care facilities and an advertisement in a local newspaper.

To be eligible, applicants had to be suffering pain from the spinal area, aged 18–60, and have less than 3 months of cumulative sick leave during the past year. Exclusion criteria were being retired or having another medical condition that contradicted participation.

Participants were then randomized to one of the three groups according to a block randomization procedure. The mean score on the Örebro Musculoskeletal Pain Screening Questionnaire for participants was 106. The results summarized here are based on those completing the study: 107 participants in the CBT group, 70 in the pamphlet group and 66 in the information package group.

Participants received a secondary preventive intervention according to a protocol, and all participants also were free to pursue ordinary treatment as usual. One group received a previously evaluated pamphlet (Symonds et al., 1995) that provides straightforward advice about how to best cope with back pain by remaining active and thinking positively. The reader is clearly encouraged to confront rather than avoid activities that may be associated with pain.

The second comparison group also received information, but in the form of a packet once a week for 6 weeks. The number and timing of the packages therefore matched the number of sessions the CBT group received. This material utilized more traditional sources of information and was based on a back school approach. Each package contained advice and illustrations of how one might cope with or prevent spinal pain such as by lifting properly and maintaining good posture. The information also encouraged participants to maintain their usual activities to speed recovery.

Finally, the experimental group received the cognitive behavioral group treatment described above. Groups were run periodically and those randomized were asked to join.

3.2. Results

The results were analyzed for a broad spectrum of variables including the key outcome variables of function and health-care utilization (Linton and Andersson, 2000). First, it should be underscored that since the patients selected suffered from acute or subacute bouts of back pain, considerable improvements would be expected according to the natural course of the problem. Indeed, for a number of variables such as pain intensity, mood, and activity levels all three groups experienced improvements, but the difference between the groups was not significant. However, a noteworthy finding concerning patient satisfaction was found. Patients rated how satisfied they were with the treatment received in terms of how helpful they found it to be. The cognitive behavioral group rated the intervention as significantly more helpful than did either of the two information groups. Second, the key variables of sick absenteeism and health-care utilization were selected since they are directly tied to long-term disability and costs.

For the key outcome variable of health-care utilization, the main result was that while the cognitive behavioral group *decreased* their number of visits from pretest to follow-up, both of the information groups reported *increases*. The cognitive behavioral group, relative to the two comparison groups, had a significantly lower level of utilization with regard to doctor's visits as well as visits to a physical therapist.

As various forms of compensation payments account for about 90% of the costs for back pain, the second key variable was sick absenteeism. Fig. 1 shows the mean number of sick days per month for each group during baseline and the last 6 months of the follow-up period. The fact that the pretest level is very low reflects the inclusion criteria; the objective was to study the prevention of long-term disability. As may be seen in the figure the number of sick days increases for both of the information groups at follow-up and then remains relatively stable. By comparison, the cognitive behavioral group lowered its rate and it remained at an average of 0.5 days per month throughout the follow-up period and the difference between the groups is significant. However, because sick leave data tend to be skewed in that a few participants have relatively long absences and many have little of no sick days, the average number of sick days does not necessarily reflect

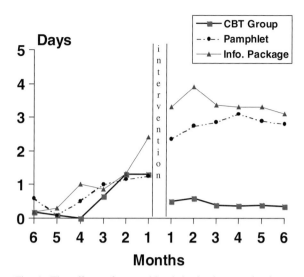

Fig. 1. The effects of a cognitive behavioral preventive intervention for patients with relatively high levels of 'yellow flags'. The mean number of sick days for back pain 6 months before the intervention and at the one-year follow-up demonstrating a significant preventive effect for the CBT group (Linton and Andersson, 2000).

long-term function. Thus, to examine the main question concerning the development of long-term sick absenteeism and to provide a nonparametric comparison, we calculated the risk of developing sick leave of more than 30 days during the follow-up period. To accomplish this we compared the cognitive behavioral group with the combined two information groups. This analysis showed that participants in the cognitive behavioral groups had a 9-fold decreased risk of being on long-term sick leave as compared to the information groups (odds ration = 9.3; 95% confidence interval = 1.2–70.8).

The results from this trial demonstrated that the cognitive behavioral group intervention resulted in significantly less disability and health-care utilization than did the control groups. Interestingly, these participants had high scores on the screening instrument, which suggests that psychological factors were quite relevant. Thus, the current intervention with its focuses on psychological aspects of the problem seemed well gauged for these participants as a preventive intervention. However, we were also curious to know if this intervention might be useful as a preventive intervention for those with only moderate levels of yellow flags, i.e. a moderate score on the screening instrument.

The aim of the next controlled trial was to evaluate the effects of the cognitive behavioral intervention for people with moderate levels of yellow flags and at an early time point, that is, prior to the need to actually seek health-care as a 'patient' (Linton and Ryberg, 2001). Therefore we recruited people from an epidemiological study who reported: (1) worst pain during the past year of ≥ 7 on a scale of 0 to 10 points; (2) ≥ 4 episodes during the past year; and (3) pain in the spinal region (back, neck, or upper back). In addition, we excluded people who had: (1) accumulated sick leave of more than 30 days during the past year; (2) comorbidity of diseases that might interfere or contraindicate the intervention. In the final analyses were 84 who were randomly assigned to a 'treatment as usual' control group and 162 assigned to the cognitive behavioral intervention. The mean score for the entire group on the Örebro Screening Questionnaire was 95 indicating a medium level of risk (medium 90–104).

For the control group 'usual' treatment was available and participants were free to pursue any ordinary treatment they deemed warranted, while the cognitive behavioral group received the six-session secondary prevention package described above.

Participants were followed for 1 year after the interventions to assess outcome (Linton and Ryberg, 2001). The mean number of sick leave days per person and month is shown in Fig. 2. It illustrates a more favorable outcome for the cognitive behavioral group. Sick leave during the baseline was very low and relatively stable the first 4 months but increased slightly during months 5 and 6. At follow-up, however, there is a significant difference as the cognitive behavioral group has leveled off its sick leave level while the usual treatment comparison group has an increase in sick leave and this difference is statistically significant (Mann–Whitney U-test, $U = 2441$, $p = 0.032$). Since the sick leave data are highly skewed in that a few participants have relatively long absences and many have no or few sick days, an odds ratio was calculated to estimate the categorical

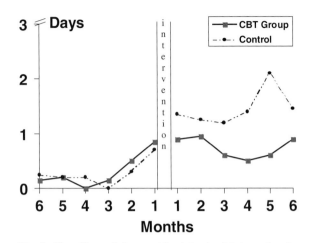

Fig. 2. The effects of the cognitive behavioral intervention for people with relatively moderate levels of 'yellow flags'. The mean number of sick days per month is shown 6 months before the intervention and at the follow-up. A significant preventive effect is shown (Linton and Ryberg, 2001)

risk. The results showed that the risk of developing an absence of 14 or more days was more than three times greater in the usual treatment comparison group (odds ratio = 3.33; 95% confidence interval = 1.19–10.2).

With regard to health-care utilization, physical function, pain and psychological variables the differences between the groups were generally quite small and not significant as both groups made similar improvements. However, the cognitive behavioral group did have significantly larger improvements on the number of pain-free days and on a measure of fear-avoidance beliefs.

Taken as a whole these results demonstrate that the cognitive behavioral intervention reduced the risk for future disability due to back pain relative to a group receiving the usual measures available. The average screening score indicated a medium risk and this seemed to coincide with the low amount of functional problems and sick leave observed at baseline. However, some participants did develop more extended problems during the follow-up and the cognitive behavioral intervention helped to prevent this development. The size of the preventive effect seemed to reflect the size of the score on the screening instrument for risk. Therefore, we wondered if the procedure might be effective for patients at a somewhat later point in time when they have more pronounced problems.

A third trial focused on return to work for those already on sick leave (Marhold et al., 2001). One effect of our previous studies was that the patient's function and workability were enhanced. It seemed that this might be utilized even for patients off work for their back pain. At the same time we reckoned from the literature and clinical experience that patients off work may need to learn certain skills in order to successfully return to work. Thus, a 12-session intervention was developed where the first six sessions consisted of the cognitive behavioral treatment described above and where the last six sessions dealt specifically with return-to-work issues. The intention was that patients should make gradual steps to return to work. These sessions dealt with generalizing coping skills to the work setting, e.g. coping with repetitive movements, heavy lifts, stress due to time urgency and insecurity about how to perform work tasks. Patients were taught skills for dealing with difficulties that might arise when returning to work such as increased pain, fatigue, or social anxiety. A plan was made and patients did homework between the sessions for taking successive steps toward a return to work. Examples of these include contacting a supervisor, visiting the workplace, and modified work.

The effects of the above-described program were tested in a randomized study that included patients with either short- or long-term work absence due to musculoskeletal pain (Marhold et al., 2001). To examine the effects of the length of the problem, patients had either long-term (>12 months, mean 26 months) sick leave or short-term (2–6 months, mean 3 months) sick leave. These patients were randomly assigned to either the cognitive behavioral return-to-work program or a 'treatment as usual' comparison group. The most common treatments for the comparison group were visits to a doctor or physical therapist.

To evaluate outcome, patients were followed for 1 year. The analyses demonstrated that the cognitive behavioral program was more effective than treatment as usual in reducing the number of days on sick leave for patients with *short-term* sick leave. In addition, the treatment program, relative to the comparison group, helped these patients to increase their activity level and gain control over their pain. However, there was no significant difference between the groups on any variable for the patients with *long-term* sick leave. These results underscore the need for an early return-to-work program that focuses on the skills needed to actually make the return. The study suggests that intervening at the right time point with this intervention is crucial for obtaining good results.

4. Conclusions

This chapter has presented and described a cognitive behavioral intervention program for early intervention that converges on the secondary prevention of disability. A particular advantage of the program may be that it keys on the psychological risk factors identified. As a result it provides a method for dealing with risk factors that traditional health-care facilities may lack and it provides an alternative to merely providing larger doses of traditional treatment when a persistent problem is imminent. The results in three randomized trials are promising as all three demonstrate advantages as compared to usual treatment. The main difference in results centered on disability and function where the participants in the cognitive behavioral program functioned significantly better than the control groups. Taken as a whole the results suggest that this intervention may be one feasible way of changing health-care routines in order to prevent the development of persistent pain and disability.

References

Compas, B.E., Haaga, D.A.F., Keefe, F.J., Leitenberg, H. and Williams, D.A. (1998) A sampling of empirically supported psychological treatments from health psychology: smoking, chronic pain, cancer, and bulimia nervosa. J. Consult. Clin. Psychol., 66: 89–112.

Kendall, N.A.S., Linton, S.J. and Main, C. (1998) Psychosocial yellow flags for acute low back pain: 'Yellow Flags' as an analogue to 'Red Flags'. Eur. J. Pain, 2: 87–89.

Linton, S.J. (2000a) Cognitive-Behavioral Therapy in the Early Treatment and Prevention of Chronic Pain: A Therapist's Manual for Groups. Author, Örebro, 40 pp.

Linton, S.J. (2000b) Psychologic risk factors for neck and back pain. In: A. Nachemsom and E. Jonsson (Eds.), Neck and Back Pain: The Scientific Evidence of Causes, Diagnosis, and Treatment. Lippincott Williams and Wilkins, Philadelphia, PA, pp. 57–78.

Linton, S.J. (2000c) A review of psychological risk factors in back and neck pain. Spine, 25: 1148–1156.

Linton, S.J. (2000d) Utility of cognitive-behavioral psychological treatments. In: A. Nachemson and E. Jonsson (Eds.), Neck and Back Pain: The Scientific Evidence of Causes, Diagnosis, and Treatment. Lippincott Williams and Wilkins, Philadelphia, PA, pp. 361–381.

Linton, S.J. and Andersson, T. (2000) Can chronic disability be prevented? A randomized trial of a cognitive-behavior intervention and two forms of information for patients with spinal pain. Spine, 25: 2825–2831.

Linton, S.J. and Ryberg, M. (2001) A cognitive-behavioral group intervention as prevention for persistent neck and back pain in a non-patient population: a randomized controlled trial. Pain, 90: 83–90.

Marhold, C., Linton, S.J. and Melin, L. (2001) Cognitive behavioral return-to-work program: effects on pain patients with a history of long-term versus short-term sick leave. Pain, 91: 155–163.

Morley, S., Eccleston, C. and Williams, A. (1999) Systematic review and meta-analysis of randomised controlled trials of cognitive behaviour therapy and behaviour therapy for chronic pain in adults, excluding headache. Pain, 80: 1–13.

Symonds, T.L., Burton, A.K., Tillotson, K.M. and Main, C.J. (1995) Absence resulting from low back trouble can be reduced by psychosocial intervention at the work place. Spine, 20: 2738–2745.

Van Tulder, M.W., Ostelo, R., Vlaeyen, J.W.S., Linton, S.J., Morely, S.J. and Assendelft, W.J.J. (2000) Behavioral treatment for chronic low back pain: a systematic review within the framework of the Cochrane Back Review Group. Spine, 25: 2688–2699.

New Avenues for the Prevention of Chronic Musculoskeletal Pain and Disability
Pain Research and Clinical Management, Vol. 12
Edited by S.J. Linton

CHAPTER 19

Multidimensional prevention

Gunnar Bergström * and Irene B. Jensen

Section of Personal Injury Prevention, Karolinska Institute, S-112 94 Stockholm, Sweden

Abstract: During the last decades a multidimensional treatment approach to chronic pain has attracted much interest among clinicians and researchers and the efficacy of such interventions has been supported in research. In this chapter we will discuss a number of important topics with regard to the multidisciplinary treatment of persistent spinal pain. We will describe an interdisciplinary approach to chronic pain, the roles of different professions in the treatment team and some important characteristics of well-functioning teamwork. The basic modules of interdisciplinary treatment are usually a combination of physiotherapeutic and cognitive behavioural interventions along with educational efforts. However, we also emphasise the importance of establishing collaboration with the workplace and involving the patients significant others in the rehabilitation process. Furthermore, the spinal pain patients referred to multidisciplinary pain centres appear to be in a poorer psychosocial condition than spinal pain patients in the general population. In the light of these facts, the positive outcome is certainly impressing. The targets for the intervention vary between the different studies on multidisciplinary treatments. We propose that at least four areas, namely pain severity, disability, affective distress and return to work, should be addressed during multidisciplinary treatment (and used as dependent variables in outcome studies). This could be seen as a minimum requirement with regard to the multidimensionality of the chronic pain experience. Based on several reviews and a number of recently published outcome studies of multidisciplinary treatments it was concluded that the support is strong for the efficacy of these interventions regarding psychosocial variables, pain reduction and return to work. However, there are several challenges for the future, which have the potential to further enhance treatment outcome and patient satisfaction after multidisciplinary treatment. For instance, despite a good outcome in many patients there are still individuals who do not benefit from these programmes, or who may have profited similarly well with a less costly and comprehensive intervention, and this necessitates a better matching of the characteristics of the patient with the content of the treatment. A further issue would also be to direct more attention to what should be determined as a clinically significant change since statistical significance based on group means does not give satisfactory information with respect to this issue. We conclude that multidisciplinary interventions are among the few treatments for persistent spinal pain for which strong support is found in empirical research for its effectiveness regarding both functional and psychosocial variables.

* Correspondence to: Gunnar Bergström, Section for Personal Injury Prevention, Karolinska Institutet, P.O. Box 127 18, S-112 94 Stockholm, Sweden. Tel.: +46 (8) 545 72648; Fax: +46 (8) 545 72630; E-mail: gunnar.bergstrom@cns.ki.se

1. Introduction

During the last decades, several countries in the western world have witnessed a proliferation of multidisciplinary pain clinics for the treatment of persistent spinal pain. This may be seen as reflecting a shift in perspective from viewing pain as being strictly of biomedical or sensory origin to the conceptualisation of pain as a multidimensional phenomenon. Theories and perspectives on pain such as the gate control theory (Melzack and Wall, 1965), the biopsychosocial model (Waddell, 1992), the operant approach (Fordyce, 1976) and the cognitive behavioural perspective (Turk et al., 1983) on pain have all contributed to this development. All these cited perspectives on pain point to the need to integrate biomedical, psychological and social factors in the assessment and treatment of pain.

The efficacy of multidisciplinary programmes as interventions for persistent spinal pain has been supported by several studies (e.g. Harkapaa et al., 1989; Alaranta et al., 1994; Loisel et al., 1997) and in several reviews (e.g. Flor et al., 1992; Cutler et al., 1994; van Tulder et al., 2000b). Moreover, the positive effects of multidisciplinary treatments have not only been confined to the reduction of pain, but have also included positive results regarding return to work and functional status. Consequently, multidisciplinary interventions have been recommended for patients with long-lasting and severe pain and disability (van Tulder et al., 2000b).

This chapter pertains to both scientific and clinical issues regarding multidisciplinary rehabilitation. We will discuss the multidisciplinary approach to persistent spinal pain, we will describe the characteristics of the patients referred to multidisciplinary interventions and possible targets for the intervention, we will give a short presentation of a number of recently published multidisciplinary treatment outcome studies together with a summary of earlier reviews on this subject and we will present some challenges for the future for both clinicians and researchers in this area.

The title of this chapter includes the term 'prevention'. Prevention can be thought of as primary, secondary or tertiary. In brief, primary prevention aims at avoiding the occurrence of an illness or disease. Secondary prevention pertains to the detection of disease at an early stage to prevent it from becoming chronic or to reduce the risk of long-term impairment and disability. Tertiary prevention focuses on enhancing function and/or minimising suffering, impairment and disability among individuals with a long-lasting illness or disease. This chapter will mainly consider tertiary prevention for individuals with spinal pain.

2. The multidisciplinary approach to chronic pain

A distinction has been suggested between multidisciplinary and interdisciplinary interventions (Gatchel and Turk, 1999). A multidisciplinary intervention requires different health professionals to be involved in the rehabilitation but it may be accomplished with relatively few contacts between the therapists and without a more elaborate integration of the targets for the intervention. In contrast, interdisciplinary rehabilitation also requires that the 'units' that constitute a treatment are highly integrated and directed at the same overall goal and that the treatment staff share a similar 'ideology' regarding the rehabilitation. Active patient participation is a key feature and, furthermore, an interdisciplinary intervention also necessitates a frequent and mutual interchange of information between the involved therapists considering the patient and the overall goal of the intervention. Consequently, a multidisciplinary composition of the treatment staff is necessary but not sufficient for an intervention to be labelled interdisciplinary.

Although this is a significant distinction, the term multidisciplinary is mostly used in this chapter because it is a wider label that can be used as a common term for the interventions reviewed here. Furthermore, there appears to be variation in the labels that different researchers use for treatments that are accomplished by different professionals. For instance, the treatment in a study by Linton et al.

(1989) on the secondary prevention of low back pain has been referred to as 'back school' (van Tulder et al., 2000c), 'functional restoration' (Bendix et al., 1998a), 'multidisciplinary' (van Tulder et al., 2000b) and behavioural (van Tulder et al., 2001b) in different reviews. Although beyond the scope if this chapter, this points to the need for a further discussion of what should be included under different treatment labels.

2.1. The interdisciplinary team

As interdisciplinary programmes involve different professions engaged in close teamwork, it is of great importance that the areas of responsibility are clearly defined. Each profession should be expert in his/her professional field and be oriented about, and respectful of, other professions and their specific knowledge. Unfortunately, our impression is that clinicians at interdisciplinary clinics sometimes either disregard the importance of other involved professionals or, alternatively, see themselves as, for instance, physiotherapist and psychologist in the same person. We believe that this is not helpful for the patients and constitutes a threat against good and fruitful cooperation. Based on the literature (Loeser and Egan, 1989a; Gatchel and Turk, 1999) and our own experience, a short summary regarding the roles of the involved professionals in an interdisciplinary rehabilitation is given in the following.

Physician. The physician's main responsibility is to carry out the medical investigation of the patients, to gather medical information from other sources (e.g. evaluations made by other medical specialists) and to be responsible for medical units in the treatment. The physician also has to communicate the medical findings to the patients and to educate the patients in basic physiology and anatomy, the effectiveness and limitations of different medical treatments for chronic pain, etc. Furthermore, as a medical authority, the physician has a salient role in reinforcing the patients in their efforts to manage their pain problem and to reassure the patients that they have not seriously damaged their spine or contracted a serious disease.

Physical therapist. The physical therapist evaluates the physical function or dysfunction of the patients and delivers treatment aimed at enhancing the physical functioning at home and at work so as to facilitate a lasting behavioural change in the individual. The physical therapist is also involved in patients' education regarding anatomy and exercise physiology, body mechanics, and the importance of physical activity in the management of chronic pain, etc.

Psychologist. The psychologist is responsible for the psychosocial evaluation and treatment of the patient. As an expert in human behaviour, the psychologist also has a certain responsibility in advising the whole treatment team regarding therapeutic strategies that facilitate behavioural change in the patients. Furthermore, the psychologist educating the patient in areas such as the role of vicious circles and how to break them, the impact of emotional and cognitive factors on the pain experience, the interplay between the patient and his/her significant others regarding the pain problem, etc.

Occupational therapist. The occupational therapist is concerned with the evaluation of the patient's functional status with respect to work duties or activities at home. These areas are subsequently targeted during treatment and patient education. The focus on physical functioning is partly similar to that of the physical therapist, but the occupational therapist is usually more focused on specific activities that are important to the patient.

Nurse. The role of the nurse is less standardised compared to that of the professionals described above. The nurse's most important function is to act as a coordinator at the clinic and be involved in patient education regarding lifestyle issues, such as smoking, dietary habits, alcohol, etc. Furthermore, the nurse can assist the physician in different ways during the medical assessment/treatment.

A minimum requirement to be expected from an intervention labelled 'multidisciplinary' or 'interdisciplinary' is that the treatment staff comprise at least a physician, a physical therapist and a psychologist. This team will be able to assess and address medical, physiotherapeutic and psychological aspects of the patients' pain experience. Based on the reviewed literature, it appears that these professionals (physicians, physiotherapists and psychologists) are regularly represented on multidisciplinary treatment staffs, whereas occupational therapists, nurses, social workers, vocational counsellors, etc., are sometimes represented and sometimes not.

2.2. Teamwork

A key feature and crucial point in an interdisciplinary intervention is the teamwork of the treatment staff. A number of important points regarding this teamwork are presented below.

- A shared treatment ideology
- Cooperativeness
- Positive reinforcement of team members
- Supervision
- The treatment staff's unique qualities as a team

The treatment staff should agree on an overall treatment ideology that defines the general goals for the treatment, the attitude that should be held between members of the treatment staff and towards patients and the methods applied during the treatment process. This 'ideology' should facilitate straightforward communication between the involved professions. The treatment team must be permeated by a genuine will to cooperate with mutual respect for other professional's specialist competence in their own field and an interest in a multidimensional perspective on pain. An interchange of positive reinforcements must be made between the members of the treatment team. The everyday work with chronic pain patients, contacts with third-party payers, the patient's significant others, referring agents, etc., can be very taxing and sometimes experienced as ungrateful, and therefore support and reinforcement from other team members is crucial.

A further point of importance is the availability of regular supervision by a professional outside the team. Despite the best intentions regarding work with both patients and team members, problems, divergent opinions and even conflicts may arise and be managed best in such a supervisory group. Finally, it is important to keep in mind that the treatment staff has unique qualities as a team, which makes it dynamic, but also vulnerable when staff members leave the team or are replaced by new personnel. This underlines the significance of keeping a well-functioning treatment staff intact.

Active patient participation. As interdisciplinary interventions are largely aimed at skills acquisition, and as these skills are to be employed in everyday situations, active patient participation is essential for a successful treatment result. However, it is unrealistic to assume that all patients are equally motivated to adhere to the treatment regimen. Therefore, to improve or maintain the patient's motivation in this respect, it is necessary for the treatment team to support and reinforce patient behaviour that constitutes constructive ways of managing pain or other described problems. It is also crucial to involve the patient in a concrete manner regarding how his/her specific pain problem can be managed in the present situation and in the future, e.g. by planning homework together with the patient, encourage the patient to contact persons important in the rehabilitation process or by giving the patient responsibility for the formulation of the rehabilitation plan described below under Treatment content. Many patients expect that their role should be passive and they attribute the responsibility for their health to rest outside themselves (with the delivery of the treatment) and even treatment personnel may view the patient as a passive and non-responsible recipient of the treatment. We believe this is unfortunate and suggest that a crucial aspect of an effective interdisciplinary treatment is an active and trustful collaboration between the patient and the clinicians.

3. Treatment content

Interdisciplinary treatments are often conducted in a group format and they may be given on an inpatient or outpatient basis. These interventions comprise different composites of several units, e.g. physical exercise, education on different aspects of pain, relaxation training, stress management, assertiveness training, etc. (Loeser and Egan, 1989b), in accordance with the conceptualisation of chronic pain as a complex, subjective and multidimensional problem. These different units would largely be subsumed under two main components, i.e. psychological or cognitive behavioural interventions and exercise-based physiotherapeutic interventions, which often constitute a large part of a multidisciplinary intervention.

The cognitive behavioural component (Turk et al., 1983; Philips, 1988) usually consists of a composite of activity planning and goal setting, problem solving, applied relaxation, cognitive coping techniques (e.g. distracting imagery, external focusing, coping self-statements), activity pacing, the role of vicious circles and how to break them, the role of significant others and assertion training. Four vital parts of the intervention can be discerned: (1) education, (2) skills acquisition, (3) cognitive and behavioural rehearsal, and (4) generalisation and maintenance (Bradley, 1996). During the education phase, the patients are taught about the psychological consequences of chronic pain, the role of psychological factors in the pain experience, etc. During the skills acquisition phase, skills (coping techniques in relation to pain or related to other situations/events problematic to the patient) are introduced to the patient who begins to practice these behaviours, and this training is further developed in the cognitive and behavioural rehearsal phase. Finally, efforts are undertaken to generalise the new skills to new situations and to prepare the patient in how to maintain new behaviours. One crucial element in the cognitive behavioural approach is the use of homework assignments in which the patients carry out their skills in everyday situations, normally beginning with more easily achievable tasks, followed by more difficult ones. Even though the inclusion of cognitive behavioural intervention (CBT) in a multidisciplinary programme is beneficial there is still limited evidence to date that any specific unit of the above-mentioned CBT strategies should be more successful than any other (Linton, 2000b).

The exercise-based physiotherapeutic component (Carlsson et al., 1999; Harms-Ringdahl et al., 1999) usually consists of a combination of gradually increased exercises or regimens such as aerobic train-ing, strength training, water exercise (pool training), muscle stretching, body awareness therapy and relaxation techniques.

Practical sessions in ergonomics may also be included as well as didactic presentations of anatomy, pain physiology and exercise physiology. Physical therapy modalities in which the patient is more or less passive (e.g. massage, manipulation) is administered to a limited degree and only when the therapist judges it to be required. The type of exercise regimen may vary as no specific exercise programme has proved to be superior to any other one (van Tulder et al., 2000b). Furthermore, the physiotherapeutic component may, similar to the cognitive behavioural component, have an emphasis on skills acquisition in which patients learn how to perform different activities (important for the patients' physical functioning) in their everyday lives.

Above and beyond what was described above regarding the integration of treatment it is crucial that a concrete and specific rehabilitation plan should be elaborated during the treatment. This plan should cover areas such as physical activities, work resumption, stress management, housework and other activities or problem areas important to the patient. Furthermore, this plan is developed by the patient together with the treatment staff and anchored with other important actors in the rehabilitation process, such as works managers, rehabilitation officials, referring agents, etc.

3.1. Education

As suggested in the former section one part of an interdisciplinary intervention consists of a basic educational programme in biomedical, physiological, ergonomic and psychosocial aspects of pain. These educational sessions may be followed by group work in which the patients are assigned a few central discussion points regarding the central theme of the session. Furthermore, these educational sessions may be seen as a comprehensive treatment rationale for, and an educational framing of, the whole intervention. In order to make the educational sessions meaningful to the patients, they should be tightly connected to the content of the other more practical parts of the treatment.

Provided that return to work is a central target for the intervention and because patients often attribute their pain problems to work factors, an active collaboration with the patient's workplace appears to be important (Loisel et al., 1997). As work supervisors could be influential in the employee's return to the workplace, programmes for training of supervisors have been developed (Linton, 1991; Håland Haldorsen et al., 1997). This training of supervisors could emphasise the supervisor's potential to contribute to a better work environment and concentrate on concrete behavioural strategies concerning how to support and facilitate work resumption among the employees (e.g. by maintaining contact with the employee during sick-listed periods or by using problem solving strategies and goal setting together with the employee). Moreover, education in the multidimensionality of the pain experience and possible physical, psychosocial and behavioural consequences of persistent pain could be included in such a programme.

Another important group to educate is the 'significant others' to the patients. This education could, after introducing the significant others to the treatment ideology and the multidimensionality of pain, concentrate on the impact of significant others on pain and well behaviours according to operant principles (Sanders, 1996; Fordyce, 1976) and to help the patients and their significant others to find actual examples of this interplay and, if deemed necessary, teach them how to change their behaviour.

4. Patient characteristics

Patients referred to multidisciplinary centres appear to have poorer health than, and differ in several aspects from, patients in the general population suffering from persistent pain (Turk and Okifuji, 1998).

For instance, Crook et al. (1986) compared persistent pain sufferers from a family medical group practice to chronic pain sufferers from a pain clinic. It was found that patients referred to a pain clinic were unemployed more often and believed that the pain was caused by an accident at work, had constant pain or pain most of the time, utilised more health care, were more restricted in their activities, spent more time in bed and reported more disability, emotional distress, negative beliefs and negative social consequences due to long-term pain. At a 2-year follow-up of these patients, nearly all differences between the pain clinic patients and the family practice patients remained, except for the experience of constant pain and health care utilisation (Crook et al., 1989).

The proportion of depressed individuals among chronic pain patients referred to pain clinics appears to be high, even though the variation in depression rates between different studies varies considerably (Romano and Turner, 1985). Becker et al. (1997) found that 40% of the patients referred to a multidisciplinary pain centre showed signs of depressive disorder and in a treatment outcome study by Kole-Snijders et al. (1999), it was reported that 30% of the patient sample were depressed. Furthermore, in a recent review, Banks and Kerns (1996) found that the reported prevalence of clinically significant depression usually ranged between 30% and 54% in clinical samples of chronic pain patients.

In a study by Garratt et al. (1993) back pain patients referred to outpatient clinics in Scotland experienced a poorer health-related quality of life than non-referred patients. Flor et al. (1992) reported that over 50% of the patients referred to multidisciplinary clinics had at least one surgery and the median for pain duration was 5 years. In an attempt to describe the profile of users of an interdisciplinary pain clinic, Weir et al. (1992) characterised the patients as socially isolated, unemployed and burdened by a host of negative psychosocial factors.

Patients with chronic non-malignant pain referred to multidisciplinary pain clinics may also perceive an equally poor or even poorer health-related quality of life and/or psychological well-being than patients with other medical conditions, e.g. gastrointestinal symptoms or hypertension (Becker et al., 1997). Patients with chronic back pain have also been shown to rate higher pain intensity and more disability than patients with cancer pain (Lin, 1998).

Altogether, it may be that multidimensional treatment is sometimes viewed as a 'last resort' among referring agents in the community and this could explain to some extent why patients referred to these clinics appear to be in a poorer psychosocial condition than non-referred patients.

5. Targets for the intervention

There is great variation in the choice of outcome variables or targets for intervention in different evaluations of multidisciplinary interventions. This makes comparisons between studies more difficult, but it may be regarded as reflecting different goals for the intervention. For instance, Melles et al. (1995) found that patients and their referring physicians rated pain control as the most important indication of successful treatment, whereas treatment staff and third-party sponsors emphasised return to work or functional improvement as the most important outcome variables.

It is of the utmost importance to decide beforehand the overall goal or goals of the treatment and to apply several targets for a multidisciplinary intervention. For instance, if return to work and functional improvement are overemphasised in the cost of pain control, the intervention may lose in credibility from the patient's point of view. In this respect, the treatment staff may be regarded as a mediator between third-party payers and patients. Since many patients referred to multidisciplinary clinics, as noted above, are in a poorer psychosocial condition than pain sufferers in general they may also feel explicitly or implicitly that referring agents, treatment staff and third-party sponsors are trying to force them to return to work regardless of their pain and suffering. This may impede their motivation for treatment and undermine adherence to treatment recommendations and collaboration with other important persons involved in the rehabilitation process.

Functional improvement and return to work are important targets for the intervention and it is a pedagogical challenge for the treatment staff at pain clinics to educate patients regarding how these variables may be related to pain control, e.g. an increase in activity may cause more pain as a short term consequence (Linton et al., 1996), but a decrease in pain in the long run. The importance of addressing pain intensity has been further elucidated in a study by Carosella et al. (1994) in which it was shown that higher pain intensity was predictive of early discharge from a multidisciplinary work rehabilitation programme.

Based on the reviews and studies presented in this chapter on the treatment outcome of multidisciplinary programmes the applied outcome variables and targets for intervention can be divided into the main areas of (1) pain intensity, (2) return to work/sick leave, (3) mood, (4) disability, (5) utilisation of health care, (6) pain behaviour, (7) cognitions, (8) coping, (9) medication intake, (10) activity level, (11) observable physical functioning, (12) social role functioning, (13) sleep quality, and (14) satisfaction with the treatment.

As a *minimum*, we believe that there should be at least four targets for the intervention and these are pain control, reduction of disability, improved mood and return to work. Pain control is of central importance to many patients and must be targeted in an efficient way. However, an exclusive focus on pain reduction is not satisfactory due to the multidimensional nature of chronic pain, and based on this perspective, at least disability and affective distress should also be considered as primary targets for the intervention.

Reduction of disability makes the patients feel less limited and handicapped and a decrease in perceived disability during treatment has also been found to be the strongest predictor of future work resumption, reduction in pain intensity and the patients' perception of treatment success (Hildebrandt et al., 1997). Pain and affective distress are associated (Linton, 2000a) and emotions like depression, anxiety, fear, anger, etc., are unpleasant and disturbing characteristics of the pain experience and may also affect adherence to treatment recommendations. Consequently, as emotional distress appears to be high among many patients referred to multidisciplinary pain clinics, improvement of the patients'

284 | *G. Bergström and I.B. Jensen*

mood should be of great value in this group. Finally, return to work is of the utmost importance because it constitutes the economic foundation in the patient's life, not to speak of society as a whole, and furthermore, it is often the main interest of the third-party payers. Moreover, to actively participate in working life has a positive meaning in and of itself for most people.

The reader is recommended to consult other sources regarding how to assess these variables (e.g. Turk and Melzack, 1992; Bergström and Jensen, 1998; Tait, 1999).

6. Outcome of multidisciplinary interventions

In the following, we have consulted reviews of the effects of multidisciplinary treatments and a number of recently published randomised controlled, or controlled clinical, trials. For the original studies reviewed, only statistically significant differences between groups at the $p < 0.05$ are presented if not stated otherwise in the text. In cases where the dropout/withdrawal/non-response rate has exceeded 30% in the active treatment or control groups, we have chosen not to report the results.

Flor et al. (1992) included 65 studies in their meta-analysis of the efficacy of multidisciplinary pain treatment centres for chronic back pain. They concluded that multidisciplinary treatments were more efficacious than no treatment or unimodal treatments and that the positive outcome covered both psychosocial (e.g. pain intensity or mood) and behavioural dimensions (e.g. back pain patients treated at multidisciplinary centres were almost twice as likely to return to work than controls and they also decreased their utilisation of health care). The results were to the advantage of the treatment at both short-term (≤6 months) and long-term (>6 months) follow-ups.

In a review and meta-analysis focusing exclusively on return to work after nonsurgical pain centre treatment for chronic pain, Cutler et al. (1994) included 37 studies. It was found that the proportion of patients actually working after nonsurgical pain cen-

tre treatments had increased from 20% pre-treatment to 54% at follow-up (time to follow-up ranged from 1 to 60 months) and that treated patients returned to work to a greater extent than those not treated.

A recent systematic review of randomised controlled trials on conservative treatment of chronic low back pain (van Tulder et al., 2000b), included 10 studies. The majority of the studies reported positive results to the advantage of the treatment in either pain, functional status or return to work. It was concluded that there existed strong support in the reviewed literature that multidisciplinary treatment is effective for the treatment of chronic nonspecific spinal pain.

Van Tulder et al. (2000c) included 15 studies in their systematic review of randomised trials of back schools for nonspecific low back pain. Moderate evidence was found for positive short-term effects for chronic low back pain when compared to other treatments and also moderate evidence for the effectiveness of back schools when employed in occupational settings and compared with placebo or waiting list controls.

In a systematic review of randomised controlled trials of nonsurgical treatment for chronic neck pain, no studies of multidisciplinary treatments were included (van Tulder et al., 2000a). In another systematic review of randomised controlled trials and non-randomised controlled clinical trials of multidisciplinary biopsychosocial rehabilitation for neck and shoulder pain, two studies were included (Karjalainen et al., 2001). The authors found limited evidence for the effectiveness of these interventions.

In a randomised controlled clinical trial by Bendix et al. (1998a,b) the outcomes 2 and 5 year after a functional restoration (FR) programme for chronic low back pain were presented for two separate research projects. At the 2-year follow-up in project A, the FR group ($n = 55$) reported less contacts with the health care system and fewer days of sick leave because of back pain than the control group ($n = 51$), but these results were not maintained at the 5-year follow-up. In project B, the 2-year follow-up revealed a larger increase in the proportion of participants considered able to work in the FR group ($n = 46$), and a lower proportion in this group had obtained pensions or had pension applications pending than in a comparison group ($n = 43$). The patients in the FR group also reported less utilisation of health care, less back pain intensity, more activities of daily living and a better total situation in relation to low back pain as compared to the comparison group. At the 5-year follow-up these results were maintained except for back pain, where no between-groups difference was found.

In a randomised controlled study by Johansson et al. (1998) a cognitive behavioural multidisciplinary intervention was compared to a waiting list control group directly after treatment and at a 1-month follow-up. The study sample consisted of 42 referred chronic pain patients (21 subjects assigned to either group) of which the majority (81%) reported multiple pain sites. Significant between-group differences in activity levels and for catastrophising thoughts were found directly after treatment in favour of the treatment group. At the 1-month follow-up the between-group differences in activity levels were maintained, but not in catastrophising thoughts. Sick leave and occupational training were assessed at the 1-month follow-up and patients in the treatment group reported more occupational training than the control group.

Kole-Snijders et al. (1999) conducted a randomised controlled study among chronic low back pain sufferers with assessment points directly after treatment (post-treatment) and 6 and 12 months after completing the treatment. The study groups underwent either an operant behavioural treatment including cognitive coping skills training (OPCO), $n = 59$, an operant behavioural treatment with a group discussion programme (OPDI), $n = 58$, a waiting list control group (WLC), $n = 31$, given a operant behavioural treatment as usual (OPUS) directly after the post-treatment assessment. Three outcome dimensions were assessed which were motor behaviour, coping control and negative affect. The results at post-treatment showed improvements in both the OPCO and OPDI as compared to the WLC in all three outcome dimensions. No between-group differences were found at the follow-ups.

Jensen and Bodin (1998) evaluated an outpatient multimodal cognitive-behavioural treatment (MM-CBT) in a controlled clinical trial with an 18-month follow-up. Eighty-eight referred patients with chronic spinal pain who had undergone MMCBT were compared with a matched control group of 35 spinal pain sufferers. Sick leave/return to work and pain intensity were chosen as priority end-points. At the 18-month follow-up, no between-groups difference was found regarding sick leave/return to work, but the treatment group showed a larger decrease in pain intensity than the control group.

In a recent randomised controlled trial with an 18-month follow-up, Jensen et al. (2001) evaluated the outcome of a behavioural medicine rehabilitation programme (BM), $n = 63$, and its two main components, behaviour-oriented physical therapy (PT), $n = 54$, and cognitive behavioural therapy (CBT), $n = 49$, compared to a 'treatment-as-usual' control group (CG), $n = 48$. The analyses were gender-differentiated and the results showed that the risk of being granted full-time early retirement was significantly lower for females in PT and CBT compared to the control group during the 18-month follow-up period. Furthermore, women in CBT and BM reported a better health-related quality of life (HRQoL) than women in the control group at the 18-month follow-up. No significant differences for men were found either in absence from work or in HRQoL.

Altogether, the efficacy of multidisciplinary treatments for persistent spinal pain is supported by the cited reviews. The positive results include pain reduction, psychosocial variables and return to work. The described original studies also pointed to positive effects of the interventions in several variables even though the positive outcome for sick leave was limited. The positive outcome reported is even more impressive against the background of the poor psychosocial adjustment to pain and the history of failed treatments in the past for many patients referred to these pain clinics.

However, a word of caution must be added as the methodological quality of the studies is often deemed to be low. For instance, in the cited systematic review by van Tulder et al. (2000b), 6 of the 10 studies (RCTs) included were judged to be of low methodological quality as evidenced in such limitations as small study groups or deficiencies in the randomisation procedure. Another example could be that in the review by Flor et al. (1992); 65% of the studies did not have a control group and, furthermore, even when a control group was used, the appropriateness of this group could often be called into question. However, despite these and other limitations the studies described in this section support the effectiveness of multidisciplinary treatments for persistent spinal pain.

7. Challenges for the future

7.1. Psychosocial and behavioural characteristics of chronic pain patients

It has been asserted that chronic pain patients have often been treated as a homogeneous group and given the same treatment regardless of their specific characteristics. Several researchers in the field of chronic pain have pointed out the need to detect distinct subgroups of patients so as to tailor treatment interventions or to control for subgroup differences when evaluating treatment outcome (Turk, 1990; Talo et al., 1992; Sanders and Brena, 1993; Rudy et al., 1995; Williams et al., 1995; Bergström, 2000). Consequently, more attention to and research regarding which patients are most in need for multidisciplinary treatment is needed. Such knowledge could enhance treatment outcome and thus be instrumental in alleviating pain and suffering in these patients. Furthermore, this could facilitate a more cost-effective use of treatment resources.

A further aspect of this issue pertains to how different units or components of the programme may be more or less effective for different patients depending on their psychosocial or behavioural characteristics. For instance, one patient may benefit from the whole programme whereas another patient may respond just as well with the physical therapy component in combination with a few measures at the workplace. The scientific knowledge enabling

a successful clinical application of such treatment matching with regard to different patient characteristics is still limited and more research is needed on this issue (Talo et al., 1996; Bergström, 2000).

Many efforts to identify subgroups or classes of pain patients based on psychosocial and/or behavioural variables have been made (Shutty and De-Good, 1987; Williams and Keefe, 1991; Main et al., 1992; Turk and Rudy, 1992; Klapow et al., 1993; Strong et al., 1995; Tait and Chibnall, 1998). One of the few instruments that have been used both in the derivation of subgroups of patients and in a following evaluation of the predictive validity of these subgroups regarding treatment outcome is the (West Haven Yale) Multidimensional Pain Inventory (MPI) (Kerns et al., 1985). Differential treatment responses have been found among temporomandibular patients (Rudy et al., 1995), fibromyalgia patients (Turk et al., 1998), and patients with persistent spinal pain (Bergström et al., 2001). The MPI has been suggested to be part of a Multiaxial Assessment of Pain (MAP) that integrates medical, psychosocial and behavioural variables (Turk and Rudy, 1987). Taxonomies similar to this may be beneficial in efforts to find the optimal treatment for a certain patient.

7.2. Gender and pain

Another issue is the possible impact of gender in the pain experience and how this could be addressed during treatment. For instance, in a review by Unruh (1996) on the topic of gender and clinical pain experience, women were found to report higher pain severity and longer duration of pain across several pain diagnoses. Unruh also recognised variation across gender in coping responses to different pain conditions and suggested that the meaning of, and adjustment to, pain may vary across gender. Women were found to seek more social support when in pain and to use more relaxation, distraction, avoidance and emotion-focused coping, whereas men were more problem-focused, relied on direct action, used more denial and attempted to look at 'the bright side of life'. Other researchers have found that females report lower pain thresholds or greater sensitivity to experimentally induced somatic stimuli (Berkley, 1997; Riley et al., 1998) and that there may be gender differences in attitudes towards pain that affect reports of pain and responses to treatment (Jensen et al., 1994a; Berkley, 1997).

Treatment outcome studies on multidisciplinary rehabilitation programmes have also shown different outcomes for men and women. Our own research has indicated that the positive effects of a multidisciplinary programme for chronic spinal pain seemed to be limited to females (Jensen et al., 1994b). In another study it was shown that the cognitive behavioural component of a multidisciplinary rehabilitation was successful in improving the health-related quality of life, and lowering the risk of early retirement among women but was less efficacious in men (Jensen et al., 2001). Furthermore, in a randomised controlled study by Lindström et al. (1992) on subacute low back pain, the results indicated that a graded activity programme (often a part of multidisciplinary programmes) reduced sick listing among males but not among females.

These findings underline the need to consider possible gender differences when evaluating multidisciplinary interventions for persistent spinal pain and to further investigate how different treatment components, and the coping strategies offered in these components, are perceived by males and females and how they may be more or less effective and credible dependent on the gender of the patient.

7.3. Motivation to change

The efficacy of an intervention may vary between different subgroups of patients or between genders but also be dependent on the patient's motivation for treatment (Jensen, 1996). Owing to the fact that multidisciplinary rehabilitation mainly relies on self-management training, the readiness of the patient to adopt these strategies is of utter importance. A structured approach regarding how to assess a patient's motivation for a specific treatment and how to work effectively with patients with different degrees of motivation could be instrumental in enhancing

adherence to treatment and to reduce dropout and relapse rates from treatment.

The transtheoretical model of change (Prochaska and DiClemente, 1998) describes how people move through motivational stages regarding whether they should change their behaviour or not. It suggests different stages of change: pre-contemplation (individuals are not ready to take action because they do not see their behaviour as a problem or, alternatively, are unwilling to change their problematic behaviour), contemplation (the individual is seriously considering changing his/her problematic behaviour), preparation (the individual has decided to take action and small changes in behaviour have already been made), action (the individual changes his/her problematic behaviour) and maintenance (the action phase is maintained over time) (Prochaska and DiClemente, 1998).

This model of change was originally developed for addictive behaviours, but it has been suggested to be applicable also to chronic pain patients (Jensen, 1996). A questionnaire based on the transtheoretical model has been evaluated and found to have an acceptable reliability and validity in chronic pain patients (Kerns et al., 1997) and, furthermore, it has been shown that different motivational profiles described by this instrument were predictive of completion versus noncompletion of a cognitive behavioural treatment for chronic pain (Kerns and Rosenberg, 2000). Additional support for the model has been found among arthritis patients where it was possible to empirically detect groups of patients generally in concordance with the mentioned stages of change (Keefe et al., 2000).

Furthermore, strategies have been developed on how to approach patients, depending on which motivational stage they are in (Miller and Rollnick, 1991). For instance, if the patient is in the preparation stage, specific advice for behavioural change and to enhance the commitment to a plan of change is recommended, whereas the therapeutic approach to a patient in the pre-contemplation stage involves elaborate strategies to enhance the motivation for behaviour change in the individual. However, research is needed regarding the clinical usefulness of this model of change and the proposed therapeutic strategies for working with individuals in different motivational stages among chronic spinal pain patients.

7.4. The point in time for the intervention

The point in time for the intervention is another issue. From a general theoretical point of view, it seems plausible that treatments should be employed before vicious circles and deconditioning have caused too much disability and emotional distress in the sufferer since this may lower his or her potential for rehabilitation. However, the research is limited regarding the impact of the duration of disability on the treatment outcome of multidisciplinary interventions (Jordan et al., 1998). In the cited study, long-term disabled patients (disabled for at least 18 months) referred to a multidisciplinary (functional restoration) programme were compared to short-term disabled patients (disabled 4–8 months) referred to the same programme. At the 1-year follow-up the short-term disabled patients showed higher work return and work retention rates than the long-term disabled patients. However, the degree of work return and work retention were surprisingly high even in the long-term disabled group and, furthermore, no significant differences were found between the groups in other socio-economic outcomes, e.g. the average number of health care visits and recurrent lost-time injury claims. The authors conclude: "Early intervention is not a panacea or a necessary condition for the successful rehabilitation of workers with disabling chronic spinal disorders" (Jordan et al., 1998, p. 2110). More research is needed concerning whether the duration of disability interacts with the outcome of multidisciplinary rehabilitation.

7.5. Clinical significance

In outcome studies of multidisciplinary treatments, mean values for the intervention are usually presented and compared to the corresponding figures for a comparison group. The difference between these mean values may or may not be statistically significant, but this does not give any conclusive information as to whether the differences are clinically significant, i.e. clinical and statistical significance do not necessarily correspond (Jacobson and Truax, 1991; Turk et al., 1993; Tait, 1999). Consequently, it is necessary to define what should be regarded as clinically significant changes among the patients. For variables such as return to work or use of medication, the criteria for success may sometimes be more easily set or understood, e.g. if the patient is working/not working at a certain point in time or uses medication or not. However, for variables that are usually based on self-reports, e.g. pain intensity or affective distress, the clinician or researcher may be more in need of statistical or mathematical procedures, or certain cut-off scores for the instrument used, to be able to discriminate between improved and non-improved patients. For instance, it is possible to compare the proportion of depressed patients before and after a treatment if an empirically derived cut-off score exists for the measure used. It is also possible to use indices as the reliable change index (Hageman and Arrindell, 1993; Rudy et al., 1995) to dichotomise patients into improved or non-improved patients or to employ estimates such as the effect size (Kazis et al., 1989; Deyo et al., 1991) to judge the size of the difference between, e.g. a treatment and a control group. A challenge for the future is to further consider the clinical significance of changes in target variables after multidisciplinary rehabilitation. This should probably facilitate the interpretation of the results in terms of meaningfulness and, consequently, be useful when presenting the efficacy of the treatment to other researchers, clinicians, third-party payers, etc.

8. Summary and conclusions

In this chapter we have discussed a number of what we consider to be important topics with regard to multidisciplinary treatment of persistent spinal pain. To begin with, we described an interdisciplinary approach to chronic pain and the roles of different professions and some important characteristics of well-functioning teamwork. This teamwork is crucial in the interdisciplinary approach and rests on such features as a shared treatment ideology, cooperativeness and respect for the specialist competence of other professions, support from other team members and supervision by a professional outside the team.

The basic modules of interdisciplinary treatments are usually a combination of physiotherapeutic and cognitive behavioural interventions along with educational efforts. In this chapter the importance of establishing collaboration with the workplace and involving the patients' significant others in the rehabilitation process was also emphasised. Furthermore, the spinal pain patients referred to multidisciplinary pain centres appear to be in a poorer psychosocial condition than spinal pain patients in the general population. In the light of these facts, the positive outcome is certainly impressing. Since the multidimensionality of chronic pain has been empirically supported in research during the last 30–40 years this should also be mirrored in the choice of the targets for the intervention in a multidimensional rehabilitation. Therefore, it was proposed that at least the four areas pain severity, disability, affective distress and return to work should be addressed during multidisciplinary treatment (and used as dependent variables in outcome studies).

Based on several reviews and a number of recently published outcome studies of multidisciplinary treatments, it was concluded that there is strong support for the efficacy of these interventions regarding psychosocial variables, pain reduction and return to work. However, there are several challenges for the future that have the potential to further enhance treatment outcome and patient satisfaction after multidisciplinary treatment. For instance, despite a good outcome among many patients, there still are individuals who do not benefit from these programmes, or may have profited similarly well with a less costly and comprehensive intervention, and this necessitates a better matching of the characteristics of the patient with the content of the treatment. A further issue would also be to direct more attention to what should be determined as a clinically significant change as statistical significance based on group means does not give satisfactory information with respect to this issue. A clinically meaningful way to report the results of outcome studies might be to give information on the proportion of improved patients (using criteria of clinical significance) and whether these patients shared certain characteristics prior to treatment (for instance MPI subgroup affiliation, motivational status or gender).

We conclude that multidisciplinary interventions are among the few treatments for persistent spinal pain where it exists strong support in empirical research for its effectiveness regarding both functional and psychosocial variables. However, we have also attempted to delineate some areas and issues that we believe are of importance in future clinical and research activities concerning multidisciplinary treatment of persistent spinal pain.

References

Alaranta, H., Rytokoski, U., Rissanen, A., Talo, S., Rönnemaa, T., Puukka, P., Karppi, S.L., Videman, T., Kallio, V. and Slätis, P. (1994) Intensive physical and psychosocial training program for patients with chronic low back pain: a controlled clinical trial. Spine, 19: 1339–1349.

Banks, S.M. and Kerns, R.D. (1996) Explaining high rates of depression in chronic pain: a diathesis-stress framework. Psychol. Bull., 119: 95–110.

Becker, N., Bondegaard Thomsen, A., Olsen, A.K., Sjogren, P., Bech, P. and Eriksen, J. (1997) Pain epidemiology and health-related quality of life in chronic non-malignant pain patients referred to a Danish multidisciplinary pain center. Pain, 73: 393–400.

Bendix, A.E., Bendix, T., Haestrup, C. and Busch, E. (1998a) A prospective, randomized 5-year follow-up study of functional restoration in chronic low back pain patients. Eur. Spine J., 7: 111–119.

Bendix, A.F., Bendix, T., Labriola, M. and Boekgaard, P. (1998b) Functional restoration for chronic low back pain. Two-year follow-up of two randomized clinical trials. Spine, 23: 717–725.

Bergström, G. (2000) The Assessment and Treatment of Long-Term, Non-Specific Spinal Pain. Behavioural Medicine, a Cognitive Behavioural Perspective. Dissertation, Department of Clinical Neuroscience, Karolinska Institutet, Stockholm.

Bergström, G. and Jensen, I.B. (1998) Psychosocial and behavioural assessment of chronic pain: recommendations for clinicians and researchers. Scand. J. Behav. Ther., 27: 114–123.

Bergström, G., Jensen, I.B., Bodin, L., Linton, S.J. and Nygren, Å.L. (2001) The impact of psychologically different patient groups on outcome after a vocational rehabilitation program for long-term spinal pain. Pain, 93: 229–237.

Berkley, K.J. (1997) Sex differences in pain. Behav. Brain Sci., 20: 371–380; discussion 435–513.

Bradley, L.A. (1996) Cognitive-behavioral therapy for chronic pain. In: R.J. Gatchel and D.C. Turk (Eds.), Psychological Approaches to Pain Management. The Guilford Press, New York, NY, pp. 131–147.

Carlsson, J., Jonsson, T., Norlander, S. and Rundcrantz, B.-L. (1999) Evidence-based physiotherapeutic treatment. Patients with neck pain. Report No. 101 (in Swedish). Statens beredning för medicinsk utvärdering (SBU) och Legitimerade sjukgymnasters riksförbund (LSR), Stockholm.

Carosella, A.M., Lackner, J.M. and Feuerstein, M. (1994) Factors associated with early discharge from a multidisciplinary work rehabilitation program for chronic low back pain. Pain, 57: 69–76.

Crook, J., Tunks, E., Rideout, E. and Browne, G. (1986) Epidemiologic comparison of persistent pain sufferers in a specialty pain clinic and in the community. Arch. Phys. Med. Rehabil., 67: 451–455.

Crook, J., Weir, R. and Tunks, E. (1989) An epidemiological follow-up survey of persistent pain sufferers in a group family practice and specialty pain clinic. Pain, 36: 49–61.

Cutler, R.B., Fishbain, D.A., Rosomoff, H.L., Abdel-Moty, E., Khalil, T.M. and Rosomoff, R.S. (1994) Does nonsurgical pain center treatment of chronic pain return patients to work. Spine, 19: 643–652.

Deyo, R.A., Diehr, P. and Patrick, D.L. (1991) Reproducibility and responsiveness of health status measures. Statistics and strategies for evaluation. Control Clin. Trials, 12: 142S–158S.

Flor, H., Fydrich, T. and Turk, D.C. (1992) Efficacy of multidisciplinary pain treatment centers: a meta-analytic review. Pain, 49: 221–230.

Fordyce, W.E. (1976) Behavioral Methods for Chronic Pain and Illness. The C.V. Mosby Company, Saint Louis, MO.

Garratt, A.M., Ruta, D.A., Abdalla, M.I., Buckingham, J.K. and Russell, I.T. (1993) The SF36 health survey questionnaire: an outcome measure suitable for routine use within the NHS. BMJ, 306: 1440–1444.

Gatchel, R.J. and Turk, D.C. (1999) Interdisciplinary treatment of chronic pain patients. In: R.J. Gatchel and D.C. Turk (Eds.), Psychosocial Factors in Pain. The Guilford Press, New York, NY, pp. 435–444.

Hageman, W.J. and Arrindell, W.A. (1993) A further refinement of the reliable change (RC) index by improving the pre–post difference score: introducing RCID. Behav. Res. Ther., 31: 693–700.

Håland Haldorsen, E.M., Jensen, I.B., Linton, S.J., Nygren, Å. and Ursin, H. (1997) Training work supervisors for reintegration of employees treated for musculoskeletal pain. J. Occup. Rehabil., 7: 33–43.

Harkapaa, K., Jarvikoski, A., Mellin, G. and Hurri, H. (1989) A controlled study on the outcome of inpatient and outpatient treatment of low back pain. Part I. Pain, disability, compliance,

and reported treatment benefits three months after treatment. Scand. J. Rehabil. Med., 21: 81–89.

Harms-Ringdahl, K., Holmström, E., Jonsson, T. and Lindström, I. (1999) Evidence-based Physiotherapeutic Treatment. Patients with Low-back Pain. Report No. 102 (in Swedish). Statens beredning för medicinsk utvärdering (SBU) och Legitimerade sjukgymnasters riksförbund (LSR), Stockholm.

Hildebrandt, J., Pfingsten, M., Saur, P. and Jansen, J. (1997) Prediction of success from a multidisciplinary treatment program for chronic low back pain. Spine, 22: 990–1001.

Jacobson, N.S. and Truax, P. (1991) Clinical significance: a statistical approach to defining meaningful change in psychotherapy research. J. Consult Clin. Psychol., 59: 12–19.

Jensen, I.B. and Bodin, L. (1998) Multimodal cognitive-behavioural treatment for workers with chronic spinal pain: a matched cohort study with an 18-month follow-up. Pain, 76: 35–44.

Jensen, I., Nygren, Å., Gamberale, F., Goldie, I. and Westerholm, P. (1994a) Coping with long-term musculoskeletal pain and its consequences: is gender a factor. Pain, 57: 167–172.

Jensen, I.B., Nygren, Å. and Lundin, A. (1994b) Cognitive-behavioural treatment for workers with chronic spinal pain: a matched and controlled cohort study in Sweden. Occup. Environ. Med., 51: 145–151.

Jensen, I.B., Bergstrom, G., Ljungquist, T., Bodin, L. and Nygren, A.L. (2001) A randomized controlled component analysis of a behavioral medicine rehabilitation program for chronic spinal pain: are the effects dependent on gender. Pain, 91: 65–78.

Jensen, M.P. (1996) Enhancing motivation to change in pain treatment. In: R.J. Gatchel and D.C. Turk (Eds.), Psychological Approaches to Pain Management. The Guilford Press, New York, NY, pp. 78–111.

Johansson, C., Dahl, J., Jannert, M., Melin, L. and Andersson, G. (1998) Effects of a cognitive-behavioral pain-management program. Behav. Res. Ther., 36: 915–930.

Jordan, K.D., Mayer, T.G. and Gatchel, R.J. (1998) Should extended disability be an exclusion criterion for tertiary rehabilitation? Socioeconomic outcomes of early versus late functional restoration in compensation spinal disorders. Spine, 23: 2110–2116; discussion 2117.

Karjalainen, K., Malmivaara, A., van Tulder, M., Roine, R., Jauhiainen, M., Hurri, H. and Koes, B. (2001) Multidisciplinary biopsychosocial rehabilitation for neck and shoulder pain among working age adults. Spine, 26: 174–181.

Kazis, L.E., Anderson, J.J. and Meenan, R.F. (1989) Effect sizes for interpreting changes in health status. Med. Care, 27: 178–189.

Keefe, F.J., Lefebvre, J.C., Kerns, R.D., Rosenberg, R., Beaupre, P., Prochaska, J., Prochaska, J.O. and Caldwell, D.S. (2000) Understanding the adoption of arthritis self-management: stages of change profiles among arthritis patients. Pain, 87: 303–313.

Kerns, R.D. and Rosenberg, R. (2000) Predicting responses to self-management treatments for chronic pain: application of the pain stages of change model. Pain, 84: 49–55.

Kerns, R.D., Turk, D.C. and Rudy, T.E. (1985) The West Haven-

Yale multidimensional pain inventory (WHYMPI). Pain, 23: 345–356.

Kerns, R.D., Rosenberg, R., Jamison, R.N., Caudill, M.A. and Haythornthwaite, J. (1997) Readiness to adopt a self-management approach to chronic pain: the Pain Stages of Change Questionnaire (PSOCQ). Pain, 72: 227–234.

Klapow, J.C., Slater, M.A., Patterson, T.L., Doctor, J.N., Atkinson, J.H. and Garfin, S.R. (1993) An empirical evaluation of multidimensional clinical outcome in chronic low back pain patients. Pain, 55: 107–118.

Kole-Snijders, A.M., Vlaeyen, J.W., Goossens, M.E., Rutten-van Molken, M.P., Heuts, P.H., van Breukelen, G. and van Eek, H. (1999) Chronic low-back pain: what does cognitive coping skills training add to operant behavioral treatment? Results of a randomized clinical trial. J. Consult. Clin. Psychol., 67: 931–944.

Lin, C.-C. (1998) Comparison of the effects of perceived self-efficacy on coping with chronic cancer pain and coping with chronic low back pain. Clin. J. Pain, 14: 303–310.

Lindström, I., Ohlund, C., Eek, C., Wallin, L., Peterson, L.E., Fordyce, W.E. and Nachemson, A.L. (1992) The effect of graded activity on patients with subacute low back pain: a randomized prospective clinical study with an operant-conditioning behavioral approach. Phys. Ther., 72: 279–290; commentary and author response, 291–293.

Linton, S.J. (1991) A behavioral workshop for training immediate supervisors: the key to neck and back injuries. Percept. Mot. Skills, 73: 1159–1170.

Linton, S.J. (2000a) A review of psychological risk factors in back and neck pain. Spine, 25: 1148–1156.

Linton, S.J. (2000b) Utility of cognitive-behavioral psychological treatments. In: A.L. Nachemson and E. Jonsson (Eds.), Neck and Back Pain. The Scientific Evidence of Causes, Diagnosis and Treatment. Lippincott Williams and Wilkins, Philadelphia, PA, pp. 361–381.

Linton, S.J., Bradley, L.A., Jensen, I., Spangfort, E. and Sundell, L. (1989) The secondary prevention of low back pain: a controlled study with follow-up. Pain, 36: 197–207.

Linton, S.J., Hellsing, A.-L. and Bergström, G. (1996) Exercise for workers with musculoskeletal pain: Does enhancing compliance decrease pain. J. Occup. Rehabil., 6: 177–190.

Loeser, J.D. and Egan, K.J.E. (1989a) History and organization of the University of Washington multidisciplinary pain center. In: J.D. Loeser and K.J.E. Egan (Eds.), Managing the Chronic Pain Patient: Theory and Practice at the University of Washington Multidisciplinary Pain Center. Raven Press, New York, NY, pp. 3–20.

Loeser, J.D. and Egan, K.J.E. (Eds.) (1989b) Managing the Chronic Pain Patient: Theory and Practice at the University of Washington Multidisciplinary Pain Center. Raven Press, New York, NY.

Loisel, P., Abenhaim, L., Durand, P., Esdaile, J.M., Suissa, S., Gosselin, L., Simard, R., Turcotte, J. and Lemaire, J. (1997) A population-based, randomized clinical trial on back pain management. Spine, 22: 2911–2918.

Main, C.J., Wood, P.L.R., Hollis, S., Spanswick, C.C. and Waddell, G. (1992) The distress and risk assessment method, a simple patient classification to identify distress and evaluate the risk of poor outcome. Spine, 17: 42–52.

Melles, T., McIntosh, G. and Hall, H. (1995) Provider, payer, and patient outcome expectations in back pain rehabilitation. J. Occup. Rehabil., 5: 57–69.

Melzack, R. and Wall, P. (1965) Pain mechanisms: a new theory. Science, 50: 971–979.

Miller, W.R. and Rollnick, S. (1991) Motivational Interviewing: Preparing People to Change Addictive Behaviour. The Guilford Press, New York, NY.

Philips, H.C. (1988) The Psychological Management of Chronic Pain. Springer, New York, NY.

Prochaska, J.O. and DiClemente, C.C. (1998) Towards a comprehensive, transtheoretical model of change: states of change and addictive behaviors. In: W.R. Miller and N. Heather (Eds.), Treating Addictive Behaviors. Plenum Press, New York, NY, pp. 3–24.

Riley III, J.L., Robinson, M.E., Wise, E.A., Myers, C.D. and Fillingim, R.B. (1998) Sex differences in the perception of noxious experimental stimuli: a meta-analysis. Pain, 74: 181–187.

Romano, J.M. and Turner, J.A. (1985) Chronic pain and depression: Does the evidence support a relationship. Psychol. Bull., 97: 18–34.

Rudy, T.E., Turk, D.C., Kubinski, J.A. and Zaki, H.S. (1995) Differential treatment responses of TMD patients as a function of psychological characteristics. Pain, 61: 103–112.

Sanders, S.H. (1996) Operant conditioning with chronic pain. In: R.J. Gatchel and D.C. Turk (Eds.), Psychological Approaches to Pain Management. The Guilford Press, New York, NY, pp. 112–129.

Sanders, S.H. and Brena, S.F. (1993) Empirically derived chronic pain patient subgroups: the utility of multidimensional clustering to identify differential treatment effects. Pain, 54: 51–56.

Shutty, M.S. and DeGood, D.E. (1987) Cluster analyses of responses of low-back pain patients to the SCL-90: Comparison of empirical versus rationally derived subscales. Rehabil. Psychol., 32: 133–144.

Strong, J., Large, R.G., Ashton, R. and Stewart, A. (1995) A New Zealand Replication of the IPAM Clustering Model for Low Back Patients. Clin. J. Pain, 11: 296–306.

Tait, R.C. (1999) Evaluation of treatment effectiveness in patients with intractable pain: measures and methods. In: R.J. Gatchel and D.C. Turk (Eds.), Psychosocial Factors in Pain. The Guilford Press, New York, NY, pp. 457–480.

Tait, R.C. and Chibnall, J.T. (1998) Attitude profiles and clinical status in patients with chronic pain. Pain, 78: 49–57.

Talo, S., Rytökoski, U. and Puukka, P. (1992) Patient classification, a key to evaluate pain treatment: A psychological study in chronic low back pain patients. Spine, 17: 998–1010.

Talo, S., Rytökoski, U., Hämäläinen, A. and Kallio, V. (1996) The biopsychosocial disease consequence model in rehabilitation, model development in the finnish work hardening programme for chronic pain. Int. J. Rehabil. Res., 19: 93–109.

Turk, D.C. (1990) Customizing treatment for chronic pain patients: who, what and why. Clin. J. Pain, 6: 255–270.

Turk, D.C. and Melzack, R. (Eds.) (1992) Handbook of Pain Assessment. The Guilford Press, New York, NY.

Turk, D.C. and Okifuji, A. (1998) Treatment of chronic pain patients: clinical outcomes, cost-effectiveness, and cost–benefits of multidisciplinary pain centers. Phys. Rehabib. Med., 10: 181–206.

Turk, D.C. and Rudy, T.E. (1987) Towards a comprehensive assessment of chronic pain patients. Behav. Res. Ther., 25: 237–249.

Turk, D.C. and Rudy, T.E. (1992) Classification logic and strategies in chronic pain. In: D.C. Turk and R. Melzack (Eds.), Handbook of Pain Assessment. The Guilford Press, New York, NY, pp. 409–428.

Turk, D.C., Meichenbaum, D. and Genest, M. (1983) Pain and Behavioral Medicine. A Cognitive-Behavioral perspective. The Guilford Press, New York, NY.

Turk, D.C., Rudy, T.E. and Sorkin, B.A. (1993) Neglected topics in chronic pain treatment outcome studies: determination of success. Pain, 53: 3–16.

Turk, D.C., Okifuji, A., Sinclair, J.D. and Starz, T.W. (1998) Differential responses by psychosocial subgroups of fibromyalgia syndrome patients to an interdisciplinary treatment. Arthritis Care Res., 11: 397–404.

Unruh, A.M. (1996) Gender variations in clinical pain experience. Pain, 65: 123–167.

Van Tulder, M.W., Goossens, M. and Hoving, J. (2000a) Non-surgical treatment of chronic neck pain. In: A.L. Nachemson and E. Jonsson (Eds.), Neck and Back Pain. The Scien-

tific Evidence of Causes, Diagnosis and Treatment. Lippincott Williams and Wilkins, Philadelphia, PA, pp. 339–354.

Van Tulder, M.W., Goossens, M., Waddell, G. and Nachemson, A.L. (2000b) Conservative treatment of chronic low back pain. In: A.L. Nachemson and E. Jonsson (Eds.), Neck and Back Pain. The Scientific Evidence of Causes, Diagnosis and Treatment. Lippincott Williams and Wilkins, Philadelphia, PA, pp. 271–304.

Van Tulder, M.W., Esmail, R., Bombardier, C. and Koes, B.W. (2000c) Back schools for non-specific low back pain. Cochrane Database Syst. Rev., 2

Van Tulder, M.W., Ostelo, R., Vlaeyen, J.W., Linton, S.J., Morley, S.J. and Assendelft, W.J. (2001b) Behavioral treatment for chronic low back pain: a systematic review within the framework of the Cochrane Back Review Group. Spine, 26: 270–281.

Waddell, G. (1992) Biopsychosocial analysis of low back pain. Baillieres Clin. Rheumatol., 6: 523–553.

Weir, R., Browne, G.B., Tunks, E., Gafni, A. and Roberts, J. (1992) A profile of users of specialty pain clinic services: predictors of use and cost estimates. J. Clin. Epidemiol., 45: 1399–1415.

Williams, D.A. and Keefe, F.J. (1991) Pain beliefs and the use of cognitive-behavioral coping strategies. Pain, 46: 185–190.

Williams, D.A., Urban, B., Keefe, F.J., Shutty, M.S. and France, R. (1995) Cluster analysis of pain patients' responses to the SCL-90R. Pain, 61: 81–91.

New Avenues for the Prevention of Chronic Musculoskeletal Pain and Disability
Pain Research and Clinical Management, Vol. 12
Edited by S.J. Linton

Problem-solving therapy and behavioral graded activity in the prevention of chronic pain disability

Johanna H.C. Van den Hout [1,2,*] and Johan W.S. Vlaeyen [1,3]

[1] *Department of Medical, Clinical and Experimental Psychology, Maastricht University, Maastricht, The Netherlands*
[2] *Institute for Rehabilitation Research, Hoensbroek, The Netherlands*
[3] *Pain Management and Research Center, University Hospital, Maastricht, The Netherlands*

Abstract: Recent findings in the back pain literature suggest that stress symptoms and negative affect are important risk factors in the development of chronic back pain disability. From a theoretical point of view, avoidance learning is postulated to be one of the mechanisms that explain the association between stress and disability levels. In back pain, two kinds of avoidance can be distinguished: fear-related avoidance and stress-related avoidance. Not only activities that elicit pain and pain-related fear, but also non-pain-related situations that are stressful, are likely to be avoided. Several studies have reported on the efficacy of interventions aimed at reducing avoidance behaviors in pain patients, of which the graded activity approach is the most known. Additionally, there is evidence that the effects of graded activity can be improved when the treatment also focuses on resolving daily hassles and stress for which the patient perceives a lack of control. In this contribution, we will highlight the value of the problem-solving therapy (PST) in the treatment and prevention of low back pain. Subsequently, the rationale and content of the PST, adjusted for its use in back pain patients, will be presented. We will also discuss the results of a randomized clinical trial investigating the supplemental value of PST when added to graded activity. Finally, recommendations and potential hindrances for clinical practice are addressed.

1. Introduction

From foregoing chapters it became more than obvious that musculoskeletal pain and associated disability, call for answers, not only with regard to the understanding of the problem, but moreover regarding the question how to deal with it. What should be done to prevent long-term disability and sick leave? Which psychological aspects should be ad-

dressed and how? The current chapter will describe a secondary preventive program that was pointed at employees with a recent new episode of sick leave as a result of non-specific low back pain. The program is innovative in that *problem-solving therapy* is combined with an operant approach, i.e. *behavioral graded activity*. The main goal of the program is to optimize return to work and to prevent long-term and/or frequent episodes of sick leave. The pro-

* Correspondence to: Anja Van den Hout, Center for Nursing Research, Maastricht University, P.O. Box 616, 6200 MD Maastricht, The Netherlands. E-mail: a.vandenhout@zw.unimaas.nl

gram is multidisciplinary; disciplines involved are general practitioner, occupational health physician, rehabilitation physician, physical therapist, occupational therapist, psychologist, and supervisor at the workplace.

The aim of this chapter is to sketch the background and the main components of the experimental intervention. Next, the randomized clinical trial and primary outcomes will be described concisely. Activating the patient is easier said than done. The use of effective techniques may be important to reach treatment goals, but still one must reckon with hindrances, inside or outside the patient, that may impede the treatment progresses. Finally, this chapter will conclude with some recommendations regarding possible hindrances for clinical practice, and how to deal with them.

2. Background of the intervention

The current intervention, i.e. problem-solving therapy and behavioral graded activity, is based on a biopsychosocial model of pain and focuses at two factors that are hypothetically related to disability in pain patients: fear–avoidance and stress-related avoidance (Fig. 1).

2.1. Fear–avoidance

An irrational fear that physical activity would instigate pain or lead to (renewed) injury, may result in the avoidance of various physical and social activities, including work (Lethem et al., 1983; Philips, 1987). In the long term, avoidance behavior is found to increase the risk of disability (Wad-

dell et al., 1993; Klenerman et al., 1995; Vlaeyen et al., 1995; Crombez et al., 1998, 1999; Vlaeyen and Linton, 2000). In line with this, pain treatments have adopted the fear–avoidance model and implemented cognitive-behavioral techniques in order to deal with pain-related fear and avoidance behavior. To this respect, the operant approach, i.e. graded activity or graded exposure, as originally introduced by Fordyce (1976), has been successfully applied in both chronic pain patients (Turner and Clancy, 1988; Turner et al., 1990; Nicholas et al., 1991; Kole Snijders et al., 1999) and sub-acute and acute low back pain patients (Fordyce et al., 1986; Linton et al., 1989; Lindström et al., 1992; Linton and Bradley, 1992). Recently, application of exposure-in-vivo techniques for patients with more elevated levels of pain-related fear was introduced (Vlaeyen et al., 2001).

2.2. Stress-related avoidance

Pain (behavior) not only allows for the avoidance of physical and painful activities, but secondly, pain behavior might legitimate the avoidance of situations that are stressful and for which the patient does not find acceptable solutions. In this context, sick leave because of back pain complaints can be considered a medical solution to a work-related problem (Knepper and Feenstra, 1991). In order to improve treatment effects in the longer term and to go into the role of stress-related avoidance, problem-solving strategies (D'Zurilla and Goldfried, 1971) have been suggested to add to the overall effectiveness of pain treatments. There are several reasons that make the application of problem-solving therapy in pain patients appealing. First, being able to come up with effective solutions in case one is confronted with daily hassles or stressful events might enable a patient to stay at work when pain relapses. Indeed, Shaw et al. (2001) found low scores on positive problem orientation and high scores on impulsiveness/carelessness style associated with more functional loss in low back pain patients. They suggest that the prolonged impact of low back pain on daily functioning may be reduced by assisting workers to conceptualize LBP as a prob-

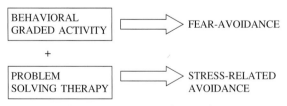

Fig. 1. A two-component intervention.

lem that can be overcome and to use active strategies in reducing risks for low back pain. Secondly, consequences of chronic pain cover a broad field of problems and more generic skills than those which focus only on pain, might be needed to cope with them. In line with this, Aldrich et al. (2000) suggest that in chronic pain, interventions should focus at the consequences of pain in everyday life rather than the pain itself. Problem-solving therapy (Nezu and Perri, 1989; Nezu et al., 1998) seems to come up to these expectations in that it can be applied in all kinds of problems, whether these are trivial or complex, and therefore might be very well applicable in those diseases where everyday functioning and well-being are at stake. Third, problem-solving therapy is said to be a particularly appropriate treatment for stress-related disorders (e.g. depression, generalized anxiety, psychosomatic disorders) because of the possible critical role of perceived uncontrollability in the etiology and/or maintenance of these disorders (D'Zurilla, 1988).

Work-related problems, e.g. strict deadlines or conflicts with co-workers, may be very inconvenient, especially when back pain is already a burden on the employee. To prevent that the employee stays at home because the burden becomes to heavy, it may help when the employee is inclined to actively solve the problems confronted with rather than to avoid, and moreover, feels confident in doing so. In line with this, a negative orientation towards problems was found to be associated with higher levels of functional disability in employees with low back pain (Van den Hout et al., 2001).

3. The experimental treatment program

In Box 1, an outline of the 8-week treatment program is given. Next, the general characteristics of the program, as well as the main components, i.e. behavioral graded activity and problem-solving therapy, will be described in more detail.

General characteristics. The treatment program took place at the rehabilitation center and consisted of 19 half-day sessions that were spread over 8 weeks. The treatment was given in small groups of at most 5 patients. The program started with an introduction of the treatment rationale. In the course of the program the team of therapists had three meetings with individual patients. During these meetings, progresses and hindrances for goal achievement and return to work were discussed. Two months after the final treatment session, a booster session was planned in which treatment components were summarized, and individual developments were discussed in the group. Patients received a workbook in which specific treatment information, handouts, graded activity graphs, and homework assignments could be collected.

Behavioral graded activity (GA). Behavioral graded activity is an operant behavioral treatment that aims to increase activity levels using quota systems. Included in the training are registration of baseline levels during the first 2 weeks, a treatment contract, positive reinforcement for activity increments, and a workplace visit (Fordyce, 1976). The physiotherapist trained a circuit of five basic exercises (bicycling, lateral pulley, steps, shoulder and abdominal exercises) in 12 1-h sessions. Three additional sessions were dedicated to back education and lifting instructions. The occupational therapist trained patients for 30 min per week on an individual basis in which principles of behavioral graded activity were applied to personal relevant activities, e.g. at work, housekeeping, and leisure activities. Furthermore, the occupational therapist contacted the occupational physician and the patient's supervisor at the workplace to agree about the return-to-work schedule and plan a workplace-visit when necessary.

Problem-solving therapy (PST). Problem-solving therapy is a cognitive behavioral therapy in which problem-solving skills are taught according to the theory as designed by D'Zurilla and Goldfried (1971). The theory describes five steps in which problems are typically solved: problem orientation, problem definition and formulation, generation of alternatives, decision-making, and implementation and evaluation. In the current trial a protocol, as originally designed by Nezu and colleagues (Nezu, 1986;

Box 1 The experimental treatment program

Week	Graded activity Physiotherapy (15 × 1 h)	Graded activity Occupational ther. (7 × 0.5 h)	Problem solving therapy (10 × 1.5 h)
1			Rationale and orientation
2	Rationale and Baseline measurements		
	Treatment contract		
3	Graded activity training and	Graded activity and	Problem-solving skills
4	3 educational lessons	workplace visit if necessary	training
5			
	Interim-evaluation		
6			
7	Generalization of skills		
8			
	Final evaluation and return-to-work scheme		

Nezu and Perri, 1989), was translated and applied as a group intervention.

Skills were taught in ten 90-min sessions and were guided by two behavior therapists. The foci of the therapy were skills training and application of skills in daily life, rather than one specific problem area. Patients were free to select their own problem areas, which did not need to be pain-related. Between sessions, homework assignments were given to practice skills in everyday life. Every session homework assignments were discussed in the group, and patients were encouraged to keep on practicing and applying problem-solving skills in everyday life. A tool that was used during the entire therapy was called the 'record of coping attempts'. An example of a solution attempt concerning a work-related problem is given in Box 2. Next to the records of coping attempts, a list of hindrances on several domains of living serves as a personal guidance during therapy.

Next, the outline of the PST will briefly be described.

3.1. Sessions 1, 2 and 3: treatment rationale and problem-orientation

The treatment rationale stresses the importance of efficient problem-solving strategies to deal with daily hassles and stress as a consequence of pain. Saving energy by solving problems efficiently, would be in favor of a prosperous recovery from pain disability. During these three first sessions, motivational processes that can stimulate or hamper efficient problem solving are addressed. Moreover, participants are stimulated to recognize personal signals of stress in order to identify problems or hindrances in time.

3.2. Session 4: problem-definition and -formulation

During this stage, the importance is stressed to: (a) collect as much information about the problem as possible, (b) describe facts in concrete and clear language, (c) distinguish relevant from irrelevant information, and facts from interpretations, (d) identify variables and circumstances that make the situation a

Box 2 The 'record of coping attempts', an example

1. What's the problem?
Since I have made a part-time return-to-work, my colleagues appeal to me with regard to several tasks I was in charge of before my disability period. The problem is that I am not able to take the responsibility for all former tasks yet.

2. What do you want to achieve?
That the tasks I can not take responsibility for at this moment, being taken care of. Gradually take responsibility for my former tasks myself again.

3. What solutions have you thought of?
Hire a part-time replacement until I have made a full return-to-work; Try to do it myself; Have an advanced full-time return-to-work; Consult colleagues; Ask colleagues to take over some tasks until I have made a full return-to-work; Leave the company; Delay some tasks until I'm fit for it again; Ask my supervisor for a temporary alternative function at the company; Go on sick leave.

4. Which solution have you chosen and why?
After consultation with my boss and colleagues, some of the tasks are taken over by my colleagues and some, with lowest priority, are delayed until later.

5. What have you done?
I gradually resumed my former activities at the workplace again. Within 3 months I had a full-time return-to-work. I did not relapse during those 3 months.

6. Was your goal achieved?
Yes, although the company had some delay with certain jobs, which have to be solved now.

7. Are you content about the solution you have chosen?
Not at all   1   2   3   **4**   5   very well

problem. Furthermore, this session pays attention to the interpretation of non-verbal behavior.

3.2.1. Session 5: goal setting
A well-formulated goal is (a) described in concrete terms, (b) positively formulated (e.g. "I want to work more", in stead of "I want to be less disabled"), (c) feasible, and (d) preferably independent of others. When goals are very large and complex, it is sensible to split them up in several smaller steps or sub-goals.

3.3. Session 6: generation of alternatives

During this stage of the problem-solving process it is stressed to generate as much solutions as possible, such that the chance of finding an appropriate solution increases. Therefore, a brainstorm technique is

taught that consists of two principles: (1) the more solutions the better, and (2) deference of judgement. Participants are encouraged to apply these principles to their personal problems, and together with the other group members solutions are generated.

3.4. Session 7: making decisions

After generating as much solutions as possible, the best solution has to be chosen during this stage of the problem-solving process. Was judgement deferred in an earlier stage, now judgement is the technique it all comes down to. A cost–benefit analysis is made in which the pros and cons of each solution are considered. The best solution is the one with the least negative consequences and the most positive consequences, and has the best chances to succeed.

3.5. Sessions 8, 9 and 10: solution implementation and verification

Self-control techniques become very important in this stage of the process, i.e. (a) the performance of the solution plan, (b) (self-) observation, (c) (self-) evaluation, and (d) (self-) reinforcement. Despite precaution and good preparations, some unforeseen hindrances may occur when the solution is carried out. When the solution does not solve the problem, the problem solver better recycles the process, to find out where it went wrong. The latter asks for a flexible use of problem-solving techniques, observing and evaluating the process and staying positive about the solvability of the problem. During the final sessions participants are encouraged to apply problem-solving skills in their personal lives. The last session anticipates on the problems and hindrances that may occur when the employee returns to work or when pain relapses.

4. The clinical trial

A randomized clinical trial was executed in order to investigate whether problem-solving therapy had a supplemental value when added to behavioral graded activity, in employees with non-specific low back pain (Van den Hout et al., 1998). A summary of study population, study design, and primary outcomes will be given in this section. For a comprehensive report of the study and results, we refer to Van den Hout et al. (submitted, 2002).

4.1. Study population

The treatment program focussed at employees who had a recent new episode of sick leave as a result of low back pain (LBP). They were referred to the study by general practitioner and/or occupational physician. In preparation of the trial, GPs and occupational physicians within a radius of 50 km from the rehabilitation center, were recruited as potential referrers to the trial. Referrers were informed about the intervention and the study protocol

TABLE I

Eligibility criteria

Inclusion
Age between 18 and 65 years
LBP for more than 6 weeks
On sick leave with LBP but no longer than 20 weeks
Fewer than 120 days of sick leave during the previous year

Exclusion
Specific back complaints (vertebral fracture, infectious disease, rheumatoid arthritis, ankylosing spondilitis, or herniated disc) (Waddell and Turk, 1992)
Predominant psychopathology
Pregnant
Not proficient in Dutch

---

beforehand. Eligibility criteria for participation in the study are displayed in Table I. In addition, potential subjects were excluded when they were in consultation and/or treated by a medical specialist for diagnosis or treatment of their LBP at the time of referral. Furthermore, subjects had to agree to stop any other treatments they were receiving for their back complaints at the start of the intervention. Subjects with medical comorbidity were excluded when the disorder interfered with the treatment program or rendered them unable to participate in every part of the program, as decided by the rehabilitation physician. Employees who were involved in any litigation regarding work conflicts were excluded as well.

In the period between September 1996 and December 1998, 115 patients were included in the trial. The final sample consisted of 84 males and 31 females, with a mean age of 39.8 years (SD = 8.9, range 21 to 55). On the average pain duration since the first pain episode was 7.8 years (SD = 8.4, range 5.6 weeks to 40.3 years). The current pain episode had a mean duration of 1.8 years (SD = 5.0, range 3 days to 40.3 years). In 68% of the patients the current pain episode had a duration of more than 12 weeks, and 69% of all patients had recurrent pain. On the average, patients were on the sick list for more than 8 weeks (57 calendar-days; SD = 53.2, median 42) before they took part in the screening procedure.

4.2. Study design

After inclusion, patients were randomly assigned to one of two treatment conditions, the first condition being graded activity plus problem-solving therapy (GAPS: $n = 58$), and the second condition being graded activity plus group education (GAGE: $n = 57$). Group education (GE) was chosen as an attention-control such that non-specific factors (i.e. attention, time, and materials) were equally provided in GAPS and GAGE conditions. GE consisted of ten 90-min sessions in which issues related to the back and to back pain were discussed. A physiotherapist, an occupational therapist, and a behavior therapist, using a protocolized manual, served as lecturers. In the GAGE condition, explicitly no skills were taught and each theme was discussed during no more than one protocolized session.

Patients were assessed just before treatment, immediately after treatment, and at 6- and 12-month follow-ups. Primary outcome measures were on functional disability, physical (health) activities, health-care utilization, days of sick leave and work status. In this chapter, a summary of the results on functional disability, days of sick leave and work status will be reported. The Roland Disability Questionnaire (RDQ; Roland and Morris, 1983) measured the level of functional disability. Next to mean RDQ-scores, the percentage of patients with a clinical relevant change on the RDQ (Stratford et al., 1998) were compared between treatment conditions. Data on sick leave and work status were retrieved from the Occupational Health Services (OHS) regarding 4 half-year time periods: 2 half-year periods preceding the intervention (periods 1 and 2); and 2 half-year periods following the intervention (periods 3 and 4). Work status could be defined in 5 classes: 100% return-to-work, <100% return-to-work, no return-to-work, disability pension as a result of back pain, disability pension not as a result of back pain.

With regard to days of sick leave in periods 2, 3 and 4, data of 84 employees were retrieved from the OHS. Baseline characteristics of this reduced sample are comparable to those described above.

4.3. Primary outcomes

4.3.1. Functional disability

RDQ-scores drop in both conditions from pre- to post-treatment and from post-treatment to 6-month follow-up. At 12-month follow-up, functional disability stabilizes in both conditions (Fig. 2). At 12-month follow-up, the GAPS condition had lower functional disability than the GAGE condition ($p < 0.05$). Because group differences may hide improvements in the individual patients, clinically relevant changes with regard to functional disability were examined on an individual level (Stratford et al., 1998). Immediately after the intervention, about 45% of the patients showed a clinically relevant improvement in both conditions. Remarkably, at 6-month follow-up, the percentage of patients with a clinically relevant improvement increases in both conditions, but most in the GAPS condition (70% vs. 55% in the GAGE condition). At 12-month follow-up, 65% and 50% of the patients improved with regard to functional disability, respectively in GAPS and GAGE conditions. Although modest, the chance of a clinically relevant improvement is highest in the GAPS condition.

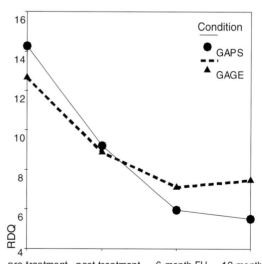

Fig. 2. Outcomes regarding functional disability (Roland Disability Questionnaire). GAPS = graded activity + problem solving therapy; GAGE = graded activity + group education; RDQ = Roland Disability Questionnaire.

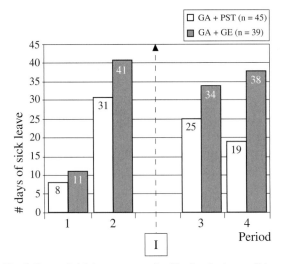

Fig. 3. Days of sick leave as a result of back pain, by condition. GA = graded activity; PST = problem-solving therapy; GE = group education; period 1 = 1 to 0.5 year pre-treatment; period 2 = 0.5 year pre-treatment; period 3 = 0.5 year post-treatment; period 4 = 0.5 to 1 year post-treatment; I = intervention.

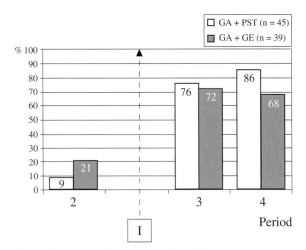

Fig. 4. Percentage of employees with 100% return-to-work, by condition. GA = graded activity; PST = problem-solving therapy; GE = group education; period 1 = 1 to 1/2 year pre-treatment; period 2 = 1/2 year pre-treatment; period 3 = 1/2 year post-treatment; period 4 = 1/2 to 1 year post-treatment; I = intervention.

4.3.2. Days of sick leave

In Fig. 3, the number of days of sick leave as a result of back pain is shown. Both conditions show an increase of days of sick leave in the half-year preceding the intervention (period 2). The first half-year following the intervention (period 3) both conditions drop days of sick leave. As in functional disability, the difference between treatment conditions becomes clear during the second half-year following the intervention (period 4): employees in the GAPS condition reported significantly less days of sick leave than patients in the GAGE condition ($p < 0.05$). The statistical analyses controlled for pre-treatment differences.

4.3.3. Work status

In Fig. 4, the percentage of patients with a 100% return-to-work is shown by condition. In the week preceding the intervention, most patients were reported to be on the sick list. Only 9% and 21% of the patients in GAPS and GAGE conditions, respectively, made a 100% return-to-work just before the treatment started. Six months after the intervention, 76% and 72% of the patients had a full return-to-

work in, respectively, GAPS and GAGE conditions. Finally, work status 1 year after the intervention is evaluated. Not only the percentage of patients with 100% return-to-work is more favorable in the GAPS condition (86% vs. 68%), but in addition, the percentage of patients receiving disability pensions, was twice as high in the GAGE condition as compared to the GAPS condition (21% vs. 9%, respectively). This may indicate that patients in the GAPS condition were more successful in their job resumption as compared to patients in the GAGE condition. The latter might be of great clinical importance, regarding the prevention of long-term work disability.

5. Conclusions and recommendations

5.1. Conclusions

From the clinical trial it was concluded that problem-solving therapy had supplemental effects when added to behavioral graded activity. First, employees who received problem-solving therapy next to behavioral graded activity, reported less functional disability 1 year after the intervention, as compared to employees not receiving problem-solving therapy. Moreover, when problem-solving therapy was added, employees not only were reported to have less days of sick leave during the second half-year after the intervention, but also work status was more favorable in that more employees had a 100% return-to-work and fewer received disability pensions.

Nevertheless, some remarks are worth mentioning. First, the trial did not compare the treatment program to a treatment-as-usual condition. We do not know what the natural course of outcomes would have been when we had not intervened shortly after the onset of sick leave. What we do know is that graded activity was shown to be more effective than treatment-as-usual on several occasions (Linton et al., 1989; Lindström et al., 1992; Linton and Bradley, 1992). As our graded activity intervention is comparable to the ones Lindström and Linton presented, with respect to contents, we may cautiously suggest that the effects we found were supplemental effects, in that they were additional to the effects graded activity had already been shown to have (Linton et al., 1989; Lindström et al., 1992; Linton and Bradley, 1992).

A second remark is with respect to the study population. The sample selected in this study consisted in the greater part of chronic low back pain patients, most of them experiencing recurrent pain. When sick leave duration was regarded, however, most employees had quit work for only a short period of time (about 8 weeks on the average). Apparently, most employees had been able to continue their jobs despite pain, what may distinguish them from chronic pain patients in general. It would be more appropriate, therefore, to consider duration of sick leave rather than duration of pain, when choosing the target population of the preventive intervention described above. A target population fit for the intervention may be employees with recurrent short episodes of sick leave as a result of back pain, including those with a recent new episode of sick leave, as to prevent them from work loss when back pain becomes less manageable in future situations.

6. Final conclusion

The results from the trial are favorable regarding the additional problem-solving therapy and indicate that the introduction of problem-solving strategies at an early stage may contribute to a prosperous return to work and prevent chronic work disability. Moreover, it is important to mention the long-term effects, in that supplemental effects of problem-solving therapy, as expected, became clear after 1 year. The latter might indicate that relapse of back pain and disability, are coped with more efficiently in future situations when problem-solving skills are put into action.

6.1. Recommendations

The implementation of a cognitive-behavioral intervention as described in this chapter, may call for some recommendations:

(1) *Make sure that the therapy is acceptable to the patient.* It may be of importance to make sure that the intervention is acceptable for the population concerned. As patients will not comply with a therapy which they can not accept or do not find plausible, it may be wise to pilot the new intervention in your own setting. Especially when patients are not prepared for a therapy from a biopsychosocial point of view, therapy outcomes may be unexpectedly poor or patients may prematurely quit the program. From the process-evaluation we conducted in the clinical trial described above, we learned that, as compared to the GAPS condition, a higher percentage of patients in the GAGE condition answered that the treatment came up to their expectations and that they had achieved treatment goals (82% GAGE vs. 51% GAPS). Furthermore, patients in both conditions chiefly noted that physiotherapy, occupational therapy and ergonomics were indispensable parts of the treatment. Although we do not know to what extent these outcomes may have influenced the effects, disappointments regarding treatment expectations may certainly not have had positive effects. Another conclusion may be that the problem-solving therapy was only accepted in this group of patients in

the presence of the graded activity part of the treatment. A solo performance of the problem-solving therapy may therefore be hard to sell in this group of patients.

There are some steps that might be taken to prevent disappointments. First, it is crucial to explain the treatment's rationale to the patient, such that it becomes acceptable and plausible to the patient. A good method to bring about the rationale is to help the patient see how it applies to his own case. With respect to the introduction of problem-solving skills, it is important to make the patient understand that the treatment will not focus at the reduction of pain, but will rather concentrate at solving the consequences of pain in everyday life (Aldrich et al., 2000). When a patient finds the treatment rationale credible and sees of what use the therapy could be for him personally, the therapy is well timed. If on the other hand, the patient is still convinced that something is wrong physically, which asks for a medical solution, it is not wise to start therapy.

(2) *Conveyance of consistent messages by all parties involved.* In line with the foregoing, it is important that all parties involved in the therapy process convey the same message to the patient. This starts with the physician who refers. In the best case, the referrer prepares the patient for the therapy, by introducing the rationale and motivating why this applies to the patient's case. This may make the patient feel confident about the therapy as appropriate for his case. Doubt on the part of the referrer, e.g. "Lets try this new therapy, but when your pain is increasing you'd better stop", may nip a prosperous therapy process in the bud. Naturally, the same advice holds for the team that is executing the treatment. Consultation and supervision on a regular basis between therapists involved in the therapy process, as well as general agreement on the therapy plan, may help to offer the patient a consistent and integrated program.

(3) *Involve the workplace in the therapy process as soon as reasonably possible.* Next to participation of therapists, it is helpful when there is involvement and cooperation on the part of the workplace. When the employee eventually returns to work, it may be very frustrating to find out that nothing has changed.

Unfortunately, this is often the case. It may therefore be advisable to involve the workplace, e.g. supervisor or on-site occupational health physician, as early as possible. In the current intervention, cooperation between the occupational health physician, the general practitioner and the multidisciplinary rehabilitation team was initiated immediately after referral. To achieve a consistent plan agreed by all parties, one party (i.e. the occupational therapist) must initiate contacts and inform about therapy appointments. Not in the last place, a plan of return-to-work must be agreed between the occupational health physician, the employer, the employee and the rehabilitation team.

(4) *Broad implementation of problem-solving skills.* Generalization of skills to daily living might be even more fruitful when all disciplines within the rehabilitation team appeal to these skills whenever the patient brings about a problem. In that way, patients might be encouraged to discuss problems and use problem-solving skills to solve them, not only within the rehabilitation setting, but also at the workplace and at home (Loscalzo and Bucher, 1999). When employees find results in their new way of dealing with work-related problems, it may facilitate the use of problem solving in future situations.

References

Aldrich, S., Eccleston, C. and Crombez, G. (2000) Worrying about chronic pain: vigilance to threat and misdirected problem solving. Behav. Res. Ther., 38: 457–470.

Crombez, G., Vervaet, L., Lysens, R., Baeyens, F. and Eelen, P. (1998) Avoidance and confrontation of painful, back-straining movements in chronic back pain patients. Behav. Modif., 22: 62–77.

Crombez, G., Vlaeyen, J.W., Heuts, P.H. and Lysens, R. (1999) Pain-related fear is more disabling than pain itself: evidence on the role of pain-related fear in chronic back pain disability. Pain, 80(1–2): 329–339.

D'Zurilla, T.J. (1988) Problem-solving therapies. In: K.S. Dobson (Ed.), Handbook of Cognitive-Behavioral Therapies. Guilford Press, New York, NY, pp. 85–135.

D'Zurilla, T.J. and Goldfried, M.R. (1971) Problem solving and behavior modification. J. Abnorm. Psychol., 78(1): 107–126.

Fordyce, W.E. (1976) Behavioral Methods for Chronic Pain and Illness. Mosby, St. Louis.

Fordyce, W.E., Brockway, J.A., Bergman, J.A. and Spengler, D.

(1986) Acute back pain: a control group comparison of behavioral vs traditional management methods. J. Behav. Med., 9: 127–140.

Klenerman, L., Slade, P.D., Stanley, I.M., Pennie, B., Reilly, J.P., Atchison, L.E., Troup, J.D. and Rose, M.J. (1995) The prediction of chronicity in patients with an acute attack of low back pain in a general practice setting. Spine, 20(4): 478–484.

Knepper, S. and Feenstra, H. (1991) Ziekte of gedrag; basisbegrippen bij de behandeling van arbeidsongeschikten. Ned. Tijdschr. Geneeskd., 135(37): 1672–1676.

Kole Snijders, A.M., Vlaeyen, J.W., Goossens, M.E., Rutten van Molken, M.P., Heuts, P.H., van Breukelen, G. and van Eek, H. (1999) Chronic low-back pain: what does cognitive coping skills training add to operant behavioral treatment? Results of a randomized clinical trial. J. Consult. Clin. Psychol., 67(6): 931–944.

Lethem, J., Slade, P.D., Troup, J.D. and Bentley, G. (1983) Outline of a fear–avoidance model of exaggerated pain perception, I. Behav. Res. Ther., 21(4): 401–408.

Lindström, I., Öhlund, C., Eek, C., Wallin, L., Peterson, L.E., Fordyce, W.E. and Nachemson, A.L. (1992) The effect of graded activity on patients with subacute low back pain: a randomized prospective clinical study with an operant-conditioning behavioral approach. Phys. Ther., 72(4): 279–290.

Linton, S.J. and Bradley, L.A. (1992) An 18-month follow-up of a secondary prevention program for back pain: help and hindrance factors related to outcome maintenance. Clin. J. Pain, 8(3): 227–236.

Linton, S.J. and Bradley, L.A. (1996) Strategies for the prevention of chronic pain. In: R.J. Gatchel and D.C. Turk (Eds.), Psychological Approaches to Pain Management: A Practitioner's Handbook. Guilford Press, New York, NY, pp. 438–457.

Linton, S.J., Bradley, L.A., Jensen, I. and Spangfort, E. et al. (1989) The secondary prevention of low back pain: a controlled study with follow-up. Pain, 36(2): 197–207.

Loscalzo, M.J. and Bucher, J.A. (1999) The COPE model: its clinical usefulness in solving pain-related problems. J. Psychosoc. Oncol., 16(3–4): 93–117.

Main, C.J., Wood, P.L., Hollis, S., Spanswick, C.C. and Waddell, G. (1992) The Distress and Risk Assessment Method. A simple patient classification to identify distress and evaluate the risk of poor outcome. Spine, 17(1): 42–52.

Nezu, A.M. (1986) Efficacy of a social problem-solving therapy approach for unipolar depression. J. Consult. Clin. Psychol., 54(2): 196–202.

Nezu, A.M. and Perri, M.G. (1989) Social problem-solving therapy for unipolar depression: an initial dismantling investigation. J. Consult. Clin. Psychol., 57(3): 408–413.

Nezu, A.M., Nezu, C.M., Friedman, S.H., Faddis, S. and Houts, P.S. (1998) A Problem Solving Approach. Helping Cancer Patients to Cope. American Psychological Association, Washington, DC.

Nicholas, M.K., Wilson, P.H. and Goyen, J. (1991) Operant-behavioural and cognitive-behavioural treatment for chronic low back pain. Behav. Res. Ther., 29(3): 225–238.

Philips, H.C. (1987) Avoidance behaviour and its role in sustaining chronic pain. Behav. Res. Ther., 25(4): 273–279.

Roland, M. and Morris, R. (1983) A study of the natural history of back pain, Part I. Development of a reliable and sensitive measure of disability in low-back pain. Spine, 8(2): 141–144.

Shaw, W.S., Feuerstein, M., Haufler, A.J., Berkowitz, S.M. and Lopez, M.S. (2001) Working with low back pain: problem-solving orientation and function. Pain, 93: 129–137.

Stratford, P.W., Binkley, J.M., Riddle, D.L. and Guyatt, G.H. (1998) Sensitivity to change of the Roland–Morris Back Pain Questionnaire: part 1. Phys. Ther., 78(11): 1186–1196.

Turner, J.A. and Clancy, S. (1988) Comparison of operant behavioral and cognitive-behavioral group treatment for chronic low back pain. J. Consult. Clin. Psychol., 56(2): 261–266.

Turner, J.A., Clancy, S., McQuade, K.J. and Cardenas, D.D. (1990) Effectiveness of behavioral therapy for chronic low back pain: a component analysis. J. Consult. Clin. Psychol., 58(5): 573–579.

Van den Hout, J.H.C., Vlaeyen, J.W.S., Kole-Snijders, A.M.J., Heuts, P.H.T.G., Willen, J.E.H.L. and Sillen, W.J.T. (1998) Graded activity and problem solving therapy in sub-acute non-specific low back pain. Physiotherapy, 84: 167.

Van den Hout, J.H.C., Vlaeyen, J.W.S., Heuts, P.H.T.G., Sillen, W.J.T. and Willen, A.J.E.H.L. (2001) Functional disability in non-specific low back pain: the role of pain-related fear and problem-solving skills. IJBM, 8(2): 134–148.

Van den Hout, J.H.C., Vlaeyen, J.W.S., Heuts, P.H.T.G., De Vet, H.C.W., Sillen, W.J.T., Willen, A.J.E.H.L., Wijnen, J.A.G. and Passchier, J. (submitted) Has problem solving therapy supplemental value when added to behavioral graded activity in non-specific low back pain patients? A randomized clinical trial.

Van den Hout, J.H.C., Vlaeyen, J.W.S., Heuts, P.H.T.G., Zijlema, H. and Wijnen, J.A.G. (2002) Secondary prevention of work-related disability in non-specific low back pain: a randomized clinical trial, evaluating problem solving therapy when added to graded activit. Clin. J. Pain, in press.

Vlaeyen, J.W. and Linton, S.J. (2000) Fear–avoidance and its consequences in chronic musculoskeletal pain: a state of the art. Pain, 85(3): 317–332.

Vlaeyen, J.W., Kole Snijders, A.M., Boeren, R.G. and van Eek, H. (1995) Fear of movement/(re)injury in chronic low back pain and its relation to behavioral performance. Pain, 62(3): 363–372.

Vlaeyen, J.W.S., de Jong, J., Geilen, M., Heuts, P.H.T.G. and van Breukelen, G. (2001) Graded exposure in vivo in the treatment of pain-related fear: a replicated single-case experimental design in four patients with chronic low back pain. Behav. Res. Ther., 39: 151–166.

Waddell, G. and Turk, D.C. (1992) Clinical assessment of low back pain. In: D.C. Turk and R. Melzack (Eds.), Handbook of Pain Assessment. Guilford Press, New York, NY.

Waddell, G., Newton, M., Henderson, I., Somerville, D. and Main, C.J. (1993) A Fear–Avoidance Beliefs Questionnaire (FABQ) and the role of fear–avoidance beliefs in chronic low back pain and disability. Pain, 52(2): 157–168.

New Avenues for the Prevention of Chronic Musculoskeletal Pain and Disability
Pain Research and Clinical Management, Vol. 12
Edited by S.J. Linton
© *2002 Elsevier Science B.V. All rights reserved*

Subject Index